# CLINICAL COACH

## *for*

# Nurse Practitioners

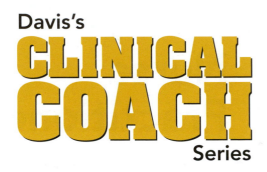

Davis's

# CLINICAL
# COACH

Series

# CLINICAL COACH

## *for*

# Nurse Practitioners

Rhonda Hensley,
EdD, APRN, BC
MSN Program Director
Grambling State University
Grambling, Louisiana

Angela Williams,
APRN, EdD(c)
Assistant Professor, Nursing
Family Nurse Practitioner
Grambling State University
Grambling, Louisiana

F.A. Davis Company • Philadelphia

F. A. Davis Company
1915 Arch Street
Philadelphia, PA 19103
www.fadavis.com

Printed in China

Last digit indicates print number: 10 9 8 7 6 5 4 3 2 1

Publisher, Nursing: Joanne Patzek DaCunha, RN, MSN
Senior Developmental Editor: William Welsh
Project Editor: Kim DePaul
Assistant Editor: Maria Price
Art and Design Manager: Carolyn O'Brien

Cover images courtesy of Blend Images, Alloy Photography, and Punchstock/Corbis

As new scientific information becomes available through basic and clinical research, recommended treatments and drug therapies undergo changes. The author(s) and publisher have done everything possible to make this book accurate, up to date, and in accord with accepted standards at the time of publication. The author(s), editors, and publisher are not responsible for errors or omissions or for consequences from application of the book, and make no warranty, expressed or implied, in regard to the contents of the book. Any practice described in this book should be applied by the reader in accordance with professional standards of care used in regard to the unique circumstances that may apply in each situation. The reader is advised always to check product information (package inserts) for changes and new information regarding dose and contraindications before administering any drug. Caution is especially urged when using new or infrequently ordered drugs.

**Library of Congress Cataloging-in-Publication Data**

Hensley, Rhonda.
  Clinical coach for nurse practitioners / Rhonda Hensley, Angela Williams.
     p. ; cm.
  Including bibliographical references and index.
  ISBN-13: 978-0-8036-2171-8
  ISBN-10: 0-8036-2171-X
1. Nurse practitioners. 2. Nursing. I. Williams, Angela, 1960- II. Title.
  [DNLM: 1. Nursing care—methods. 2. Nurse Practitioners. 3. Nurse's
Role.  WY 100 H526c 2010]
  RT82.8.H47 2010
  610.7306'92—dc22

                                                          2009038830

There are so many people who have provided assistance in bringing this project to completion. To all the wonderful editors and technical people at F. A. Davis, know that you have our heartfelt gratitude for your guidance and direction in this work. To the graduate nursing faculty at Grambling State University who carried an extra load or offered words of encouragement to help us get through this work, thank you.
To our families who watched over many late nights of writing, researching, and rewriting, thank you for understanding and patience.

As a personal dedication to the person who always encouraged us professionally, constantly instilled in us the desire to achieve "excellence without exception," and in whose footsteps we strive to follow, we dedicate this work to your honor and memory, Dr. Betty E. Smith, R.N.
Dr. Smith served as Dean of the School of Nursing at Grambling State University for more than 20 years. Because of her vision, the graduate nursing program became a reality, and because of her inspiration the graduate nursing program continues to be a program that strives and attains excellence on a daily basis.

# Reviewers

**Susan L. Berg, MSN, FNP-BC**
Director, Family Nurse Practitioner Program
Assistant Professor
Missouri State University
Springfield, Missouri

**Michelle Cook, MS, RN**
Professor
Massachusetts Bay Community College
Framingham, Massachusetts

**Connie Cooper, EdD, MSN, RN**
Instructor
DePaul University
Louisville, Kentucky

**Judith L. Draper, MSN, CRNP**
Clinical Assistant Professor
Drexel University
Philadelphia, Pennsylvania

**Cherie Gilbert, MSN, MBA, GNP**
Assistant Professor
Dalhousie University
Halifax, Nova Scotia, Canada

**Joellen W. Hawkins, RN, PhD, WHNP-BC**
Professor Emeritus
William F. Connell School of Nursing
Boston College
Chestnut Hill, Massachusetts

**Jane Flanagan, PhD, ANP-BC**
Assistant Professor
Connell School of Nursing, Boston College
Chestnut Hill, Massachusetts

**Lea R. Hall, RN, MSN, FNP-BC**
Assistant Professor of Nursing
Indiana State University
Terre Haute, Indiana

## Cherie Howk, PhD, FNP-BC
Assistant Professor
Indiana State University
Terre Haute, Indiana

## Esperanza Villanueva Joyce, EdD, CNS, RN
Associate Dean for Academics
The University of Texas at El Paso
El Paso, Texas

## Teri Kaul, PhD, APRN-BC, ANP/FNP
Director Graduate Nursing Program
Concordia University Wisconsin
Mequon, Wisconsin

## Diane Nunez, RN, MS, ANP-C
Clinical Associate Professor
Arizona State University
Phoenix, Arizona

## Martha Olson, RN, BSN, MS
Nursing Instructor, Assistant Professor
Iowa Lakes Community College
Emmetsburg, Iowa

## Alberta Peters-Herron, FNP-BC, MSN, DNP-student
Assistant Professor
Goldfarb School of Nursing at Barnes-Jewish College
St. Louis, Missouri

## Judith Pine, PhD, ANP-BC
Nurse Practitioner—Pulmonary, Critical Care Medicine
North Shore University Hospital
Manhasset, New York

## Kerry Risco, PhDc, MSN, CRNP, NP-C, WCC
Assistant Professor
Slippery Rock University
Slippery Rock, Pennsylvania

## Lynne Welch, EdD, APRN, FNP-BC
Family Nurse Practitioner, Professor & Dean Emeritus
Marshall University
Huntington, West Virginia

# Acknowledgments

The following persons provided authorship and critical review of specific content for this work:

Dr. Brenda Thomason, PNP, assistant professor of nursing at Grambling State University, provided her expertise in writing and review of the content related to pediatrics. Dr. Thomason has had extensive experience in her career as an advanced practice nurse in pediatric cardiology.

Penny Cain, FNP, assistant professor of nursing at Grambling State University, provided substantial content for the geriatric material included in this work. Mrs. Cain has worked in the field of geriatrics for many years. For the past ten years, she has been employed as an advanced practice nurse in an internal medicine clinic, in addition to her teaching responsibilities.

# Table of Contents

# 1 Getting Started

# CHAPTER 1

# Getting Started

S tarting out in advanced nursing practice can be an overwhelming experience. The first year of practice is possibly the most difficult transition, with all of its many post-graduation examinations, licensure procedures, and job search activities. This chapter is dedicated to assisting the new graduate in maneuvering through the first year of practice with success. Included in this chapter is a wealth of information on areas including:

- Preparing a professional portfolio
- Making an impression in the job interview
- Negotiation skills for success in practice
- Establishing a new practice
- Collaborative practice agreements
- Application for billing numbers
- Prescriptive authority and DEA applications

## Preparing a Professional Portfolio

The final semesters in graduate school in preparing for the role of an advanced practice nurse are filled with a multitude of activities including:

- Completion of research activities
- Examinations
- Preparation for certification examinations
- Planning for graduation
- Deciding where you will be working after graduation

Many graduate programs prepare their graduates in the fine art of marketing themselves in their new roles by helping them write a formal business plan or prepare a professional portfolio. It is critical for nurse practitioners (NPs) who are just entering the arena of advanced practice nursing to be fully prepared to "sell" themselves and their professional potential to an employer. One of the first steps in this is the preparation of a professional portfolio. A portfolio that is sharp, organized, and complete will be an asset for any NP looking for a job. The following list presents items that novice NPs should consider keeping in their portfolios:

- College or university transcripts
- Certification as an advanced practice nurse
- Copies of nursing and advanced nursing licenses
- A statement of career goals and special interests
- Letters of recommendation
- Articles written
- Certificates of continuing education or training
- Drug Enforcement Administration (DEA) number and state controlled substances prescriber number
- National Provider Identifier (NPI) number and other provider numbers for reimbursement
- Copy of the state law addressing the NP scope of practice, requirements for collaborative practice agreements, and prescriptive authority
- Productivity data from previous employments as an NP
- Data on performance measures from personal clinical experiences
- Testimonials or letters of appreciation from patients

New NP graduates have plenty of activities to undertake in the first month after graduation, including:

- Passing the national certification examination
- Obtaining advanced practice licensure
- Beginning interviewing for a position
- Requesting provider numbers (NPI, Medicare, Medicaid, private insurance companies)
- Applying for prescriptive authority
- Applying for a DEA number and a controlled substances prescriber number in the state in which the NP hopes to practice
- Obtaining malpractice insurance coverage

## Making an Impression in the Interview

The interview process is perhaps the most important step in the establishment of professional relationships for future employment. The old adage that "you only get one chance to make a first impression" is important to remember in a professional job interview. Therefore, it is imperative to be prepared. The NP should have an individual professional portfolio organized and ready for review, have a list of questions for the potential employer, be prepared to answer questions, and have a clear understanding of what the NP desires from this new employment opportunity (see Box 1–1). Above all, take a few extra minutes to prepare physically for the interview: to dress professionally and be well groomed, well rested, and confident.

Some clinical sites may have had considerable experience in working with NPs, while others may be at the novice level. As a potential employee, the NP should be able to articulate the NP scope of practice as well as particular state requirements for collaborative practice agreements, required physician supervision, and sources of reimbursement for NP services.

Questions the NP may want clarified by the potential employer include:
- What type of patients are typically seen in this clinic?
- What is an average number of visits per day for this clinic?
- What level of supervision can the NP expect in this practice? Is the supervision direct or by documentation review only?
- What are the hours of operation for this practice?
- Are there weekend or on-call expectations for the NP?
- If there are on-call expectations, is there physician backup for this?
- Is the NP expected to make hospital or nursing home visits for the practice?
- What is the policy of the practice with regard to continuing education?
- Are there opportunities for partnerships or profit sharing in this practice?

---

**Box 1–1  Anticipated Interview Questions**

The NP should be prepared to answer any of the following questions in an interview:
- What can an NP bring to this practice?
- What can you personally bring to this practice?
- What are your greatest job strengths? Weaknesses?
- What previous experiences have you had in this field?
- What are the legal parameters in this state for NP practice?
- How many patients are you used to seeing in an average clinic day?
- What level of supervision have you had in previous clinic employments?
- Where do you see yourself professionally in 5 years? In 10 years?

## Negotiating Skills for Landing a Great Job

These basic negotiating rules will be helpful in landing a new job or negotiating for advancement in a current position.

- **Be prepared:** Know your market value. Search the internet and current research on NP opportunities before the interview. Research the practice economics: the most common visit level billed, most frequently billed current procedural terminology (CPT) codes, percentage of practice income required to cover operating expenses, collection rate for the practice. (Office managers should be able to share this information with you.)

**COACH CONSULT**

If you get the position, you will be working with the person interviewing you, and thus do not want your image to be portrayed incorrectly from the start.

- **Recognize that employment negotiations are different from one employer to the next:** Focus on portraying your image honestly
- **Understand your needs and priorities:** Salary; bonuses, quarterly and production linked; partnerships; time off for vacation, holidays, sick time; continuing education expenses; payment of licensure and malpractice fees, professional dues; and payments for health insurance and retirement plans.
- **Recognize what the employer can and cannot do economically and ethically before pressing in the wrong direction:** What kind of support staff personnel is there and how many will be available to you in this practice? How many patients will you be expected to see per hour or per day? How much physician consultation time will you have available to you in the beginning of this employment?
- **Know if calls are required:** If so, how often? Are there expectations for evening or weekend hours in this position? Is call time reimbursed?
- **Understand the dynamics of the particular negotiations:** Sizing up the situation and understanding the relative position of each party will help you determine when to press your advantage and when to back off.
- **Always be honest:** Recognize areas of concern so you can rehearse how to handle them when they inevitably come up.
- **Recognize the role of fairness in negotiations:** You should be able to justify every request you make in terms of fairness.

- **Be creative:** Consider the value of the total package. Be willing to make tradeoffs to increase the total value of your employment package.
- **Focus on your goals, not on winning:** Keep your career goals in mind.
- **Know when to quit bargaining:** Don't be greedy.
- **Never forget that employment is an ongoing relationship:** Job negotiations are the starting point for your career with an employer. Start on a positive note.

Understanding these principles will allow you to effectively negotiate the terms of your new job. Just as there are positive hints for success in negotiations, there are also certain things one should never do in negotiating for a new job. Do not:

- Show up late for an interview
- Forget your interviewer's name
- Fail to do your research on the position
- Talk too much or too little
- Lose eye contact with the interviewer
- Be dishonest during the interview process
- Assume you have landed the job
- Ask if you got the job
- Fail to follow up

If you are an NP who has been working in a clinical site for some time and are ready to negotiate for improvements in your employment package, consider doing the following before approaching your employer.

- Making a list of what you have contributed to the practice in the past year. Have data to support your contributions
- Having a list of your total number of patient visits for the year, along with the dollars billed and received
- Making a list of any administrative projects on which you have worked and determining a dollar value for each project
- Including data from patient satisfaction surveys if these are collected
- Including patient communications regarding your practice management if these are available

**COACH CONSULT**

A personal note thanking those who interviewed you for their time can have a positive impact. Even if you are not offered the position or do not accept it, you will have left a positive professional image of yourself in the minds of the interviewers.

- Listing your activities within the community that have directly and indirectly influenced your practice environment. Include items such as involvement in community health fairs, community health agencies, and on-site education in local schools and churches. Demonstrate how, if any, these activities have enhanced the practice environment

## Establishing Your Practice

Once you land a position, you will need to follow your state guidelines for establishing your practice. For example, in Louisiana, the NP must have a collaborative practice agreement to apply for prescriptive authority. Some states have time frames for applying for prescriptive authority. Check your state practice act for specific information.

Some things you will need to do in your new practice setting are:
- Design and order prescription pads with your name and provider numbers
- Advertise that you have joined the practice
- Have business cards printed
- Have your name added to the office signage and stationery

Some activities you may want to consider to boost your patient population in your new practice position include:
- Offering free classes for patients in your clinic on specific health topics such as diet and foot care for diabetes, lifestyle modifications for various disorders, osteoporosis, and prevention of sexually transmitted diseases
- Offering to write a health column for the local newspaper, with timely health-related information for members of the community
- Getting involved in community agencies dealing with health-care issues in the community's area
- Organizing and participating in local health fairs for community residents
- Getting involved in your local NP professional organizations to help you stay current on practice issues, job market information, and continuing education programs
- Setting up a tracking system for your own practice to include number of patient visits, income generated, and quality improvement indicators that reflect your practice patterns. This information will be critical for future employment negotiations

## Collaborative Practice Agreements

Many states require NPs to have written agreements with physicians in order to practice or have prescriptive privileges. These agreements are legal mandates, but also are used as guides for providing care. In order to adapt the guidelines so that they meet a particular state's mandates, it is imperative to review the state practice act to see what information must be included in any required documents. Some state boards of nursing now have templates for use in the preparation of collaborative practice agreements. Examples of information that may need to be incorporated include a description of the practice setting, types of patients seen in the practice, procedures for medical record reviews including physician signatures, details of physician availability, an explanation of after-hours call policies, and an explanation of the referral process used by the practice. Other NP functions that might be addressed in the agreement include:

### COACH CONSULT

An NP in a new employment setting can establish long-term relationships with employers and the community by getting involved in the community, especially in areas related to health care. Involvement can take many directions, from providing health education in the NP's clinic, working in local health fairs, and writing health columns in the local newspapers to serving on area health and policy-making boards (see Box 1–2).

- Needs for in-hospital care
- Needs for suturing and minor surgical procedures
- Whether the NP will have a nursing home practice

Collaborative practice agreements should delineate the practice guidelines that the NP will be utilizing in patient care. Deviation from the guidelines may be used against NPs in malpractice suits unless there is clear documentation that the deviation was discussed with the collaborating physician in the management of the patient who brings the suit. All adaptations based on these guidelines should include the date of revision and the signatures of the providers. Each revision should include an update of references when a variation is clinically sound.

## Billing Numbers

After having established a place of practice and obtaining licensure and practice agreements, the NP is ready to begin work. Initially, NPs may see patients "incident to" their care by the physician with whom the NP has a practice agreement, billing third party payers under the physician's billing numbers for Medicare, Medicaid, and private insurance companies. The

A physician friend shared his philosophy for establishing a successful new practice environment. His philosophy is called the "three-touch method." Patients need to feel accepted in your clinic as valued clients and as part of their own health-care team. As health-care providers, physicians and nurses engage patients in a variety of ways. One such way includes a conscious effort to physically touch a patient three times while the patient is at the clinic for professional services:

- At the beginning of the visit, extend your hand to the patient in a handshake, greet the patient as a visitor to the practice, and introduce yourself
- During the office visit, utilize touch as you perform a physical examination. Check every patient's heart and lung sounds at every visit regardless of complaints. You can also check the patient's ear, nose, and throat to further engage in the touch philosophy. It never hurts to look and listen: doing so may reveal something that needs attention
- Before the patient leaves the room, reach out and give the patient another handshake or pat the patient on the shoulder as a sign of reassurance. It may even be appropriate to give some patients a hug

Patients who feel engaged by the health-care practitioner feel more accepted by the practitioner; are more likely to leave a visit in a satisfied state of mind; and, most importantly, are more likely to return when they need further care.

NP needs to be aware that in billing for services on this basis, the following regulations apply:

- The physician must evaluate the patient on the patient's initial visit to the office
- The physician must see and evaluate the patient on subsequent visits often enough to reflect the physician's active participation in the patient's management
- The physician must be involved in any new diagnoses for an established patient
- The physician must be present in the office or immediately available to provide assistance and direction in the patient's care
- Billing that is incident to a physician's care cannot be used in a hospital for inpatient or outpatient services unless the physician's office suite is located within the hospital

NPs need to apply for their own Medicare, Medicaid, and NPI numbers. They may also be required to apply for privileges with local private insurance carriers. Office managers for clinic practices are generally excellent resources for getting all of these applications processed in an efficient and timely manner.

## National Provider Identifier Number

If you bill for services, you will need an NPI number. Getting an NPI number is easy and free. Once you obtain your NPI number, it is estimated that it will take 120 days to do the remaining work required for using it. This includes working on your internal billing systems; coordinating with billing services, vendors, and clearinghouses; and testing with payers. As outlined in the federal regulation implementing the Health Insurance Portability and Accountability Act (HIPAA), you must also share the NPI number with other providers, health plans, clearinghouses, and any entity that may need it for billing purposes. Delays in applying for an NPI create risks for cash flow in the NP's clinical practice.

As of March 1, 2008, Medicare Fee-For-Service 837P and CMS-1500 claim forms must include an NPI number in the primary fields, such as the billing, pay-to, and rendering fields. Since January 1, 2008, Medicare has required NPI numbers to identify the primary providers of a patient's care—the billing and pay-to providers—in Medicare electronic and paper institutional claims such as the 837I and UB-04 claims.

**COACH CONSULT**

Additional information and education about the NPI number can be found at the Centers for Medicare and Medicaid Services (CMS) NPI page at www.cms.hhs.gov/National ProvIdentStand. Providers can apply for an NPI number online or can call the NPI enumerator to request a paper application.

## Medicare Provider Enrollment

All providers who will be providing services to Medicare beneficiaries must complete the Medicare Enrollment Application (CMS-855I). Providers will need to have an NPI number prior to applying for Medicare Provider enrollment. Providers will utilize the CMS 1500 form when billing for services provided to Medicare beneficiaries.

To facilitate the Medicare enrollment process, the provider must submit the latest version of the Medicare enrollment application, found on the CMS Web site (www.cms.hhs.gov). NPs must be certain to complete the application form in its entirety and include any requested supporting documentation. Examples of supporting documents may include professional licenses, business licenses, verification of education, and an authorization agreement for Electronic Funds Transfer (CMS-588).

## Medicaid Provider Enrollment

Each state's Medicaid program has different enrollment requirements. Typically, providers are required to submit a valid license, registration, or certification that is in accordance with their state's laws and regulations.

A directory of state Medicaid programs is available online at the CMS website. Billing for Medicaid services is generally done with form UB 04, which has replaced the uniform billing (UB 92) form.

### Private Insurance Enrollment

Providers may elect to enroll in one or several private insurance companies' list of providers. Requirements for enrollment vary from one insurance company to another. The NP's clinical practice can identify third-party payers who will be utilized by patients in that practice setting.

Tips in applying for billing numbers and avoiding returned application forms include:

- Using one's legal name consistently on the application forms
- Completely providing all requested information
- Making certain that all signature lines contain original signatures and are dated; blue ink should be used
- Submitting all required supporting documentation
- Providing notary seals where indicated

## Prescriptive Authority and Drug Enforcement Administration Numbers

The co-signature of a collaborating physician is not required in any state on any prescription that an NP is authorized to write. Any prescription written for a controlled substance will include the NP prescriber's federal DEA number, denoting the NP's independent or plenary authority to prescribe in accordance with the state's scope-of-practice specifications.

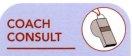

**COACH CONSULT**

Other useful resources may include a listing of each state's Board of Nursing, found at the National Council of State Boards of Nursing (http://www.ncsbn.org/) and the National Association of Boards of Pharmacy (http://www.nabp.net/).

All prescriptions should include the standard information expected from all authorized prescribers, such as the prescriber's name, title, license/specialty, ID/Rx number as applicable, practice address, and phone number; the patient's name; the date of the prescription; and the name of the drug being prescribed and its strength, dosage, route of administration, specific directions for its use, quantity, number of refills, and instructions regarding generic substitution. Check the state advanced practice act for information about receipt of samples of both controlled and non-controlled drugs. Box 1–3 provides helpful hints in prescribing.

## Box 1-3 Helpful Hints for Prescribing Practices

- Keep all prescription pads stored in a secure location. Never leave pads in a drawer in a patient examination room
- Write legibly. For clarity, use caution with decimal points, fractions, and symbols. Never leave blank spaces at the bottom of a prescription. Draw a line between the name of the medication being ordered and your signature line
- For clarity about the quantity of a drug dosage form to be dispensed, write the numeric form of the quantity (#20) and then spell out the number (twenty). This is important with any controlled substances. It would be quite easy for a patient to change #15 to #150 if you do not spell out the number completely
- Do not write prescriptions for persons who are not established patients in your practice
- Write all prescriptions in the clinic setting. Leave prescription pads at work
- Note all medicines prescribed and their amounts and dosages in the patient's chart
- Duplicate prescription pads can be helpful in preventing prescription abuse by patients
- Completely fill out all required information on the patient prescription form, including the patient's name and age and the date on which the prescription is written
- Indicate the number of refills for a prescription and whether generic substitutions are permitted

# 2 Symptom Management

# CHAPTER 2

# Symptom Management

On every clinic day, patients present with symptoms—some easy to identify, and others more vague or problematic. This chapter is designed to identify the most common complaints presented in a primary-care office and to explore the possible differential diagnoses for each complaint so as to reach the correct final diagnosis for the patient. Common patient complaints included for discussion in this chapter constitute a long list of complaints, each of which may be a part of multiple possible final diagnoses. Discussion of each symptom is presented in an alphabetical format for ease of use. For each symptom presentation, this chapter provides a discussion of the differential diagnoses, with helpful guides to associated symptoms and diagnostic procedures to aid in ruling out or supporting a particular diagnosis.

## Abdominal Pain in Adults

Abdominal pain can arise from any number of organ-system problems, including gastrointestinal (GI), musculoskeletal, reproductive, genitourinary, and vascular disorders. It can also be an effect of medications, of the ingestion of toxins, or even of viral or bacterial infections. The first step in diagnosing the cause of abdominal pain is to identify and manage those of its causes that are life-threatening, such as abdominal aortic aneurysm (AAA), acute appendicitis, adrenal crisis, cholelithiasis, acute pancreatitis, ectopic pregnancy, intestinal obstruction, acute GI bleeding, sickle cell crisis, peritonitis, and acute pyelonephritis.

### Assessment

When assessing abdominal pain, make sure to use a pain scale and to identify pain by its type; as dull, sharp, stabbing, or burning. Determine alleviating and aggravating factors for the pain, and check the patient's history regarding substance use; history of GI, reproductive, or vascular diseases; and recent changes in appetite or weight. Also assess for the presence of associated symptoms. When performing a physical examination:

- Inspect for distention, peristaltic waves, and abdominal girth
- Assess bowel sounds and the character of bowel motility
- Percuss for abdominal sounds and liver span
- Palpate for rigidity, masses, tenderness, rebound tenderness, guarding, and costovertebral angle tenderness (CVAT)
- Perform an obturator test and psoas test
- Assess for Murphy's sign
- Assess for hernias
- Perform a digital rectal examination for GI bleeding

A number of physical assessment tests are specific to the abdomen, mainly for identifying appendicitis and peritoneal irritation. Table 2–1 presents a summary of assessment tests that may aid in identifying the cause of an acute abdomen.

### Table 2–1  Abdominal Assessment Tests

| TEST | DESCRIPTION | CONDITIONS |
|------|-------------|------------|
| Aaron's | Pain in patient's epigastric area upon palpation of McBurney's point | Appendicitis |
| Balance | Fixed dullness to percussion in L flank; dullness in R flank that decreases with changes in position | Peritoneal irritation |
| Blumberg's | Rebound tenderness | Peritoneal irritation Appendicitis |
| Cullen's | Umbilical ecchymosis | Hemoperitoneum Pancreatitis Ectopic pregnancy |
| Dance's | No bowel sounds in RLQ | Intussusception |
| Grey Turner's | Flank ecchymosis | Hemoperitoneum Pancreatitis |

## Table 2–1 Abdominal Assessment Tests—cont'd

| TEST | DESCRIPTION | CONDITIONS |
|---|---|---|
| Iliopsoas | Patient raises R knee against resistance, extension of R hip with patient on L side | Pain = appendicitis |
| Kehr's | Radiation of abdominal pain to L shoulder | Splenic rupture Renal calculi Ectopic pregnancy |
| Markle's | Patient stands with straightened legs and raises up on toes; jams body on heels in returning to floor | Pain = Peritoneal irritation or Appendicitis |
| McBurney's | Rebound tenderness with palpation of McBurney's point | Appendicitis |
| Murphy's | Inspiration halts on palpation of gallbladder, pain to right shoulder | Cholecystitis |
| Obturator | Pain on flexion and internal rotation of R leg with knee bent | Appendicitis |
| Romberg-Howship's | Pain extending down medial aspect of thigh to knee | Strangulated obturator muscle Hernia |
| Rovsing's | RLQ pain intensifies with pressure applied to LLQ | Peritoneal irritation Appendicitis |

Adapted from Hansen, J. Practitioner's Pocket Pal. Miami: MedMaster, Inc., 2001, pp 16–17.

## Diagnostic Testing

Diagnostic procedures indicated to assist in identifying the cause of every case of abdominal pain include a complete blood count (CBC) with a differential count and urinalysis. The following diagnostic procedures should also be considered:

- With vomiting: Electrolytes, blood urea nitrogen (BUN), and creatinine
- For suspected pregnancy: Serum human chorionic gonadotropin (hCG)
- If the patient's history indicates: Testing for gonorrhea and chlamydia
- To identify free air, ileus, bowel obstruction, or calcification: A flat-plate x-ray of the abdomen

- For suspected obstruction, peritonitis, or bowel ischemia: An ultrasound examination or computed tomographic (CT) scan of the abdomen
- For suspected ovarian torsion, pelvic abscess, or ectopic pregnancy: A transvaginal ultrasound examination

Table 2–2 provides an overview of acute and chronic causes of abdominal pain in adults.

| Table 2–2 **Acute and Chronic Causes of Abdominal Pain** | | |
|---|---|---|
| **DIAGNOSIS** | **HISTORY** | **FINDINGS ON PHYSICAL EXAMINATION** |
| **LIFE-THREATENING CAUSES OF ABDOMINAL PAIN** | | |
| Peritonitis | Severe pain, fever, chills; movement worsens pain | Fever, abdominal tenderness and guarding, rigidity, rebound tenderness, decreased bowel sounds, hypotension, tachycardia, pallor, diaphoresis |
| Perforation of viscus | Severe, generalized pain | Similar to peritonitis findings |
| Bowel infarction | Diffuse pain, possible bloody diarrhea, patient age generally >50 years | Hypotension, tachycardia, pallor, sweating, signs of peritonitis, abdominal distention |
| Bowel obstruction | Nausea, vomiting, abdominal distention, history of constipation, history of abdominal surgery | Abdominal distention, tympanic percussion of abdomen high-pitched, rushing bowel sounds early, decreased later; restlessness |
| Myocardial infarction | Severe epigastric pain, possible nausea and vomiting | Diaphoresis, no abdominal tenderness |
| Rupture of AAA | Acute abdominal pain, low back or flank pain | Pulsatile abdominal mass, hypotension, tachycardia, asymmetrical—pulses |
| **ACUTE ABDOMINAL PAIN** | | |
| Gastroenteritis | Nausea, vomiting | — |
| Appendicitis | Epigastric or periumbilical pain that progresses to RLQ, worsens over hours | Low-grade fever, tenderness in RLQ, bowel sounds variable, positive psoas/obturator signs, rebound tenderness |

## Table 2–2 Acute and Chronic Causes of Abdominal Pain—cont'd

| DIAGNOSIS | HISTORY | FINDINGS ON PHYSICAL EXAMINATION |
|---|---|---|
| **ACUTE ABDOMINAL PAIN** | | |
| Hepatitis | General malaise, myalgia, nausea, pain in RUQ | Hepatic tenderness or enlargement Jaundice |
| Diverticulitis | Pain in LLQ, constipation, nausea, vomiting, possible minor rectal bleeding | Fever, tenderness in LLQ, occasional rectal mass, decreased bowel sounds, localized signs of peritonitis |
| Cholecystitis | Colicky pain in epigastric area, may radiate to scapula. Nausea, vomiting, jaundice, dark urine, changes in stool color | Fever, tenderness in RUQ with guarding, decreased bowel sounds |
| Pancreatitis | Upper abdominal pain that may radiate to the back, nausea, vomiting. Possible history of alcoholism or cholelithiasis. Pain intensifies with sitting up or leaning forward | Periumbilical tenderness, possible hypotension, tachycardia, pallor, and sweating. Decreased bowel sounds. |
| Salpingitis (PID) | Lower quadrant pain (right and left sides), fever, chills, dyspareunia, vaginal discharge | Fever, tenderness with guarding, rebound. Adnexal tenderness, cervical motion tenderness, purulent vaginal discharge |
| Ectopic pregnancy rupture | Menses late by more than 2 weeks, severe, acute onset of pain | Adnexal tenderness, palpable mass, postural hypotension, tachycardia |
| Ureteral stone | Pain in flank, radiates to groin; painful urination; hematuria | Flank tenderness, decreased bowel sounds. Fever if UTI present |
| Prostatitis | | |

*Continued*

## Table 2–2  Acute and Chronic Causes of Abdominal Pain—cont'd

| DIAGNOSIS | HISTORY | FINDINGS ON PHYSICAL EXAMINATION |
|---|---|---|
| **CHRONIC ABDOMINAL PAIN** | | |
| Reflux esophagitis | Burning, epigastric, or substernal pain radiating to jaws; worse when lying flat; relieved by antacids or sitting upright | Normal GI examination, patient often obese |
| Peptic ulcer | Recurrent epigastric pain from 1–4 hours after meals. Pain intensifies with alcohol, aspirin or other NSAIDs, steroids; relieved by antacids or food | Deep epigastric tenderness |
| Ulcerative colitis | Rectal urgency; recurrent defecation of small amounts of semiformed stool, pain worse before bowel movement, blood in stool | Low-grade fever, colon and rectal tenderness, blood in stool, weight loss |
| Irritable bowel | Recurrent abdominal pain, change in bowel habits, alternating diarrhea and constipation is common, anxiety worsens symptoms | No fever, minimal abdominal tenderness, no blood in stool |
| Regional enteritis | Pain in RLQ or periumbilical area, may be relieved by defecation, soft stools | Low-grade fever, periumbilical or RLQ tenderness, possible weight loss |

Adapted from Wasson, J. The Common Symptom Guide, ed. 5. New York: McGraw-Hill, 2002.

## Differential Diagnoses

The differential diagnosis of abdominal pain includes peptic ulcer, biliary tract disorder, gastritis, peritonitis, diverticulitis, referred renal pain, urinary tract infection, pelvic inflammatory disease (PID), hernia, myocardial infarction (MI), inflammatory bowel disorders, testicular torsion, and rectus sheath hematoma. Table 2–3 identifies common causes of GI complaints according to the quadrant in which the complaints are noted.

## Referred Abdominal Pain

Referred abdominal pain occurs fairly frequently with GI complaints. Be aware that GI conditions may also have referral areas for pain. Thus, for example:

- Cholecystitis is often referred laterally to the right scapula
- Pancreatitis may produce referred pain through the mid-back
- Pain from the inferior diaphragm may present on the superior surface of the ipsilateral shoulder
- Duodenal ulcer may be accompanied by mid-back discomfort
- Disorders of the biliary tree may have pain referred to the right shoulder or right posterior chest
- Back pain may be observed in patients with peptic ulcer, pancreatitis, cancer, prostatitis, endometriosis, or a dissecting aortic aneurysm

**COACH CONSULT**

To manage sudden and severe abdominal pain, follow these guidelines:
- Monitor vital signs, observing for tachycardia and hypotension
- Palpate pulses below the waistline
- Examine to identify any of the following symptoms:
  - Mottled skin below the waist
  - Pulsating epigastric mass
  - Rebound tenderness
  - Rigidity of the abdominal wall

Table 2–3 **Common Gastrointestinal Complaints by Quadrant**

| RIGHT UPPER QUADRANT | LEFT UPPER QUADRANT |
| --- | --- |
| Duodenal ulcer | Gastritis |
| Pancreatitis | Gastric ulcer |
| Peritonitis | Cardiac ischemia |
| Cholecystitis | Peritonitis |
| Retrocecal appendicitis | Splenic infarct |
| Right heart failure | Left-lower-lobe pneumonia |
| Cardiac ischemia | Pancreatitis |
| Hepatitis | Splenic rupture |
| Right-lower-lobe pneumonia | Colonic pain |

*Continued*

## Table 2–3  Common Gastrointestinal Complaints by Quadrant—cont'd

| RIGHT LOWER QUADRANT | LEFT LOWER QUADRANT |
|---|---|
| Appendicitis | Intestinal obstruction |
| Mittelschmerz | Mittelschmerz |
| Perforated cecum | Psoas abscess |
| Intestinal obstruction | Salpingitis |
| Salpingitis | Ectopic pregnancy |
| Ectopic pregnancy | Left inguinal hernia |
| Right inguinal hernia | Diverticulitis |
| Psoas abscess | Testicular torsion |
| Diverticulitis | Enteritis |
| Testicular torsion | |
| Enteritis | |
| **DIFFUSE ABDOMINAL PAIN** | |
| Peritonitis | Small-bowel obstruction |
| Streptococcal pharyngitis (children) | Pancreatitis |
| Mesenteric thrombus | Abdominal aortic aneurysm |
| Early appendicitis | Gastroenteritis |
| Metabolic causes | |

Lee, B. Medical Notes. Philadelphia: F.A. Davis, 2009.

## Abdominal Pain in Children

Acute abdominal pain in children requires immediate attention and accurate diagnosis and treatment. As with any condition of acute onset, a detailed history is essential, including the time of onset; aggravating and palliative measures; associated symptoms of nausea, vomiting, diarrhea, and bleeding; and the relationship of onset to food, stress, trauma, or medications.

Principal causes of acute abdominal pain vary with age. Common causes of abdominal pain in infancy are colic, incarcerated hernia, intussusception, bowel perforation, intestinal malrotation, volvulus, and Hirschsprung's disease. Intussusception presents with a sudden, paroxysmal onset of colicky pain; may be accompanied by "currant jelly" stools, vomiting, decreased bowel sounds and a palpable mass in the right upper quadrant (RUQ); and is more common in children between the ages of 5 months and 2 years of age. Intestinal malrotation is suspected when a previously healthy infant does not eat, vomits, does not produce stool, is inconsolable, and presents with abdominal distention. Incarcerated hernias may present with a tender abdominal mass as well as abdominal pain.

During childhood, causes of abdominal pain include appendicitis, gastroenteritis, pancreatitis, urinary tract infection, hemolytic uremic syndrome, right lower lobe pneumonia, constipation, and Henoch–Schönlein syndrome. Gastroenteritis is generally viral and presents with crampy pain, diarrhea, vomiting, and malaise, and possibly with fever. Appendicitis presents with periumbilical pain that later radiates to the right lower quadrant (RLQ) and may be accompanied by vomiting, diarrhea, and fever.

In adolescence , causes of abdominal pain include inflammatory bowel disease (IBD), peptic ulcer disease, PID, dysmenorrhea, pregnancy, mittelschmerz (ovulatory pain), testicular torsion, and ovarian torsion. Mittelschmerz presents with pain of sudden onset in the right or left lower quadrant at the midpoint of the menstrual cycle that persists for more than 24 hours. Table 2–4 shows common causes, histories, and clinical findings in cases of pediatric abdominal pain.

## Assessment

To begin an assessment of the acute abdomen, obtain a careful history. Questions for children and parents about the characteristics of abdominal pain may provide essential clues to making appropriate diagnoses. For example, abdominal pain of sudden onset may be seen in cases of perforation, intussusception, testicular torsion, and ruptured ectopic pregnancy. Severe abdominal pain may be indicative of IBD or sickle cell crisis. Abdominal pain of gradual onset may indicate various inflammatory processes, including appendicitis, pancreatitis, or cholecystitis. Intermittent abdominal pain is typically noted with disease or trauma to a muscular viscus such as the pancreatic duct, uterus, fallopian tubes, biliary tree, or intestinal wall.

## Table 2–4 Pediatric Abdominal Pain

| DIAGNOSIS | HISTORY | FINDINGS ON PHYSICAL EXAMINATION |
|---|---|---|
| Acute: Appendicitis | Epigastric or periumbilical pain that progresses to RLQ. Gradual onset. Possible vomiting and fever. Patient generally over 3 years of age. | Low-grade fever<br>RLQ tenderness<br>Positive psoas/obturator tests |
| Acute: Mesenteric adenitis | Similar to that in appendicitis | Temperature over 101°F |
| Acute: Intussusception | Acute, sudden onset of abdominal pain, vomiting, decreased bowel movements | Mild temperature elevations<br>Palpable abdominal mass<br>Bowel sounds with high-pitched, rushing sound alternating with absence of bowel sounds<br>Possible rectal blood on examination |
| Acute: Bowel obstruction | No bowel movement<br>Vomiting, dehydration | Hyperactive bowel sounds, abdominal distention, hyperresonance |
| Lactose intolerance | Bloating, recurrent abdominal pain | Normal |
| Constipation | General abdominal aches | Palpable stool |
| Peptic ulcer | Nonspecific abdominal pain/aches | Positive occult blood possible |
| Worm infestation (*Ascaris*, hookworm, *Taenia*, *Strongyloides*) | Diffuse pain, weight loss, anemia, diarrhea. May have nighttime awakening with abdominal pain complaints | Hookworm: Possible pallor |
| Colic | 2 weeks to 4 months of age, pain often in early evenings | Normal |
| Lead poisoning | Diffuse abdominal pain | Usually normal |

| Table 2–4 **Pediatric Abdominal Pain—cont'd** | | |
|---|---|---|
| **DIAGNOSIS** | **HISTORY** | **FINDINGS ON PHYSICAL EXAMINATION** |
| Sickle cell crisis | Family history of sickle cell disease | Ileus of right abdominal wall |
| Cholecystitis | Epigastric colicky pain, may radiate to shoulder or scapula, nausea, vomiting, fever, jaundice, dark urine, clay-colored stools | Fever, RUQ tenderness, decreased bowel sounds |

Adapted from Olson, L., DeWitt, T., First, L. and Zenel, J. Pediatrics. St. Louis: Elsevier-Mosby, 2008.

Danger signs in the assessment of pediatric abdominal pain include:
- Age under 5 years
- Fever, weight loss, growth delays, joint pain, and rash
- Abdominal pain that awakens a child from sleep
- Pain that radiates to the back, shoulder, or lower extremities
- Steatorrhea
- Blood in the stool
- Bilious vomiting
- Perianal skin tags, fissures, or fistulas
- Family history of severe GI disease

**ALERT**

Critical findings related to abdominal pain in children and warranting serious concern include:
- Abdominal guarding
- Abdominal mass
- Bilious or fecaloid vomiting
- Borborygmi/absent bowel sounds
- Hematemesis or melena
- Hepatosplenomegaly

## Diagnostic Testing
In cases of abdominal pain, consider the following diagnostic procedures:
- Evaluate all complaints of abdominal pain with a CBC and differential count; assays for serum electrolytes, glucose, and creatinine; and a urinalysis
- With upper GI pain, consider checking laboratory values for amylase and lipase, and ordering liver function tests
- If hemolytic anemia or sickle cell crisis is suspected, a peripheral smear may aid in making a diagnosis
- A pregnancy test is necessary prior to any x-ray studies for all female patients of childbearing age
- If PID is suspected, order cervical and vaginal cultures

A plain abdominal x-ray film may identify air–fluid levels, free air, bowel obstructions, foreign bodies, and masses

- Abdominal ultrasound examination will aid in the diagnosis of liver, gallbladder, pancreas, kidney, uterus, and adnexal abnormalities
- A CT scan is indicated with abdominal trauma or masses
- A chest radiograph can help rule out lower-lobe pneumonia
- A testicular blood flow scan should be done for acute pain in the scrotum

## Differential Diagnoses
### *Acute Appendicitis in Children*
The incidence of appendicitis in children generally peaks between 10 and 15 years of age. The triad of classic signs of appendicitis—abdominal pain, vomiting, and fever—applies. Pain may initially present in the umbilical area but radiates to the RLQ as inflammation progresses. If perforation occurs, pain will be more generalized. Pain from appendicitis may awaken a child from sleep. Appendicitis in children may also present with vomiting accompanied by pain; often, however, children with appendicitis will have anorexia. Initially a low-grade fever may be present, escalating if perforation occurs. The onset of pain before vomiting is a key to differentiation between appendicitis and infectious enteritis. Obtain a CBC and urinalysis, and consider an abdominal ultrasound examination to aid in the diagnosis. Any child in whom appendicitis is highly suspect requires immediate surgical referral. Any child with acute abdominal pain of undetermined origin should be hospitalized for further observation and evaluation.

**COACH CONSULT**

If you suspect FAP, investigate the characteristics of the abdominal pain and obtain a complete review of systems and a dietary history, history of illness patterns, and sexual history. Identify potential risk factors for parasitic or bacterial infections. Perform diagnostic procedures including a CBC with a differential count, erythrocyte sedimentation rate (ESR), chemistry profile, urinalysis, and stool cultures for parasites. If chronic diarrhea is present, consider evaluating for *Clostridium difficile* toxins.

### *Functional Abdominal Pain of a Chronic Nature*
Chronic abdominal pain in children is generally allocated on the basis of the Rome II criteria to one of the three categories of functional abdominal pain (FAP), dyspepsia, or irritable bowel syndrome (IBS). Features common to all of these presentations include:

- Physical or psychosocial stress
- Illness-related behaviors such as school absences, avoidance of normal activities,

and possible parental tolerance of behavioral problems in a child resulting from the parental perception of illness

• A family history of gastrointestinal disorders

FAP presents with a clustering of episodes of pain that may persist for several weeks, is generally periumbilical or midepigastric, and is typically of a colicky nature. FAP demonstrates no relationship to food, exercise, or bowel movements, but may be associated with nausea, headache, pallor, or weakness.

Dyspepsia presents with pain, bloating, heartburn, nausea, and vomiting. There may also be a presentation of reflux, hiccups, or flatulence. In many cases dyspepsia has a symptomatic relationship to meals.

IBS presents with abdominal pain that may be relieved with defecation. Other symptoms may include frequent stooling, bloating, passage of mucus per rectum, and dyspepsia.

## Abdominal Aortic Aneurysm

A life-threatening AAA may present as dull lower abdominal pain, lower back pain, or severe chest pain. The pain is generally constant, worsens when the patient is supine, and lessens somewhat when the patient sits up or leans forward.

### Assessment
Assessment of a nonruptured AAA will reveal a pulsating, palpable epigastric mass. Additional symptoms evident with AAA include:

• Mottled skin below the waist
• Absent femoral and pedal pulses
• Blood pressure (BP) readings lower in the legs than in the arms
• Abdominal tenderness, guarding, and possible rigidity
• Signs of shock

### Diagnostic Testing
Diagnostic procedures to consider for suspected AAA include ultrasound examination, magnetic resonance imaging (MRI), and CT scan. Of the three, the CT scan and MRI are the most accurate in defining a possible aneurysm.

### Differential Diagnoses
#### Abdominal Rigidity
Abdominal rigidity may be voluntary or involuntary. Voluntary rigidity is usually symmetrical,

> **ALERT**
>
> Any patient with a pulsatile abdominal mass and hypotension should be sent immediately to the emergency department for surgical evaluation and intervention.

greater on inspiration than on expiration, and eased by relaxation techniques. It is generally related to a patient's fear or nervousness about a potential diagnosis or examination. Involuntary rigidity most commonly results from GI diseases, but may also be related to pulmonary or musculoskeletal disorders. Involuntary rigidity is often asymmetrical, unaffected by respiration, and present when the patient sits up. It is accompanied by nausea, vomiting, tenderness, distention, and abdominal pain. Involuntary rigidity is observed with AAA, mesenteric artery ischemia, peritonitis, and in certain cases of insect stings, especially black widow spider bites.

## Mesenteric Artery Ischemia

Mesenteric artery ischemia may present with 2 to 3 days of low-grade pain followed by an episode of diarrhea and severe abdominal pain. Signs of shock, vomiting, and anorexia may also be present. Mesenteric artery ischemia is more commonly seen in middle-aged patients with a history of heart failure, arrhythmia, or hypotension.

## Peritonitis

Peritonitis may present with generalized or localized rigidity. Other signs and symptoms of peritonitis include sudden, severe abdominal pain with tenderness; guarding; rebound tenderness; hypoactive or absent bowel sounds; fever; chills; tachycardia; tachypnea; and hypotension. Diagnostic procedures for peritonitis include plain abdominal radiography and CT scanning. Plain radiographic films will reveal any free air under the diaphragm resulting from perforation of the viscera. The CT scan will identify fluid collections, abscesses, and strangulated obstructions.

## Back Pain

Back pain is a common symptom treated in family practice and primary-care settings. It is often related directly to work or physical stress, but may also result from a genitourinary problem, GI disease, cardiovascular problem, neoplastic disorder, or postural changes like those associated with pregnancy.

**COACH CONSULT**

Insect toxins may produce a generalized, cramping abdominal pain leading to rigidity. The patient may also present with fever, nausea, vomiting, tremors, and a burning sensation in the hands and feet. Children may demonstrate an expiratory grunt and will keep their legs flexed.

**ALERT**

If the patient has severe back pain with an acute presentation, quickly rule out life-threatening causes such as a dissecting AAA, appendicitis, cholecystitis, intervertebral disk rupture, acute pancreatitis, and acute pyelonephritis.

Characteristics of specific types of back pain include:

- Pain unaffected by activity and rest may be referred from the viscera
- Referred spondylogenic pain worsens with activity and improves with rest
- Pain of neoplastic origin worsens at night and is usually relieved by walking
- AAA may present as deep lumbar pain unaffected by activity and accompanied by a pulsating epigastric mass
- A perforated ulcer or acute pancreatitis may mimic back pain, beginning as severe epigastric pain that radiates to the back, accompanied by abdominal rigidity and tenderness

Table 2–5 differentiates back pain by site of origin as musculoskeletal, visceral, or radicular.

## Assessment

In cases of back pain, obtain a complete history, review of systems, and physical examination. Include the following:

- Note spinal curvatures
- Have the patient bend forward, backward, and laterally and observe for paravertebral muscle spasms
- Check for point tenderness in the dorsolumbar area of the spine
- Have the patient walk on the heels and then on the toes of the feet to assess for spinal nerve root irritation or muscular disorders
- Have the patient perform straight leg lifts in the seated and supine positions. Pain along the sciatic nerve may indicate disk herniation or sciatica
- Check for CVAT

## Diagnostic Testing

Diagnostic procedures for specific back pain complaints vary according to the nature of the cause. For low back pain of mechanical origin, consider the following diagnostic suggestions:

- Low back pain lasting longer than 4 weeks: CBC, ESR, x-radiography, or a bone scan

**COACH CONSULT**

When a child complains of back pain, evaluate with a thorough review of systems, a physical examination, and spinal x-ray films. If the diagnosis is unclear, continue the evaluation with a bone scan, CT scan, and MRI. A diagnosis of growth-related pain, back strain, or overuse syndromes in children should be made only after a complete evaluation rules out other causes of back pain.

## Table 2–5  Differentiation of Back Pain by Site of Origin

| DIAGNOSIS | HISTORY | FINDINGS ON PHYSICAL EXAMINATION |
|---|---|---|
| **MUSCULOSKELETAL SOURCES OF BACK PAIN** | | |
| Spinal fracture | Trauma; severe, persistent pain | Localized spinal or paraspinal tenderness, possible neurological changes |
| Osteomyelitis | History of recent infection, constant back pain progressing over weeks | Spinal percussion produces pain, little or no fever |
| Malignant tumor | Severe progressive pain, patient often elderly with history of weight loss or malignancy | Direct spinal tenderness to palpation or percussion |
| Muscle strain | History of lifting or strain, no radiation of pain | Paraspinous muscle spasm, negative straight leg test |
| Osteoarthritis | Multiple joint pains | Limited range of motion |
| Ankylosing spondylitis | Stiffness and low back pain, usually in young males | Sacroiliac tenderness, reduced flexion of spine on forward bending; loss of lumbar lordosis |
| **VISCERAL SOURCES OF BACK PAIN** | | |
| Peptic ulcer | History of peptic ulcer; pain in lumbar area, relieved with antacids | Stool positive for blood, epigastric tenderness |
| Pancreatitis | Upper epigastric discomfort, history of alcoholism or gallstones | Epigastric or generalized abdominal tenderness, decreased bowel sounds |
| Abdominal aortic aneurysm | Upper abdominal discomfort | Absent femoral pulses, palpable pulsatile mass |
| Kidney stone | Flank pain radiating to perineum, dysuria, hematuria | Flank or upper abdominal tenderness |
| Gynecological diseases | Lower abdominal to sacral discomfort (See section on vaginal discharge) | Abnormal pelvic examination |
| Prostatitis | Change in urination, painful urination, lower abdominal pain | Tender, enlarged prostate |

| Table 2–5 **Differentiation of Back Pain by Site of Origin—cont'd** | | |
|---|---|---|
| **DIAGNOSIS** | **HISTORY** | **FINDINGS ON PHYSICAL EXAMINATION** |
| **RADICULAR BACK PAIN** | | |
| Major neurological deficit | Trauma, possible bladder dysfunction, paresthesias in lower extremities | Bladder enlarged after voiding, flaccid anal sphincter, sensory loss in perineum, absent DTRs, weakness |
| Herniated intervertebral disk | Pain in back with radiation into leg(s) or buttocks, worsens with coughing, sneezing | Decreased DTRs in lower extremities, straight leg lift causes back pain |
| Spinal stenosis | Low back pain, may radiate to thighs, may be relieved by bending forward | Thigh weakness, unsteady gait |
| **OTHER CAUSES OF BACK PAIN** | | |
| Herpes zoster | Unilateral pain along dermatome(s) | Usually a rash following dermatome band |

Adapted from Wasson, J. The Common Symptom Guide. ed. 5.New York: McGraw-Hill, 2005.

- Spinal fracture: Plain lumbosacral x-ray films; if the x-ray results are negative but pain persists, consider a bone scan
- Herniated disks and tumors: MRI
- Osteoarthritis: CT scan to visualize cortical bone
- Osteomyelitis and neoplasms: Bone scans
- Spinal stenosis: MRI or CT scan, especially if plain x-ray films are not diagnostic
- With sciatica symptoms lasting longer than 4 weeks: MRI or CT scan, or an electromyogram (EMG) to identify the location of a nerve root injury

## Differential Diagnoses

Mechanical low back pain in adults comprises more than 95% of all etiologies of adult back pain. Included in the category of mechanical back pain are lumbosacral strain, herniated intervertebral disks, spinal stenosis, spondylolysis, and degenerative processes. Medically serious sources of back pain include fracture, tumor, cauda equina syndrome, and AAA. Table 2–6 presents serious sources of back pain.

## Table 2–6 Serious Sources of Back Pain

| FRACTURE | TUMOR OR INFECTION | CAUDA EQUINA SYNDROME | ACUTE ABDOMINAL AORTIC ANEURYSM |
|---|---|---|---|
| Major trauma Strenuous lifting Use of corticosteroids History of osteoporosis in elderly patient | Age >50 or <20 years History of cancer Fever, chills, weight loss Risk factors for infection Pain that worsens when supine Severe nighttime pain Rest pain Pain that fails to improve with therapy | Saddle anesthesia Recent urinary retention, increased urinary frequency, or overflow incontinence Severe or progressive neurological deficit in legs Unexpected laxity of anal sphincter Perianal sensory loss Knee-extension weakness or foot drop | Age >60 years Abdominal pulsating mass Other atherosclerotic vascular diseases Resting or night pain Tearing pain |

Adapted from Desai, S. Clinician's Guide to Diagnosis. Cleveland: Lexi-Comp Inc., 2001.

### Ankylosing Spondylitis

Ankylosing spondylitis causes chronic, progressive sacroiliac pain radiating up the spine, aggravated by lateral pressure on the pelvis, and unrelieved by rest. It may cause local tenderness, fatigue, fever, anorexia, and weight loss. Severe morning pain is more common than pain at other times of the day. Other signs and symptoms of ankylosing spondylitis may include progressive limitation of back mobility and chest expansion, peripheral arthritis, and anterior uritis. Onset generally occurs in the late teen years or early 20s. Diagnostic findings that support the presence of ankylosing spondylitis include:

- Elevated ESR
- Absence of rheumatoid factor
- Possible mild anemia. Check the patient's CBC and serum iron level
- Human leukocyte antigen (HLA) B27 factor, found more often in whites than in African Americans
- Plain radiographs showing changes in the sacroiliac joint
- MRI to help detect early changes in the sacroiliac joint and ischial tuberosities

Treatment of ankylosing spondylitis includes:

- Management of pre-existing chronic arthritis; nonsteroidal anti-inflammatory drugs (NSAIDs) may slow progression of the disease

- Refractory cases may respond to:
  - Etanercept (Enbrel): 50 mg SQ weekly, or
  - Adalimumab (Humira): 40 mg SQ weekly, or
  - Infliximab (Remicade): 5 mg/kg monthly, by injection

## Appendicitis

Appendicitis typically presents with right lower quadrant pain accompanied by anorexia, nausea, fever, and rebound tenderness over McBurney's point. The pain may also be retrocecal and radiate to the back. Diagnostic procedures for ruling out appendicitis include a CT scan, MRI, and ultrasound examination. The CT scan is preferred for all men and for women who have had a hysterectomy; ultrasound examination will aid in identifying PID as a cause of pain.

## Cholecystitis

Cholecystitis presents with pain in the right upper quadrant (RUQ) that may radiate to the right shoulder or back, accompanied by anorexia, fever, vomiting, tenderness, abdominal rigidity, pallor, and sweating. Diagnostic procedures for ruling out cholecystitis include ultrasound examination and cholescintigraphy. MRI may be helpful when the ultrasound examination is not diagnostic.

## Pancreatitis

Pancreatitis presents as fulminating, continuous pain in the upper abdomen that may radiate to the back and both flanks. Associated symptoms include abdominal tenderness, nausea, vomiting, fever, pallor, tachycardia, abdominal guarding, rigidity, and diminished bowel sounds. Diagnostic procedures to consider with pancreatitis include a CT scan for identifying the spread of inflammation, and ultrasound examination to identify enlargement of the pancreas, cholelithiasis, or dynamic ileus. Laboratory studies that aid in the diagnosis include:

- Serum amylase and lipase assays, the results of both of which may be elevated to more than three times their normal values
- Leukocytosis (10-30 x $10^3/\mu L$)
- Urinalysis showing proteinuria, granular casts, and glycosuria
- Elevated serum levels of BUN and serum alkaline phosphatase

Management of acute pancreatitis includes a clear liquid diet, gradually progressing to soft solids to rest the pancreas; bed rest; and management of pain. Severe cases may require surgical intervention. Table 2–7 presents the Ranson criteria for the diagnosis of acute pancreatitis.

## Pyelonephritis

Pyelonephritis presents with progressive flank and lower abdominal pain together with back pain or CVAT. It may also present with fever, nausea,

## Table 2–7 Ranson Criteria for Pancreatitis

| THREE OR MORE PREDICT SEVERE CASES | DEVELOPMENT WITHIN 48 HOURS INDICATES WORSENING |
| --- | --- |
| Age >55 years<br>WBC >16,000<br>Blood glucose >200 mg/dL<br>Serum LDH >350 IU/L<br>AST >250 IU/L | 10% drop in hematocrit<br>Rise in BUN >5 mg/dL<br>Arterial $PO_2$ <60 mm Hg<br>Serum calcium <8 mg/dL |

Lee, B. Medical Notes. Philadelphia: F.A. Davis Company, 2009.

vomiting, urinary frequency, and urinary urgency. Imaging studies are generally ordered for patients who fail to respond to treatment. Some studies to order in suspected pyelonephritis include:

- CT scan to identify a renal or perirenal abscess
- Ultrasound examination to visualize an abscess and hydronephrosis
- CBC to reveal a left shift and leukocytosis
- Urinalysis to show pyuria, bacteriuria, hematuria, and white cell casts
- Urine culture to aid in identifying responsible pathogens

Treatment for pyelonephritis includes the use of quinolone antibiotics or nitrofurantoin for 14 days; if the condition does not respond to these, consider hospitalization and IV antibiotic therapy.

### *Chordoma*

A chordoma is a slowly developing malignant tumor commonly found in the sacrum, coccyx, or at the base of the skull. Its symptoms may include constipation and bowel incontinence as the tumor enlarges.

### *Endometriosis*

Endometriosis presents with severe, cramping, deep sacral and lower abdominal or pelvic pain that worsens with the onset of menses and is aggravated by defecation. Diagnostic procedures for endometriosis include ultrasound examination to identify cysts or masses and MRI. Treatment includes:

- Hormone treatment to inhibit ovulation for a period of 4 to 9 months
- Gonadotropin releasing hormone (GnRH) analogues, danazol, oral contraceptive therapy, or medroxyprogesterone therapy
- Analgesic medication during menses

### Intervertebral Disk Rupture

Intervertebral disk rupture presents with lower back pain that may or may not radiate into the legs. The pain is worsened with activity, coughing, and sneezing, and may be relieved by rest. Assessment may reveal decreased reflexes, paresthesias in the lower legs, and changes in posture and gait. Patients will typically lean toward the affected side, walk slowly, and express difficulty in rising from a seated position. Diagnostic procedures to rule out intervertebral disk rupture include MRI, which is the most sensitive imaging study for detecting bulging or protrusion of disks and impingements of fragmented disks on other structures, and CT scanning, which may identify herniated disks and stenosis.

### Sprains and Strains of Lumbosacral Muscles

Sprains and strains of lumbosacral muscles present as a localized ache accompanied by pain and tenderness. Flexion of the spine intensifies the pain.

### Metastatic Tumors and Myelomas

Myelomas present with pain of abrupt onset that worsens with exercise and may also be accompanied by joint swelling, tenderness, malaise, fever, and weight loss. Diagnostic procedures for suspected myeloma include MRI as the preferred study modality, with skeletal radiographs to identify punched out lesions.

### Perforated Ulcer

A perforated ulcer presents with sudden, intense epigastric pain that may radiate to the back. Assessment may reveal abdominal rigidity, tenderness with guarding, absence of bowel sounds, and shallow respirations. Diagnostic procedures to consider include an upper GI series and endoscopy.

### Prostate Cancer

Prostate cancer may produce a chronic, aching back pain. It may also present with hematuria and a decreased urine stream or difficulty in initiating the urine stream. Diagnostic procedures that aid in the diagnosis of prostate cancer include transurethral ultrasound examination and measurement of the serum level of prostate specific antigen (PSA).

### Renal Calculi

Renal calculi produce colicky pain along the costovertebral angle, flank, and suprapubic and external genital areas. They may also produce nausea,

**CLINICAL COACH**

Monitor the patient with suspected prostate cancer for changes in PSA values. Even if the initially measured level is within the normal range, any elevation in the PSA level over time should be investigated further, even if the level is still within the normal ranges. Some prostate cancers do not secrete PSA. It is important to note that PSA values may be altered by prostatic massage.

vomiting, urinary urgency, and hematuria. Diagnostic procedures to rule out renal calculi include a CT scan, which is the most sensitive study for these accretions, excretory urography following a plain x-ray film, and ultrasound examination to visualize stones.

## Sacroiliac Strain

Strain of sacroiliac structures produces pain that radiates to the buttock, hip, and lateral aspect of thigh. The pain may be aggravated by weight bearing and by abduction of the leg.

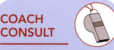

**COACH CONSULT**

When diagnosing spinal stenosis, MRI is better than plain films for identifying disk-space narrowing and disk impingement.

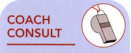

**COACH CONSULT**

Children with back pain should be assessed with a bone scan or CT scan for possible spondylosis, which is common in teenage gymnasts and football players. It occurs when a superior vertebra slips forward on an adjacent inferior vertebra. Its typical presentation is as low back pain that worsens with activity. The treatment is rest with analgesic drugs and surgery if the condition remains unresolved.

### Spinal Stenosis

The pain of spinal stenosis resembles that of a ruptured disk, commonly affects both legs, radiates to the toes, and may produce numbness and tingling. Diagnostic procedures for ruling out spinal stenosis include plain spinal x-ray films and MRI.

### Spondylolisthesis

Spondylolisthesis presents with lower back pain with or without nerve-root involvement. Paresthesia, buttock pain, and pain radiating down the legs may also be present. Spondylolisthesis is best identified with MRI.

### Transverse Process Fracture

A transverse process fracture presents with severe localized pain with muscle spasms.

### Vertebral Compression Fracture

A vertebral compression fracture may initially be painless, presenting several weeks later with back pain that is aggravated with movement and weight-bearing and local tenderness in the area of the fracture. Diagnostic procedures for ruling out compression fractures include plain spinal cord radiography and CT scanning to detect more subtle bone changes.

### Vertebral Osteoporosis

Vertebral osteoporosis usually occurs in older children and may cause chronic, aching back pain, aggravated by activity. It may also cause tenderness in the affected area. Diagnostic procedures for vertebral osteoporosis include a bone density test and plain radiography to identify anterior wedging of vertebral bodies.

### *Diskitis*

Diskitis is a low-grade infection of the disk spaces between two adjacent vertebra that leads to severe back pain; the patient may also present with fever, fatigue, and anorexia. Diagnostic procedures for diskitis includes blood cultures, a white blood count (WBC), and ESR, with *Staphylococcus aureus* being the most common causative pathogen of this condition. Treatment includes antibiotics for 3 to 6 weeks for patients with severe pain; positive findings on a bone scan or a positive blood culture; and bed rest for significant spasms. A back brace may be helpful for supporting the spine.

**COACH CONSULT**

Other differential diagnoses for back pain include lumbosacral strain; scoliosis, which is generally not painful but may cause discomfort for some children; and tumors, juvenile ankylosing spondylitis, and spinal tuberculosis, although these last three conditions are generally rare causes of back pain.

### Treatment

Low back pain of mechanical origin is treated pharmacologically as well as with physical therapy and physical activity. Its pharmacological management includes:

- NSAIDs and cyclo-oxygenase-2 (COX-2) inhibitors
- Muscle relaxants
- Cyclobenzaprine (Flexeril): 10 mg from qd to tid
- Methocarbamol (Robaxin): 750- to 1000 mg qid

Physical management of back pain may include manipulation if there is no radiculopathy, hot/cold therapy to provide temporary relief, and physical activity such as low-stress aerobic exercise. Patients whose back pain severely limits their mobility may be given 2 to 3 days of bed rest followed by progressive involvement in low-stress aerobic exercise.

Patients should also be taught to minimize stress to the back through proper lifting and supportive postures when sitting and sleeping, and to avoid sitting for prolonged periods.

**ALERT**

Muscle relaxants may be helpful in treating back pain, but they have an adverse effect of drowsiness.

## Breathing Problems, Acute Onset

Adult patients who present with breathing problems of acute onset of may be experiencing an acute respiratory illness or an exacerbation of a chronic respiratory disease. Respiratory symptoms of acute onset may be precipitated by any number of factors, among which are chest trauma, allergens, dust, positioning, overexertion, aspiration of a foreign object, prolonged bedrest or inactivity, or recent surgery. In assessing the situation, always consider alleviating factors such as changes in position and use of bronchodilators. Always inquire about the patient's history of tobacco use, occupational exposures, and recent travel. Table 2–8 provides an overview of the most common breathing problems of acute onset in adults.

Acute exacerbations of asthma are a fairly common respiratory complaint in primary care. Key indicators of asthma include wheezing; a cough that worsens in the evening; chest tightness; difficulty in breathing; and symptoms that are worsened by physical activity, changes in the weather, allergen exposure, and emotions. Patients with asthma may also present with comorbid complaints of gastroesophageal reflux disease (GERD) or atopic dermatitis in the

## Table 2–8 Acute-Onset Breathing Problems in Adult Patients

| DIAGNOSIS | HISTORY | PHYSICAL EXAMINATION | DIAGNOSIS AND TREATMENT |
|---|---|---|---|
| Asthma | Episodic dyspnea, cough, wheezing May have exposure to irritants (dust, pollen, other allergens) | Diffuse hyperresonance Wheezes, rhonchi, prolonged expiration Classifications by steps 1–4 by severity of asthma | Spirometry Chest x-ray, CBC Peak expiratory flow Stepped approach to treatment Develop an asthma treatment plan for patient Environmental and allergy control |
| Foreign body | Usual onset while eating, inebriated, or semiconscious | Complete obstruction: Respiratory distress, cyanosis Incomplete obstruction: Tachypnea, stridor, wheezing, diminished breath sounds on one side | Heimlich maneuver to expel foreign object |
| Hyperventilation | Acute onset, anxious, may have circumoral or extremity paresthesia Lightheadedness, chest discomfort | Tachypnea, deep sighing respirations, normal examination findings between attacks | Paper bag breathing Antianxiety drugs |

## Table 2–8 Acute-Onset Breathing Problems in Adult Patients—cont'd

| DIAGNOSIS | HISTORY | PHYSICAL EXAMINATION | DIAGNOSIS AND TREATMENT |
|---|---|---|---|
| Pneumonia | Onset hours to days, sputum production, fever, chills, may have hemoptysis, pleurisy | Tachypnea, fever, localized dullness, rales/wheezes, purulent sputum, asymmetric chest expansion | Chest x-ray, sputum culture, CBC, glucose, electrolytes pulse oximetry, PPD (purified protein derivative) TB skin test Treatment: antibiotics macrolides, fluoroquinolones, or beta-lactam options |
| Pneumothorax | Sudden dyspnea, pleuritic chest pain, may have history of trauma or may be postoperative | Unilateral hyperresonance, decreased chest movement, tracheal deviation to opposite side | — |
| Pulmonary edema | Severe dyspnea, worse when lying down, frothy sputum | Gasping for breath, tachypnea, moist rales, wheezes, jugular vein distention, cool moist skin, gallop rhythm | Chest x-ray |
| Pulmonary embolus | Sudden-onset dyspnea, dull chest pain, sweating, apprehension, cough, hemoptysis History of recent surgery or immobilization | Tachypnea, tachycardia rales, S3 or S4, pleural friction rub, calf tenderness | Chest x-ray |
| Respiratory failure | Confusion, lethargy, somnolence | Shallow, rapid respiration, decreased breath sounds, cyanosis May have pneumonia | Chest x-ray |
| Anemia | History of bleeding, fatigue, postural dizziness | Pallor, tachycardia, postural hypotension, stool guaiac positive | CBC, serum iron, ferritin, TIBC |

*Continued*

Table 2–8 **Acute-Onset Breathing Problems in Adult Patients—cont'd**

| DIAGNOSIS | HISTORY | PHYSICAL EXAMINATION | DIAGNOSIS AND TREATMENT |
|---|---|---|---|
| Lung tumor | Change in cough pattern, hemoptysis, chest ache. History of cigarette smoking | Usually normal | Chest x-ray, CT scan |
| Tuberculosis | Fever, night sweats, weight loss, chronic cough, hemoptysis | Usually normal. May have apical rales, weight loss, and fever | Chest x-ray, Mantoux/PPD test, sputum smears. Treatment of active disease: Isoniazid (INH), rifampin, pyrazinamide and ethambutol, or streptomycin |

Adapted from Wasson, J. The Common Symptom Guide, ed. 5.New York: McGraw-Hill, 2001.

flexural areas. Patients with asthma should be educated about the proper use of a peak flow meter and provided with a personal asthma management plan based on changes in respiratory performance indicated by the peak flow meter. A stepwise approach is recommended for managing asthma patients. Table 2–9 provides an analysis of a stepwise approach to managing adult asthma.

## Exacerbations of Pediatric Asthma

Many of the same considerations are necessary with pediatric asthma patients as with adult patients, including the identification of aggravating and alleviating factors. Mothers of infants will often express concerns about "rattling" noises they hear during the breathing of an infant younger than 6 months of age. Reassure these parents that infants may experience noisy breathing as their airways enlarge during the first 6 months of life.

Physical examination of the pediatric patient with pulmonary disease may reveal certain pediatric-specific warning signs, such as:

- Nasal flaring
- Rib retractions
- Cyanosis
- Grunting respirations
- Dullness or hyperresonance
- Adventitious breath sounds, including rales, rhonchi, and wheezes

## Table 2–9  Stepped Approach to Management of Adult Asthma

| STEP | SYMPTOMS | LUNG FUNCTION INDICATORS | TREATMENT |
|------|----------|--------------------------|-----------|
| Step 4 Severe persistent | Continual symptoms Limited physical activity Frequent exacerbations Frequent nighttime symptoms | $FEV_1$ <60% predicted PEF (peak expiratory flow) variability >30% | High-dose inhaled corticosteroid and long-acting inhaled beta2 agonist and if needed: Corticosteroid tablets |
| Step 3 Moderate persistent | Daily symptoms Daily use of inhaled short-acting beta-2 agonist Exacerbations affect activity Exacerbations more than twice a week Nighttime symptoms >1 time/week | $FEV_1$ 60%–80% predicted PEF variability >30% | Low- to medium-dose inhaled corticosteroid and long-acting inhaled beta 2 agonist Alternative: Low- to medium-dose inhaled corticosteroid and leukotriene modifier or theophylline |
| Step 2 Mild persistent | Symptoms >2 times/week, but <1 time/day Exacerbations may affect activity Nighttime symptoms >2 times/month | $FEV_1$ >80% predicted PEF variability 20%–30% | Low-dose inhaled corticosteroid Alternative: Cromolyn, leukotriene modifier, or sustained-release theophylline |
| Step 1 Mild intermittent | Symptoms <2 times/week Asymptomatic and normal PEF between exacerbations Exacerbations brief (few hours–few days) Nighttime symptoms <2 times a month | $FEV_1$ >80% predicted PEF variability <20% | No daily medications needed Quick relief 2–4 puffs short-acting beta-2 agonist May respond to short course of systemic corticosteroids |

Adapted from Nurse Practitioner Prescribing Reference Winter 2008–2009. New York: Haymarket Media Publications, 2009.

Some specific pediatric respiratory diseases states that can produce breathing problems of acute onset are asthma, bronchiolitis, croup, epiglottitis, foreign body obstruction, hyperventilation, pneumonia, and pneumothorax. Histories and physical symptoms of each of these conditions are presented in Chapter 8.

# Bruising

Some patients report bruising easily even in the absence of any obvious disease. This is especially true for older patients with thinner skin and less subcutaneous tissue for protection. Disease-related causes of bruising stem from a dysfunction of blood coagulation factors, platelet dysfunction, or excessive vascular fragility.

Disorders of coagulation may lead to large superficial bruises and even to spontaneous bleeding into deep tissues and joints. Typically, bleeding of this nature can be attributed to hemophilia, severe liver disease, or warfarin therapy. Platelet dysfunctions that may reduce platelet counts and produce consequent bruising include leukemia, Henoch–Schönlein disease, lupus erythematosus, Rocky Mountain spotted fever, bacterial endocarditis, and disseminated meningococcal disease.

## Differential Diagnoses
### Leukemia
There are two types of leukemia: acute myeloid leukemia (AML) and acute lymphoblastic leukemia (ALL). Acute symptoms of leukemia include fatigue, fever, epistaxis, mucosal bleeding, heavy menstrual bleeding, and pancytopenia. Patients with ALL and AML have less than 20% blasts in their bone marrow. Laboratory findings in leukemia include pancytopenia with circulating blasts—a hallmark of the disease—a decreased fibrinogen level, disseminated intravascular coagulation (DIC), a prolonged prothrombin time (PT), a mediastinal mass on a chest radiograph (in ALL), and Auer rods in the cytoplasm of leukemic blast cells (in AML). Both AML and ALL are treated with chemotherapy.

### Henoch–Schönlein Disease
Henoch–Schönlein disease is an allergic vascular disease that produces purpura, abdominal pain, and hematuria as presenting symptoms in both adults and children. The lesions of purpura may appear on the lower extremities, buttocks, arms, hands, and trunk. Diagnostic testing reveals leukocytoclastic vasculitis with immunoglobulin A (IgA) in laboratory tests and glomerulonephritis with crescents on biopsy of the kidneys. Treatment consists of corticosteroids.

## Lupus Erythematosus

Assessment of a patient with lupus erythematosus reveals localized red plaques (often on the face), scaling, follicular plugging, atrophy, telangiectasia, and depigmentation of the skin. Laboratory tests reveal antinuclear antibodies (ANA) in high titer. Treatment includes options for both local and systemic management:

Local options include:

- Topical application of high-potency corticosteroid cream to skin lesions, followed by the covering of treated lesions with plastic film
- Monthly local infiltration of lesions with a triamcinolone acetonide suspension

Systemic options include:

- Antimalarial drugs: only for patients without a history of seizures
- Hydroxychloroquine sulfide: 0.2 to . 0.4 mg PO qd  for 3 months
- Chloroquine sulfate: 250 mg qd
- Quinacrine: 100 mg qd; this may cause yellow staining of the skin
- Isotretinoin: 1 mg/kg/day
- Thalidomide for refractory disease: 300 mg qd; monitor for neuropathy

> **ALERT**
>
> Antimalarial drugs should be used only for patients without a history of seizures. Quinacrine may cause yellow staining of the skin. Patients treated with thalidomide should be monitored for neuropathy.

## Rocky Mountain Spotted Fever

Rocky Mountain spotted fever is acquired from the bite of an infected tick in an area where the disease is endemic. From 2 to 14 days after the bite, the person bitten develops a flulike prodrome with chills, headache, myalgia, and restlessness, and occasionally delirium and coma. Between days 2 and 6 of the fever, the patient may present with a red, macular rash, generally beginning on the wrists and ankles. The patient may also develop a cough, facial flushing, and injected conjunctiva. Laboratory findings include thrombocytopenia, hyponatremia, increased serum levels of ALT (alanine aminotransferase), hyperbilirubinemia, and changes in the cerebrospinal fluid (CSF). Treatment consists of doxycycline or, in pregnant patients, chloramphenicol.

## Bacterial Endocarditis

Bacterial endocarditis presents with fever, underlying valvular disease, and a heart murmur indicating valvular regurgitation. Symptoms following embolization may include a cough, dyspnea, arthralgia, diarrhea, and pain in the flank or back. Other signs and symptoms include petechiae on the conjunctiva and nailbeds (splinter hemorrhages); lesions of the fingers, toes, and feet; and Janeway lesions of the palms and soles. Laboratory and imaging studies used to help in the diagnosis of bacterial endocarditis include three blood cultures to identify the causative agent and chest radiography to visualize right-sided endocarditis and pulmonary infiltrates. Treatment involves empiric use of vancomycin until culture results are returned; prophylactic use of antibiotics before dental and respiratory procedures and to prevent skin or musculoskeletal infections; and penicillin, which is the antibiotic of choice for treating the disease, although clindamycin, cephalexin, or azithromycin may also be used.

### *Disseminated Meningococcal Disease*

Assessment for disseminated meningococcal disease begins with the presentation of fever, headache, vomiting, confusion, delirium, and convulsions. The patient may also present with a petechial rash on the skin and mucous membranes, with lesions varying from pinpoint size to large and ecchymotic, and positive Kernig's and Brudzinski's signs. Lumbar puncture shows a cloudy, purulent cerebrospinal fluid (CSF). Treatment consists of aqueous penicillin at G 24 million units/24 hours, diuretic therapy, and use of adrenal steroids.

## Chest Pain

Chest pain generally results from an abnormality or disorder that affects the thoracic or abdominal organs, but can also be related to hematologic disease, musculoskeletal disorders, anxiety, stress, exertion, deep breathing, the ingestion of certain foods, and even drug therapy. Chest pain can be of sudden or insidious onset; constant or intermittent; and mild or severe. The location of the pain may vary from midsternal to epigastric, and the pain may radiate to the arms, neck, jaw, or back. Table 2–10 shows the relation of chest pain to disease processes in various body systems.

### Assessment

The assessment of chest pain should begin with the patient's history. The location, duration, character, and quality of the pain and its triggering and relieving factors are important. Past cardiac disorders; use of drugs that can trigger coronary artery spasm, such as cocaine, triptans, and phosphodiesterase inhibitors; and the presence of risk factors for coronary artery disease (CAD) or pulmonary embolism may be important. The presence or absence of risk factors for CAD, such as hypertension, hypercholesterolemia, smoking, and a positive family history of CAD influences the probability of underlying CAD but does not help in diagnosing the cause of acute chest pain.

**ALERT**

An initial evaluation of chest pain is critical to determine the severity of the pain and the potential for imminent risk of cardiac events such as a myocardial infarction.

Symptoms produced by serious thoracic disorders overlap and vary greatly, but the following distinctions can sometimes be made:

- Crushing pain radiating to the jaw or arm suggests acute ischemia or MI. Patients often ascribe myocardial ischemic pain to indigestion
- Exertional pain relieved by rest indicates angina pectoris. Tearing pain radiating to the back suggests thoracic aortic dissection

## Table 2–10  Chest Pain Related to Disease Processes by Body Systems

| BODY SYSTEM | DISEASE CONDITIONS THAT MAY PERSIST WITH CHEST PAIN |
| --- | --- |
| Cardiovascular | Myocardial infarction, angina, pericarditis, aortic stenosis, aortic dissection, pulmonary embolism, cardiomyopathy, myocarditis, mitral valve prolapse, pulmonary hypertension, hypertrophic obstructive cardiomyopathy, carditis, acute rheumatic fever, aortic insufficiency, right ventricular hypertrophy |
| Pulmonary | Pneumonia, pleuritis, bronchitis, pneumothorax, tumor |
| Gastrointestinal | Biliary disease, esophageal spasms, esophageal rupture, GERD, Mallory-Weiss tears, peptic ulcer disease |
| Musculoskeletal | Disk disease (cervical or thoracic), costochondritis, subacromial bursitis |
| Other | Anxiety, panic attacks, herpes zoster, chest wall tumors, thoracic outlet syndrome, mediastinitis, breast disorders |

Adapted from Fauci, A, et al. Harrison's Principles of Internal Medicine, ed.17. New York: McGraw-Hill, 2009.

- Burning pain radiating from the epigastrium to the throat, exacerbated by lying in the supine position and relieved by antacids, suggests GERD
- Fever, chills, and cough suggest pneumonia
- Significant dyspnea suggests pulmonary embolism or pneumonia

When beginning your assessment, check the patient's vital signs. Observe for tachypnea, tachycardia, fever, paradoxical pulse, and changes in BP. Check the BP in both of the patient's arms. Check pulses in all extremities, because poor perfusion of a limb may be due to an aortic dissection that has compromised the flow to an artery. Fever and rales suggest pneumonia, while fever alone may be seen in pulmonary embolism, acute MI, esophageal rupture, and pericarditis.

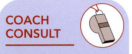

**COACH CONSULT**

Chest pain can be exacerbated by respiration, movement, or both in serious or minor disorders; these triggers are not specific. Brief (<5 sec), sharp, intermittent pains rarely result from serious disorders.

Perform a thoracic assessment of the patient's lung sounds; listen for a friction rub, crackles, rhonchi, wheezes, and diminished breath sounds. Assess the patient's respiratory rate and oxygen situation, and examine the patient for jugular venous distention.

Also assess the patient's heart sounds for murmurs, clicks, gallops, and a pericardial friction rub. Palpate for thrills, gallops, tactile fremitus, and abdominal masses or tenderness. An S4 sound or systolic murmur may be present in MI. An aortic regurgitation murmur and paradoxical pulses suggest thoracic aortic dissection. Table 2–11 presents conditions causing cardiac-related chest pain, with the type of pain and its duration, location, quality, and other features of the pain in each condition.

## Diagnostic Testing

Minimal testing for any patient with chest pain includes pulse oximetry, an electrocardiogram (ECG), and chest radiography. For adults, blood tests for cardiac markers are often done. Results of these tests should be integrated with findings from the patient's history and physical examination, and specific diagnoses should be pursued. Blood tests are not valuable as primary screening procedures for a specific cause of chest pain. In particular, a single normal set of cardiac markers should not be used to rule out a cardiac cause of chest pain. If myocardial ischemia is likely, testing should include serial measurement of cardiac markers with accompanying ECGs and possibly with stress ECGs or stress imaging tests.

## Table 2–11 Clinical Features of Cardiac-Related Chest Pain

| CONDITION | DURATION | QUALITY | LOCATION | OTHER FEATURES |
|-----------|----------|---------|----------|----------------|
| Angina | 2–10 min | Pressure Tightness Squeezing Heaviness Burning | Retrosternal, may radiate to neck, jaw, shoulders, arms (radiation to L arm common) | May be precipitated by stress, exertion, cold S4 gallop or mitral regurgitation murmur during pain |
| Unstable angina | 10–20 min | More severe than simple angina | Like angina | Like angina, but can occur with minor exertion or at rest |
| Acute MI | May be more than 30 min | More severe than simple angina | Like angina | Unrelieved by NTG May also have heart failure or arrhythmia |
| Aortic stenosis | Recurrent episodes | Like angina | Like angina | Late-peaking systolic murmur, radiates to carotid arteries |
| Pericarditis | Hours to days | Sharp | Retrosternal or toward cardiac apex, radiates to L shoulder | Sitting up, leaning forward may relieve Pericardial friction rub |
| Aortic dissection | Abrupt onset, constant pain | Tearing or ripping, knifelike | Anterior chest, radiates to back | May have hypertension, connective tissue disease (Marfan syndrome) Murmur of aortic insufficiency, pericardial rub, weak peripheral pulses |
| Pulmonary embolism | Abrupt onset, minutes to hours long | Pleuritic | Often lateral on affected side | Dyspnea, tachypnea, tachycardia, hypotension |

NTG: nitroglycerin.
Adapted from Fauci, A., et al. Harrison's Principles of Internal Medicine, ed. 17. New York: McGraw-Hill, 2009.

A diagnostic trial of sublingual nitroglycerin or an oral liquid antacid does not adequately differentiate myocardial ischemia from GERD or gastritis. Either drug may relieve symptoms of either disorder.

## Differential Diagnoses

### *Angina Pectoris*

Symptoms of angina pectoris include tightness or pressure in the chest that may be described as indigestion. Pain may radiate to the arms, neck, jaw, and back. Anginal pain usually lasts from 2 to 10 minutes. Angina can be provoked by stress, exertion, or a heavy meal. Other symptoms may include nausea, vomiting, dyspnea, tachycardia, dizziness, diaphoresis, and palpitations. Prinzmetal's angina may produce pain at rest, as well as nausea, vomiting, palpitations, and shortness of breath. The pain of stable angina can develop with exertion, emotional excitement or stress, or after a heavy meal. Rest and sublingual nitroglycerin can bring relief within minutes.

### *Anxiety*

Chest pain related to anxiety is generally intermittent, sharp, and stabbing, lasting from only a few seconds to several minutes and followed by a dull aching sensation that may continue for hours to days.

### *Aortic Aneurysm*

Aortic aneurysm presents with intense stabbing pain of sudden onset in the chest and neck that may radiate to the back, abdomen, and lower back. Other symptoms include a palpable abdominal mass, loss of consciousness, diaphoresis, and hypotension.

### *Asthma*

An acute asthma attack will present with diffuse and painful chest tightness, with a dry cough and wheezing. The cough gradually progresses to a productive cough with severe dyspnea. Other findings may include rhonchi, prolonged expirations, intercostals muscle retractions, nasal flaring, accessory muscle use, and tachypnea. Patients experiencing such attacks may be restless, anxious, diaphoretic, and flushed or cyanotic.

### *Bronchitis*

Bronchitis may present with burning chest pain or substernal tightness. The patient may also have a cough that worsens the chest pain and that may or may not be productive.

### *Costochondritis*

Costochondritis is characterized by chest wall pain of insidious onset that is aggravated by movement, deep inspiration, or exertion. The pain may be aching or pressure-like, is generally localized, and may wax and wane. Pain upon palpation is a typical finding, commonly in the second through the fifth costochondral junctions. It is managed with NSAIDs such as ibuprofen or Naprosyn. Local heat may provide relief, and gentle stretching of the pectoralis major muscles two or three times a day may be helpful.

### Interstitial Lung Disease

With the advancement of interstitial lung disease, the patient experiences progressive dyspnea and pleuritic chest pain. There may also be clubbing of the fingers and toes, a nonproductive cough, and cyanosis.

### Lung Abscess

Patients with lung abscesses may have pleuritic chest pain. Other symptoms include a purulent, blood-tinged sputum; diaphoresis; anorexia; fever; chills; weakness; fatigue; dyspnea; and clubbing of the fingers and toes.

### Lung Cancer

Chest pain associated with lung cancer is generally intermittent and deep within the chest.

### Mitral Valve Prolapse

Mitral valve prolapse may or may not be accompanied by pain. If pain is present, it is usually reported as a sharp, stabbing pain. Other symptoms include weakness, dizziness, tachycardia, and palpitations.

### Myocardial Infarction

The chest pain associated with MI is a crushing substernal pain, unrelieved by nitroglycerin or rest. The pain may radiate to the jaw, neck, arm, shoulder, or back. Other symptoms include pallor, clammy skin, dyspnea, hypo- or hypertension, nausea, vomiting, and anxiety.

### Pericarditis

Pericarditis typically presents with a sharp or cutting type of pain in the precordium or retrosternal area. The pain is exacerbated by deep breathing or coughing, grows worse in the supine position, and is relieved by sitting upright and leaning forward. Patients with pericarditis may also present with a pericardial friction rub, fever, tachycardia, and dyspnea.

### Pleurisy

Pleurisy may present as sharp, unilateral pain of abrupt onset that is aggravated by deep breathing, coughing, or movement of the chest wall.

### Pneumonia

Patients with pneumonia experience pleuritic chest pain that is worse on inspiration than on expiration. Other symptoms include fever, chills, a dry cough that later becomes productive, crackles, rhonchi, diaphoresis, cyanosis, and tachycardia.

### Pneumothorax

Pneumothorax typically presents as sudden, sharp, severe, and unilateral chest pain with decreased breath sounds, subcutaneous crepitation, and decreased vocal fremitus. It may also present with anxiety, restlessness, tachycardia, and tachypnea.

### Pulmonary Embolism

A pulmonary embolism is suspected with the sudden occurrence of dyspnea with chest pain resembling that of severe angina and that worsens with deep breathing or chest-wall movement. Other symptoms include tachycardia, tachypnea, crackles, wheezing, restlessness, cough, hypotension, and cyanosis.

### Sickle Cell Crisis

The pain of a sickle cell crisis may begin as vague pain, progressing to severe pleuritic pain. Patients may also have abdominal distention, fever, jaundice, and dyspnea.

### Thoracic Outlet Syndrome

Thoracic outlet syndrome presents with angina-like pain upon lifting of the hands over the head; the pain disappears when the arms are lowered. Other symptoms include paresthesia along ulnar-nerve distribution of the arm and skin pallor.

### Tuberculosis

Tuberculosis (TB) typically causes pleuritic chest pain after coughing. Besides a cough, the symptoms are weight loss, fever, malaise, dyspnea, and hemoptysis. Patients with tuberculosis may also present with dullness to percussion, increased tactile fremitus, and anorexia.

### Tularemia

Tularemia presents with pleuritic chest pain after inhalation of the bacteria *Francisella tularensis*, which cause this disease. The patient may also have fever, chills, headache, a nonproductive cough, dyspnea, and empyema.

## Confusion

Confusion is the inability to think clearly and spontaneously. The onset of states of confusion may be insidious or sudden, depending on their cause. Confused states may also be temporary or transient, or in the worst-case scenario they may be marked by a permanent decline in cognitive status. Confusion can be aggravated by stress and sensory deprivation: a classic example of this is that of the hospitalized patient in an intensive care setting with little stimulation to help the patient's orientation to the date and time, much less to the patient's situation.

In cases of severe confusion of sudden onset, accompanied by hallucinations and motor hyperactivity, the NP must consider a state of delirium. By contrast, confusion of more progressive onset, particularly in an aging patient, may indicate dementia, such as that of Alzheimer's disease.

Potential medical causes of confusion could include:

- Brain tumor
- Cerebrovascular accident (stroke)
- Diminished cerebral perfusion
- Medication effect/side effect
- Fluid and/or electrolyte imbalance
- Head trauma
- Infection/fever
- Hypoxemia
- Hypo-/hyperthermia
- Nutritional deficiencies
- Seizure disorder
- Metabolic encephalopathy

Features of these potential causes of confusion are shown in Table 2–12.

## Table 2–12 **Causes of Confusion**

| POTENTIAL CAUSE | ASSOCIATED SYMPTOMS |
| --- | --- |
| Brain tumor | Confusion worsens as tumor progresses<br>Personality changes, sensory and motor deficits, visual deficits, aphasia, headaches |
| Cerebrovascular disorders | Confusion may be insidious or transient (TIA), acute, or permanent (stroke)<br>Vital-sign changes |
| Decreased cerebral perfusion | Early symptom is mild confusion<br>Hypotension<br>Tachycardia, irregular pulse<br>Edema<br>Cyanosis |
| Drugs | Withdrawal from opioids and barbiturates<br>Other drugs that may cause confusion: lidocaine, indomethacin, chloroquine, atropine, cimetidine<br>Herbals: St. John's wort |
| Fluid/electrolyte imbalances | Other signs: dehydration, oliguria, low-grade fever |
| Head trauma | May have periodic changes in LOC, papillary changes, vomiting, sensory and motor deficits |

*Continued*

## Table 2–12 Causes of Confusion—cont'd

| POTENTIAL CAUSE | ASSOCIATED SYMPTOMS |
|---|---|
| Heat stroke | Dizziness, irritability, temperature changes, may have seizures and changes in LOC |
| Hypo-/hyperthermia | Skin changes, pulse rate increases, BP drops, progressive worsening of confusion state<br>Respiratory rate increases |
| Hypoxemia | Acute illness: Mild to severe confusion<br>Chronic illness: Persistent confusion |
| Infection/fever | In severe infections may have progressively worsening confused states<br>Headache, nuchal rigidity |
| Nutritional deficiencies | Thiamine, niacin, vitamin $B_{12}$ |
| Seizure disorder | Postictal confusion |
| Metabolic disturbances | Hyperglycemia<br>Hypoglycemia<br>Uremic or hepatic encephalopathy<br>May have tremors, restlessness |

LOC: level of consciousness; TIA: transient ischemic attack.

Adapted from Munden, J. and Schaeffer, L. (Ed). Portable Signs and Symptoms. Philadelphia: Lippincott Williams & Wilkins, 2008.

## Constipation

Constipation is marked by small, infrequent, or difficult bowel movements. A diagnosis of constipation is based on a deviation from the patient's history of normal elimination patterns. A pertinent history should include recent and normal elimination patterns, recall of typical diet habits, and an assessment of normal daily fluid intake. Patients should also be asked about their alcohol intake, changes in diet, changes in medications, and physical activity patterns.

### Assessment

The physical examination for constipation should include a meticulous GI examination including auscultation for bowel sounds, percussion, palpation for tenderness or masses, and hepatosplenomegaly. A rectal examination should be done to identify inflammation and determine anal sphincter tone, and a stool specimen should be sent for occult blood testing. Danger signs associated with constipation include:

- A distended, tympanic abdomen
- Vomiting
- Blood in the stool
- Weight loss
- Severe constipation of recent onset
- Worsening constipation in elderly patients

**ALERT**

A tense, distended tympanic abdomen, especially when associated with nausea and vomiting, suggests a mechanical obstruction of the GI tract.

## Diagnostic Testing

Diagnostic testing in cases of constipation includes both laboratory studies and imaging studies. Among the laboratory studies used are:

- Assay of thyroid-stimulating hormone (TSH) levels to rule out hypothyroidism
- Assays of serum electrolytes, including potassium, calcium, glucose, and creatinine for patients with constipation of recent onset and those with chronic constipation that has not responded to therapy
- Fecal occult blood tests for all cases of chronic constipation in middle-aged or elderly patients
- A WBC count in patients with abdominal pain or fever to rule out ileus as the cause of constipation

Imaging studies are indicated in patients with acute abdominal pain, fever, and leukocytosis. Studies that may be utilized include:

- A chest film with the patient in the upright position and flat and upright abdominal x-ray films, which may reveal a colon full of stools
- An abdominal CT scan for abdominal abscesses
- Lower GI endoscopy
- An x-ray film following a Gastrografin enema in patients with acute abdominal pain or suspected colon cancer
- Air contrast barium enemas
- Colonoscopy
- Cases of anal obstruction
- Defecography to demonstrate changes in the anorectal angle

## Differential Diagnoses

Constipation may originate primarily from within the colon and rectum or may originate externally. Causes of constipation directly attributable to the colon or rectum include:

- Left colon obstruction, such as from a neoplasm, volvulus, or stricture
- Slow colonic motility, particularly in patients with a history of chronic laxative abuse
- Hirschsprung's disease
- Chagas' disease
- Outlet obstruction

Outlet obstruction may be anatomical or functional. Anatomical outlet obstruction may be due to intussusception of the anterior wall of the rectum on straining at stool, to rectal prolapse, and to rectocele. Functional causes of outlet obstruction include puborectalis or external sphincter spasm or both upon bearing down, short-segment Hirschsprung's disease, and damage to the pudendal nerve, which is typically related to chronic straining at stool or vaginal delivery.

Characteristics of outlet obstruction include difficulty in evacuating the bowels despite straining, often even with soft stools.

Extracolonic causes of constipation include:

- Poor dietary habits (most common)
- Medications:
  - Narcotics
  - Iron supplements
  - Nonmagnesium antacids
  - Calcium-channel blockers
  - Inadequate thyroid hormone supplementation
  - Many psychotropic drugs
  - Anticholinergic agents
- Systemic endocrine or neurological diseases
- Psychological factors
- Dietary issues
  - Inadequate water intake
  - Inadequate fiber intake
- Overuse of coffee, tea, or alcohol
- Recent change in bowel habit paralleled by changes in the diet
- Systemic diseases
- Endocrine disorders, most commonly hypothyroidism

**COACH CONSULT**

Although laxatives are frequently used to treat constipation, chronic laxative use becomes habituating and may lead to a dilated atonic colon that requires increasing laxative use with decreasing efficacy.

- Neurological disorders, including diabetic autonomic neuropathy, spinal cord injury, head injury, cerebrovascular accident, multiple sclerosis, and Parkinson disease

## Treatment

Patients with simple constipation may respond to increases in fluid intake and dietary fiber. Those with more complicated constipating disorders may require bowel-training regimens, including osmotic laxatives, enemas, and glycerin suppositories as needed. Patients who do not respond to this level of management may require long-term treatment with potent laxatives, with caution taken to monitor for laxative abuse syndrome.

Dietary and behavioral adjustments useful in managing constipation include:

- A high-fiber diet (15 to 20 g/day) to increase stool bulk
- Bran at up to 1 cup a day (although this may cause bloating, flatulence, and malabsorption of iron and calcium)
- Adequate fluid intake
- Prune juice
- Moving the bowels at the same time daily, usually after meals, since the ingestion of food stimulates colonic motility

Stool-bulking preparations used to treat constipation include:

- Psyllium: 10 to 15 g/day (which may cause bloating and flatulence)
- Methylcellulose: Up to 6 to 9 g/day in divided doses: tends to cause less bloating than other fiber agents
- Stimulant laxatives, which:
  - Directly stimulate peristalsis and reduce colonic absorption of water and generally work within 6 to 12 hours
  - Senna (Senokot): 2 to 8 tablets PO bid

**COACH CONSULT**

Often, what appears to be acute or subacute constipation may represent a colonic ileus from systemic or intra-abdominal infection or other intra-abdominal emergencies.

**ALERT**

Patients who present with complaints of constipation accompanied by weight loss, rectal bleeding, or anemia, especially if they are older than age 40, should have flexible sigmoidoscopy and either a barium series of the lower GI tract or colonoscopy to rule out structural diseases such as cancer or strictures.

**COACH CONSULT**

The dose of a fiber supplement should be gradually increased to the recommended dose over a period of several weeks.

- Bisacodyl: 5 to 15 mg/day PO or PR (as 10-mg suppositories). May cause fecal incontinence, hypokalemia, abdominal cramping, rectal burning
- Osmotic laxatives, which attract and retain water in the GI tract, include:
  - Sorbitol: 15 to 30 mL of a 70% solution qd or bid (may produce transient abdominal cramping and flatulence)
  - Polyethylene glycol: 17 g qd (may induce dosage-related fecal incontinence)
  - Lactulose: 15 to 30 mL PO q4–8h (this works in one day, but may cause flatulence or bloating).
  - Magnesium hydroxide (milk of magnesia): 15 to 30 mL qd (works in 6 hours)
  - Magnesium citrate: 15–30 mL qd (works in 6 hours)
- Stool softeners work by increasing water secretion and as detergents that increase water penetration into the stool; they work within 1 to 3 days
  - Sodium docusate (Colace): 300 to 600 mg qd (not as effective in severe constipation)
  - Calcium docusate: 300 to 600 mg qd
  - Mineral oil: 15 to 45 Lm qd PO (may cause malabsorption of fat- soluble vitamins, dehydration, or fecal incontinence)
- Suppositories and enemas
  - Bisacodyl suppositories: 10 to 15 mg rectally qd PRN
  - Fleet's enema: 4.5 oz
  - Sodium phosphate enema
  - Glycerin suppositories: one 2- to 3-g suppository qd, may produce rectal irritation

## Cough

A cough provides the body with a defensive mechanism for removing foreign matter such as mucus and foreign bodies from the airways. Diagnostic procedures that aid in identifying the cause of a cough include a plain chest radiograph, which can reveal infection and neoplasms and will also differentiate pulmonary from parenchymal diseases. Other diagnostic procedures of benefit in identifying the cause of a cough include CT scanning, MRI, and bronchoscopy.

A discussion of cough must include identification of the various types of cough. Table 2–13 provides an overview of common acute and chronic causes of cough to consider in making a differential diagnosis.

## Table 2–13 Differential Diagnoses for Acute and Chronic Cough

| DIAGNOSIS | HISTORY | PHYSICAL EXAMINATION FINDINGS |
|---|---|---|
| **ACUTE ONSET OF COUGH** | | |
| Adult upper respiratory infection | Rhinitis, sore throat, facial pain, malaise, minimal sputum | Chest examination normal, pharyngitis, sinus tenderness may be present |
| Asthma | Dry cough, wheezing, dyspnea Aggravated by noxious stimuli, exercise, use of beta blockers | Wheezing, retractions, prolonged expirations |
| Bacterial and mycoplasma infections | Onset over hours, sputum productive (yellow or green), fever, chills, may have hemoptysis, pleuritic chest pain | Tachypnea, fever, asymmetric expansion, localized dullness, increased breath sounds, rales/crackles |
| Pediatric croup | 6 months–3 years, follows URI, barking cough, hoarseness, wheezing | Minimal fever, inspiratory stridor, wheezes |
| Pediatric whooping cough | Inspiratory whooping, staccato cough, nausea, vomiting | Fever, stridor, wheezing |
| **CHRONIC COUGH** | | |
| Pediatric: foreign body, lung collapse, fibrocystic lung disease, chronic infections | Chronic cough, weight loss, foul sputum | Weight loss, localized lung abnormalities possible |
| Cigarette smoking | Minimal sputum | May lead to chronic lung disease |

*Continued*

## Table 2–13 Differential Diagnoses for Acute and Chronic Cough—cont'd

| DIAGNOSIS | HISTORY | PHYSICAL EXAMINATION FINDINGS |
|---|---|---|
| **CHRONIC COUGH** | | |
| Chronic lung disease | Dyspnea, sputum production worse in morning | Hyperresonant lungs, distant breath sounds, scattered rhonchi or wheezes, prolonged expiration |
| Medication induced | ACE inhibitor cough Beta blockers may potentiate asthma cough | Normal |
| Gastroesophageal reflux disease | Heartburn | Normal chest examination |
| Psychogenic | Mainly daytime symptoms | Barking, loud cough, normal examination |
| Lung tumor | Hemoptysis, chest ache | Normal chest examination, enlarged supraclavicular nodes |
| Tuberculosis | Fever, night sweats, weight loss, hemoptysis | Apical rales, crackles, weight loss, fever |
| Congestive heart failure | Nocturnal cough, orthopnea, dyspnea | Moist rales/crackles, ankle edema, may have S3 gallop, diastolic murmur or loud pulmonic component of S2 heart sound |

ACE: angiotensin converting enzyme.
Adapted from Wasson, J. The Common Symptom Guide, ed. 5. New York: McGraw-Hill, 2002.

## Depression and Anxiety

Depression and anxiety may present with a combination of symptoms including anhedonia, sadness, changes in appetite, changes in sleep patterns, somatic complaints, anxiety, and even suicidal thoughts or ideations. The history is often complicated by patterns of alcoholism, drug abuse, physical or sexual abuse, trauma, chronic medical illness, or suicide attempts. The following medications may precipitate feelings of depression or anxiety:

- Birth control pills
- Methyldopa

- Steroids
- Reserpine
- Antidepressants
- Sedatives
- Tranquilizers
- Thyroid medications
- Amphetamines
- Beta blockers

## Major Depression

Major depression is a chronic, relapsing disorder that can start at any age but is most commonly diagnosed in adults between the ages of 20 and 45 years. Depressive episodes may persist for as long as 6 months, especially if untreated. Major depression often coexists with anxiety disorders, substance abuse disorders, and eating disorders. Risk factors for depression include a prior depressive episode, family history of depression, medical comorbidity, stressful life events, recent childbirth, poor social support, prior suicide attempt, female sex, and current substance abuse. Practitioners need to ask specific questions to elicit an adequate history from patients with depression. Box 2–1 contains a list of appropriate questions for patients who have potential suicidal tendencies or thoughts.

Symptoms of major depression include:
- Sadness
- Discouragement or feeling "down in the dumps"
- Lack of interest in activities
- Irritability, anxiety
- Apathy
- Somatic complaints

---

### Box 2–1  Clinical Questions for Patients With Depression

- Have you had thoughts about death or about killing yourself?
  - If the patient answers yes, ask:
    - Do you have a plan?
    - Are there means to carry out the plan (gun, bullets, poison, etc)?
    - Have you actually rehearsed or practiced how you would kill yourself?
    - Do you tend to be impulsive?
    - Can you resist the impulse to hurt or kill yourself?
    - Have you heard voices telling you to hurt or kill yourself?
- Ask about previous attempts, especially the degree of intent
- Ask about suicides among family members

- Sleep disturbances
- Fatigue
- Musculoskeletal complaints of a nonspecific nature, such as back pain or motor tension
- Shortness of breath
- Nonspecific gastrointestinal complaints

A number of medical conditions are associated with depressive symptoms. Generally speaking, any patient with a chronic disease may experience depressive symptoms, especially if the disease state is progressive or poorly controlled. Some medical conditions that can be accompanied by depressive symptoms are identified in Table 2–14.

## Treatment

Goals in treating of depression are to reduce its signs and symptoms, restore the patient to the presymptomatic level of functioning, and reduce the likelihood of relapse. If the patient responds to acute therapy, continuation therapy is used to prevent a relapse, which is defined as the return of symptoms within 6 months after the acute episode. If the patient remains symptom free for a period of at least 6 months while receiving continuation therapy, the therapy can be stopped. However, if new episodes of depressive

| Table 2–14 **Depressive Symptoms Associated With Medical Diagnoses** | |
|---|---|
| **BODY SYSTEM** | **MEDICAL CONDITIONS WITH DEPRESSIVE FEATURES** |
| Cardiovascular | Cardiomyopathy, CHF, MI |
| Neurological | Alzheimer's disease, multiple sclerosis, Parkinson's disease, head trauma, narcolepsy, brain tumors, Wilson's disease |
| Cancer | Pancreatic cancer, lung cancer |
| Endocrine | Hypo and hyper-thyroid disease, Cushing's disease, Addison's disease, hypo- and hyperparathyroid disease, hypoglycemia, pheochromocytoma, ovarian or testicular problems |
| Infectious diseases | Syphilis, mononucleosis, hepatitis, AIDS, tuberculosis, influenza, encephalitis, Lyme disease |
| Nutritional deficiencies | Folate, B vitamins, iron |

Adapted from Nemeroff, C. and Schatzberg, A. Recognition and Treatment of Psychiatric Disorders. Washington DC: American Psychiatric Press, Inc., 1999.

symptoms occur months or years later, it is necessary to consider maintenance therapy to prevent further recurrence of symptoms. A treatment
timeline for major depressive symptoms may follow the steps listed here:

- Evaluate the patient, assess for suicide risk and the presence of
  psychosis
- Consider concurrent medical or psychiatric disorders, prior
  responses to antidepressant therapy, and substance abuse
- Initiate pharmacological therapy with a selective serotonin
  reuptake inhibitor (SSRI) or serotonin–norepinephrine reuptake inhibitor (SNRI), or a tricyclic antidepressant (TCA)
- Assess the patient's response to medications within 1 to 2 weeks;
  if the patient is being treated with a TCA, monitor plasma levels
  of the drug
- If the patient has a full response to treatment, have patient return
  in 6 weeks
- If partial response to treatment, increase the dose of medication
  and reassess in 1 to 2 weeks
- If the patient has no response to treatment, increase the dose
  of medication and reassess in 1 week. If no response occurs at
  3 weeks, change to another antidepressant and monitor the
  patient at 1- to 2-week intervals
- Reassess the treatment responses at 6 weeks
- If the patient has a full response, continue the antidepressant medication at the same dose for 4 to 9 months and then discontinue it
  by tapering the dose over a 4-week period. If the patient has a partial response or no response, change to another antidepressant
- If the patient has more than three depressive episodes, consider
  maintenance therapy
- Consider psychiatric therapy, counseling, or both for difficult
  cases of depression, such as those of:
  - Patients who remain nonresponsive after treatment with two
    antidepressant medications
  - Patients whose condition deteriorates or who have suicidal
    thoughts, frequent relapses, manic symptoms, or a history of
    substance abuse develop comorbid mental disorders.

All antidepressant medications are effective in managing symptoms of
depression but have differences in their side-effect profiles, dosing schedules, and effects on concurrent medical or psychiatric disorders. It is essential to use full therapeutic dosing to achieve a full clinical response to
treatment. Table 2–15 provides data on antidepressant medications, including their dosing, side effects, and other considerations.

# Table 2–15  Antidepressant Drugs

| DRUG | INDICATION | | | | CONTRAINDICATIONS | PRECAUTIONS | SIDE EFFECTS |
|------|------------|--|--|--|-------------------|-------------|--------------|
|      | DEPRESSION | ANXIETY | PMDD | OTHER | | | |
| Cymbalta (duloxetine) | √ | √ | | √ | MAOI | Severe renal or hepatic Pregnancy Category B | N, DM, constipation, S, ↓ appetite, mania, syncope Weight change, F, BV, I, decreased libido, ↑ BP, hepatotoxicity, hyponatremia, seizure |
| Effexor Effexor SR (venlafaxine) | √ | √ | | √ | MAOI | Severe renal, ESRD, hepatic insufficiency Hx seizures | GI upset, DZ, S, I, HA, nervous DM, vasodilation, abnormal dreams, sexual dysfunction, anorexia, SIADH |
| Celexa (Citalopram) | √ | | | | MAOI | Hx seizures, hepatic or renal disease, recent MI, avoid abrupt cessation Potentiated by cimetidine; inhibits CYP34A and CYP2C19 | GI upset, DM, S, I, anorexia, rhinitis, sexual dysfunction, agitation, F, arthralgia, myalgia, hyponatremia, SIADH, abnormal bleeding |
| Lexapro (citalopram) | √ | √ | | √ | MAOI | Hx seizures, hepatic or severe renal Pregnancy C, avoid abrupt cessation | N, I, S, ejaculation disorder, F, decreased libido, anorgasmia, decreased appetite, DZ |

# Table 2–15 Antidepressant Drugs—cont'd

| DRUG | INDICATION | | | | CONTRAINDICATIONS | PRECAUTIONS | SIDE EFFECTS |
|---|---|---|---|---|---|---|---|
| | DEPRESSION | ANXIETY | PMDD | OTHER | | | |
| Prozac (fluoxetine) | √ | | | √ | MAOI | Renal or hepatic disease Recent MI, Hx seizures Monitor weight, avoid abrupt cessation, Pregnancy C | N, CNS stimulation, S, HA, mania, sexual dysfunction, sweating, GI upset, respiratory symptoms, motor impairment, serum sickness, rash. Children: thirst, agitation, personality disorder, epistaxis, urinary frequency |
| Sarafem (fluoxetine) | √ | | √ | | MAOI | Same as Prozac | Asthenia, N, anorexia, DZ, nervousness, I, decreased libido, HA, impaired concentration, rash |
| Paxil Paxil CR (paroxetine) | √ | | √ | √ | MAOI Pimozide thioridazine | Hx seizures, mania, narrow acute-angle glaucoma, suicidal tendencies, Pregnancy C | Asthenia, sweating, decreased appetite, DZ S, HA, decreased libido, tremor, GI upset, DM, impotence, Hyponatremia, abnormal bleeding |
| Zoloft (sertraline) | √ | | √ | √ | MAOI Pimozide, oral disulfiram | Monitor for mania, seizures, suicidal tendencies, cardiac disease, Pregnancy C | GI upset, I, S, sexual dysfunction, tremor, DM, anorexia, weight loss, anxiety, decreased libido, hyponatremia |

*Continued*

## Table 2–15 Antidepressant Drugs—cont'd

| DRUG | INDICATION | | | | CONTRAINDICATIONS | PRECAUTIONS | SIDE EFFECTS |
|------|------------|---|---|---|-------------------|-------------|--------------|
| | DEPRESSION | ANXIETY | PMDD | OTHER | | | |
| Remeron (mirtazapine) | √ | | | | MAOI | Hepatic or renal disease Hx mania, suicide, Hx MI, angina, ischemic stroke. Pregnancy C | S, increased appetite, weight gain, DZ, N, DM, C, CNS effects, BP changes, elevated cholesterol, agranulocytosis |
| Amitrityline | √ | | | | MAOI Acute post-MI | Hx seizures, urinary retention, glaucoma Hepatic, renal, thyroid, or diabetes. Pregnancy Category C | DR, anticholinergic effects, CNS overstimulation Arrhythmias, stroke, coma, EPS (extra pyramidal side effects), BP changes, N, F, R, HA, PH, libido changes, breast enlargement |
| Sinequan (doxepin) | √ | | | √ | MAOI, post MI glaucoma, urinary retention | Cardiovascular disease Epilepsy, suicide. Psychosis, diabetes Pregnancy | CNS effects, anticholinergic effects, hypotension, GI upset, PH, endocrine effects |
| Tofranil (imipramine) | √ | | | √ | MAOI, post-MI | Urinary retention, glaucoma, mania, bipolar disorder, cardiovascular disease, Pregnancy Category C | DR, anticholinergic effects, CNS overstimulation, BP changes, N, F, HA, changes in blood sugar, PH |

# Table 2-15 Antidepressant Drugs—cont'd

| DRUG | INDICATION | | | | CONTRAINDICATIONS | PRECAUTIONS | SIDE EFFECTS |
|------|-----------|---|---|---|-------------------|-------------|--------------|
| | DEPRESSION | ANXIETY | PMDD | OTHYER | | | |
| Pamelor (nortriptyline) | √ | | | | MAOI, post-MI | Urinary retention, glaucoma, epilepsy, mania, ECT, diabetes, bipolar, liver disease, Pregnancy Category C | DR, anticholinergic effects, CNS overstimulation, BP changes, N, F, HA, changes in blood sugar, PH, jaundice |
| Wellbutrin SR and XL (bupropion) | √ | | | | Seizure, bulimia Anorexia, MAOI | Seizure risk. Bipolar, unstable heart disease, CHF, recent MI, hepatic or renal disease, Pregnancy Category C | CNS stimulation, mania, DM, HA, migraine, GI effects, edema, R, palpitations, urinary frequency, sweating, tinnitus, hypertension |
| Equetro (carbama-zepine) | | | | √ | Bone marrow depression, MAOI | Hx cardiac, renal, liver disease. Baseline CBC, lipids. Pregnancy Category D | DZ, S, GI upset, ataxia, pruritus, R, aplastic anemia, agranulocytosis, bone marrow depression |
| Depakote ER (divalproex Na) | | | | √ | Hepatic disease | Discontinue if hepatic dysfunction, pancreatitis Thrombocytopenia Monitor liver function Pregnancy Category D | DZ, HA, GI upset CNS effects, R, cardiovascular effects, arthralgia, liver abnormalities Clotting abnormalities |
| Lamictal (Lamotrigine) | | | | √ | | Discontinue with rash Avoid abrupt cessation Pregnancy Category C | GI upset, I, DZ, S, R, abdominal pain, abnormal dreams, blood dyscrasias |

*Continued*

## Table 2–15 Antidepressant Drugs—cont'd

| DRUG | INDICATION | | | | CONTRAINDICATIONS | PRECAUTIONS | SIDE EFFECTS |
| | DEPRESSION | ANXIETY | PMDD | OTHER | | | |
|---|---|---|---|---|---|---|---|
| Lithobid (lithium carbonate) | | | | | Renal or cardiac disease. Not with diuretics, sodium depletion | Seizure disorder, Maintain fluid and salt intake, monitor lithium levels. Monitor thyroid, renal function. Pregnancy Category D | Polyuria, polydipsia, DR, tremor, hypothyroid, EPS, GI upset, renal toxicity, seizures, hypotension, lethargy, metallic taste, DM, BV |
| Desyrel (trazodone) | √ | | | | | | DR, F, I, HA, BV, DM, confusion, N, akathisia, anemia, flatulence |
| BuSpar (azaspirone) | | √ | | | MAOI | Severe renal or hepatic Pregnancy Category C | DZ, GI upset, HA, Nervousness, CNS or emotional effects, nonspecific chest pain, tinnitus, dream disturbances |
| Ativan (lorazepam) | | √ | | | Acute narrow-angle glaucoma | Avoid abrupt cessation Drug or alcohol abuse. Depression. Suicidal tendencies. Renal, hepatic, or pulmonary disease. Not in pregnancy | CNS depression, DZ, weakness, unsteadiness, transient memory loss, N, HA I, agitation, abuse potential |

BV: blurred vision; C: constipation; D: diarrhea; DM: dry mouth; DR: drowsiness; DZ: dizziness; ECT: electroconvulsive therapy; ESRD: end-stage renal disease; F: fatigue; HA: headache; Hx: history; I: insomnia/sleep disturbances; MAOI: monoamine oxidase inhibitor; N: nausea; PH: photosensitivity; PMDD: premenstrual dysphoric disorder; R: rash; S: somnolence; SIADH: syndrome of inappropriate diuretic hormone secretion; V: vomiting.

Adapted from Nurse Practitioner Prescribing Reference Winter 2008–2009. New York: Haymarket Media Publications, 2009.

## Behavioral Management

In addition to medication therapy for depression, the NP should consider cognitive and behavioral approaches to its management. Examples of some approaches that can be utilized include:

- Bibliotherapy: Check the self-help section of local bookstores for book titles that may be helpful to patients in your practice. Keep copies of selected texts on your bookshelf. Give patients reading assignments from selected books to read before their next appointments, and review key concepts with them during these visits
- Relaxation exercises: Progressive muscle relaxation is an excellent exercise for improving relaxation, sleep, and rest quality. In this exercise the patient is encouraged to find a quiet setting with relaxing music. Next, the patient is encouraged to tighten and then relax specific muscle groups for 10 seconds each, beginning slowly and methodically and moving from the toes to the top of the head. For example, the patient can begin with deep, cleansing breaths and then tighten muscles of the feet for 10 sec and continue the deep cleansing breaths while totally relaxing these same muscles. This is followed by upward progression of slow muscle group relaxation until all areas of the body have been engaged in this activity. The exercise concludes with a 10-sec tightening of the entire body musculature followed by a 10-sec total relaxation of the entire body
- Biofeedback: This relaxation technique is helpful in easing hypertension, chronic pain, tension headaches, and migraine headaches. Essentially, biofeedback uses electromyography to feed brain-wave activity back to the patient as the cue for a conscious relaxation response
- Counseling (individual, family, and group): If there are few or no professional counselors in your clinical area, consider engaging local pastors with whom you are familiar. Many pastors have been trained in basic counseling skills and this can supplement medication therapy and your own in-office counseling
- Music therapy: Playing or listening to music before bedtime can be a relaxing endeavor that improves the quality of sleep.
- Date nights: Encourage patients who report problems with their significant others to schedule and engage in simple date nights once a week. This gives patients a goal, lets them have time to relax away from daily stressors, and reinforces a relationship with their significant others. Even patients with limited resources can

have date nights. Encourage them to have a neighbor babysit any children they have, pack a picnic lunch, and go for a long walk with their partner
- Game playing: Many patients with depression and anxiety do not engage in game-playing activities, which can be relaxing as well as providing a setting for engaging with other people. Encourage patients to purchase a deck of cards or a game board of some type and to play at least once a week

### *Comorbid Psychiatric Diagnoses*

- If a patient with depression presents with a comorbid psychiatric disorder, it is sometimes better to treat one disorder before treating the other. If for example, a patient who presents with depression and substance dependence is treated first for the substance dependence, the treatment may also resolve the features of depression. If this does not work, the depression can be treated. Patients with eating disorders or obsessive–compulsive disorders should have these conditions treated first, and if the depressive features remain, these can be treated. The opposite scenario is true for patients with comorbid generalized anxiety disorder (GAD), in whom the treatment of depression often resolves the anxiety symptoms
- If the patient with depression has comorbid medical disorders with his or her depression, considerations must be given to each disorder in the management of the other. Table 2–16 provides guidance for selecting an antidepressant medication for patients with medical comorbidities

## Anxiety

Disorders characterized by anxiety are very common psychiatric conditions seen in primary care settings. There are a number of such disorders, including panic disorder, obsessive-compulsive disorders, post-traumatic stress disorder, social anxiety, and GAD. Table 2–17 presents characteristics of each.

Management of anxiety involves a stepwise approach:
- Evaluate the patient, considering the urgency of treatment, previous benzodiazepine use, and potential for substance abuse
- Initiate pharmacological therapy with:
  - A benzodiazepine (diazepam, oxazepam) if there has been:
    - Previous benzodiazepine use or a rapid response is needed
    - No previous benzodiazepine use or if there is a history of substance abuse

## Table 2–16 Antidepressant Selection With Comorbid Medical Diagnoses

| CONDITION | PREFER | AVOID |
|---|---|---|
| Cardiac disease (CAD, orthostatic hypotension, arrhythmias) | SSRI, bupropion, mirtazapine | TCAs, MAOIs, trazodone |
| Seizures, head trauma | SSRI, MAOI, desipramine, venlafaxine, mirtazapine | Maprotiline, clomipramine, bupropion, TCAs |
| Stroke | SSRI, nortriptyline | — |
| Dementia | SSRI, trazodone, bupropion | Amitriptyline, clomipramine, protriptyline, amoxapine, TCAs |
| Parkinson's disease | SSRI, amitriptyline, doxepin | Amoxapine, MAOIs |
| Asthma | SSRI, nortriptyline | Amoxapine, MAOIs |
| Angle-closure glaucoma | SSRI, bupropion, trazodone, nefazodone | Amitriptyline, clomipramine, protriptyline, amoxapine |
| Cancer | SSRI, bupropion, mirtazapine, venlafaxine | TCA, MAOIs |

MAOI = monoamine oxidase inhibitor.
Adapted from Nemeroff, C. and Schatzberg, A. Recognition and Treatment of Psychiatric Disorders. Washington DC: American Psychiatric Press, Inc., 1999.

- Buspirone if there is comorbid depression
- Antidepressants (imipramine, or an SSRI)
- Assess the response:
  - If symptoms do not resolve, increase the dose of benzodiazepine or buspirone every 2 or 3 days until symptoms resolve
  - If there is a full response, treat for 4 to 6 months and then gradually taper the dose of medication. If symptoms return, restart therapy and continue indefinitely
  - In cases of partial or no response, confirm the diagnosis, assess the comorbid diagnosis, change to another treatment agent, or consider psychiatric referral
- Consider psychiatric referral for combination drug therapy for difficult cases that resist resolution

## Table 2–17 Characteristics of Anxiety Disorders

| ANXIETY DISORDER | COMMON CHARACTERISTICS | DIAGNOSIS/SCREENING |
|---|---|---|
| Panic disorder | Palpitations, pounding heart, tachycardia, sweating, choking sensation<br>Nausea, abdominal distress, feelings of detachment from body<br>Fear of dying, feelings of losing control, shortness of breath, smothering<br>Chest pain, discomfort, trembling, shaking<br>Numbness, tingling, dizziness, light-headedness, fainting<br>Chills or hot flashes | Diagnosis with four or more symptoms during a spontaneous or discrete period of intense fear or discomfort, must reach peak intensity within 10 min<br>Discrete cases: cognitive behavioral<br>Persistent or severe cases: SSRIs<br>Must rule out medical causes such as angina, hyperthyroidism, pheochromocytoma, or substance abuse as a cause |
| Obsessive–compulsive disorder | Obsessions: Contamination, doubt, somatic concerns, need for symmetry/order, aggressive or sexual impulses<br>Compulsions: Checking, washing, cleaning, counting, repeatedly asking or confessing, ordering, hoarding | Patient symptom presentation<br>Tools: Florida Yule–Brown OCD Scale or MINI<br>Treatment:<br>Behavioral psychotherapy<br>Pharmacological: TCA (clomipramine) or SSRI |
| Post-traumatic stress disorder | Persistent re-experiencing of traumatic event, flashbacks, hallucinations<br>Feelings of detachment, estrangement<br>Diminished interest in activities<br>Sleep disturbances, anger outbursts, hypervigilance, difficulty concentrating<br>Exaggerated startle response | Must have triad of intrusive, avoidant, and hyperarousal symptoms<br>Diagnostic tools: MINI (Mini Mental Status Examination) or Treatment Outcome PTSD Scale<br>Treatment: Low-dose SSRI |
| Social anxiety | Nongeneralized: Predictable, limited to one or a few public situations (speaking)<br>Generalized: Most or all interactional situations produce anxiety | Minor episode: Consider beta blocker or benzodiazepine prn<br>Severe: SSRI or benzodiazepine; often treatment resistant |

| Table 2–17 | **Characteristics of Anxiety Disorders—cont'd** | |
|---|---|---|
| **ANXIETY DISORDER** | **COMMON CHARACTERISTICS** | **DIAGNOSIS/SCREENING** |
| Generalized anxiety disorder | Excessive anxiety and worry more days than not for >6 months<br>Unable to control worry<br>Impaired social/occupational functioning<br>Three or more of the following symptoms:<br>Restless or on edge<br>Easily fatigued<br>Difficulty concentrating, blank mind<br>Irritability<br>Muscle tension<br>Sleep disturbances | Diagnosis with uncontrollable worry accompanied by three or more symptoms, and anxiety is not related to another disorder<br>Diagnostics to rule out medical disorders as cause<br>Treatment:<br>Psychotherapy<br>Benzodiazepines, buspirone, or an SSRI<br>Assess drug response 2–3 days, may take 2–3 weeks for maximum response |

PTSD: post-traumatic stress disorder.
Adapted from Nemeroff, C. and Schatzberg, A. Recognition and Treatment of Psychiatric Disorders. Washington DC: American Psychiatric Press, Inc., 1999.

# Diaphoresis

Diaphoresis is profuse sweating in response to stimulation of the autonomic nervous system by physical, thermal, or psychological stressors. The sweating is either generalized or localized to specific areas of the body such as the palms, soles, and forehead. Diaphoresis may be accompanied by tachycardia and an increase in BP. Recurrent episodes of diaphoresis accompany many chronic illnesses; isolated episodes may be evident with acute pain or fever.

Symptoms that may accompany diaphoresis, depending on its cause, include:

- Insomnia
- Headache
- Disturbances of vision
- Hearing problems
- Palpitations
- Cough
- Difficulty in breathing
- Muscle cramps or stiffness

- Nausea or vomiting
- Abdominal pain
- Recent changes in drug use, including prescription, over-the-counter (OTC), and street drugs

## Assessment

Questions that help guide the clinical decision-making process in patients with diaphoresis include:
- What is the extent of the diaphoresis?
- Does the diaphoresis occur during the day, at night, or both?

When performing the physical assessment, assess the patient's skin turgor and mucous membranes, observe the nails for splinter hemorrhages and Plummer's nails, and check the patient's eyes for exophthalmos and excessive tearing.

Urgent assessment of diaphoresis is indicated when there is evidence of:
- Hypoglycemia
- Heat stroke
- MI
- Heart failure

Emergency management of each of the preceding conditions is identified in Table 2–18.

## Differential Diagnoses

### *Acquired Immune Deficiency Syndrome*

Night sweats are common in acquired immune deficiency syndrome (AIDS) and may also accompany fatigue, unexplained weight loss, diarrhea, and a persistent cough.

### *Acromegaly*

Acromegaly presents with excessive growth of the hands, feet, jaw, and internal organs. Other symptoms include amenorrhea, headaches, vision loss, and sweatiness of the hands. With increased hypersecretion of growth hormone, patients exhibit increased diaphoresis.

Laboratory and diagnostic findings in patients with acromegaly include:
- Elevated levels of insulin-like growth factor-1 (IGF-1)
- Elevated serum glucose level
- Elevated serum levels of liver enzymes
- Elevated levels of BUN and creatinine
- MRI reveals a pituitary tumor in 90% of cases
- Plain radiography reveals a thickened skull

## Table 2–18 Emergency Management of Diaphoretic Crises

| CRISIS EVENT | PATIENT MANAGEMENT |
|---|---|
| Hypoglycemia | Check vital signs: Hypotension? Tachycardia?<br>Check glucose level<br>Observe for irritability, anxiety, tremors<br>Administer IV glucose 50%<br>Cardiac monitor, maintain airway |
| Heatstroke | Vital signs: BP, pulse<br>Move to cool room, remove clothing<br>Start IV for fluid and electrolyte replacement<br>Monitor output |
| Autonomic hyperreflexia | Post-spinal cord injury<br>Symptoms: Headache, restlessness, blurred vision, nasal congestion<br>Vital signs: May have bradycardia, elevated BP<br>Examine eyes for intraocular hemorrhage<br>Examine for slurred speech, paralysis, weakness<br>Check for bladder distention<br>Start IV |
| Myocardial infarction | Cardiac monitor, make sure airway is patent, start IV, transfer to ED |

ED: emergency department.
Adapted from Portable Signs and Symptoms. Philadelphia: Lippincott Williams & Wilkins, 2008

### Anxiety

Diaphoresis may be seen in acute or chronic anxiety states, mainly on the palms, soles, and forehead. Patients with acute or chronic anxiety may also have palpitations, tachycardia, tremors, and GI distress.

### Withdrawal From Drugs or Alcohol

Generalized diaphoresis may occur in withdrawal syndromes. The patient may also have pupillary dilation, tachycardia, tremors, and an altered mental status.

### Hodgkin's Disease

Early findings in Hodgkin's disease may include night sweats. The patient may also have fever, fatigue, pruritus, weight loss, and painless swelling of lymph nodes. The microscopic finding of Reed–Sternberg cells is characteristic of Hodgkin's disease.

### Infective Myocarditis

Infective myocarditis commonly follows an upper respiratory infection (URI), with symptoms including chest pain, signs of heart failure,

tachycardia, and a gallop rhythm. Diagnostic findings in infective myocarditis include:

- ECG: Sinus tachycardia and nonspecific repolarization changes
- Chest radiography: Cardiomyopathy and enlarged pulmonary vessels
- Echocardiography: Cardiomyopathy and contractile dysfunction
- Laboratory findings include an:
  - Elevated WBC
  - Elevated ESR
  - Elevated serum level of troponin I in 30% of patients
  - Elevated serum level of creatinine kinase-MB fraction (CK-MB) in 10% of patients

Treatment for infective myocarditis includes management of heart failure, rest, and antimicrobial therapy.

## *Malaria*

Suspect malaria in patients who have recently traveled to areas where this
disease is endemic. Profuse diaphoresis occurs during the late stages of
malaria, but early signs and symptoms include chills, high fever, headache,
arthralgia, and hepatosplenomegaly. The patient may also have nausea, vomiting, anemia, and thrombocytopenia. Laboratory tests for malaria include a
Giemsa-stained blood smear to identify the intraerythrocytic parasites that
cause the disease and serology for leukocytosis, leukopenia, abnormal liver
function, thrombocytopenia, and anemia. Treatment consists of giving antimalarial drugs.

## *Pesticide Poisoning*

Patients with pesticide poisoning may have diaphoresis as well as nausea,
vomiting, diarrhea, blurred vision, miosis, excessive tearing, muscle
cramps, and paralysis.

## *Pheochromocytoma*

The patient with pheochromocytoma may present with intermittent
diaphoresis. Hypertension is the primary clinical sign of this condition,
with other symptoms including palpitations and headaches. Diagnostic
tests for pheochromocytoma include CT scanning to detect tumors of
adrenal medulla and MRI to locate extra-adrenal tumors not seen on
CT scanning. Laboratory tests should reveal normal levels of thyroid
hormones, elevated glucose levels, and leukocytosis; the patient's ESR
may also be elevated. The most sensitive laboratory test for pheochromocytoma is a 24-hour urine specimen for the assay of total and
fractionated metanephrine, urinary catecholamines, and creatinine.

Treatment involves removing the adrenal tumor and treating the hypertension that occurs in the condition, preferably with atenolol also given to control tachycardia.

## Pneumonia

The patient with pneumonia may present with intermittent diaphoresis and may also have chills, fever, pleuritic chest pain, tachypnea, dyspnea, cough, headache, and cyanosis. Chest radiography confirms this disease.

## Tetanus

Patients with tetanus may have a history of wound contamination. They typically present with profuse sweating and may also have a low-grade fever, tachycardia, and hyperactive deep-tendon reflexes (DTRs). Other symptoms of tetanus include jaw stiffness, spasms, dysphagia, and irritability. Diagnosis is by clinical presentation. Treatment of acute tetanus involves human tetanus immune globulin, bedrest to diminish seizures, and IV penicillin given daily.

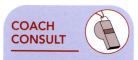

**COACH CONSULT**

Tetanus can be prevented by administering the tetanus–diphtheria (Td) vaccine.

## Thyrotoxicosis

Diaphoresis is common in thyrotoxicosis. The patient may also present with weight loss or gain, heat intolerance, sweating, tachycardia, palpitations, a forceful heartbeat, dyspnea, diarrhea, Plummer's nails, and menstrual irregularities. Diagnostic procedures include a thyroid scan for radioiodine uptake, CT scans of the orbits for Graves' ophthalmopathy, testing for an elevated ESR, and examination of the ECG for changes in cardiac function, particularly premature atrial contractions and atrial fibrillation. Treatment includes propranolol, thiourea drugs, and iodinated contrast agents.

## Pulmonary Tuberculosis

Night sweats are the hallmark symptom of pulmonary TB. Patients with this disease may also present with a low-grade fever, fatigue, weakness, anorexia, and weight loss. A productive and possibly bloody cough may be present. Diagnostic procedures for TB include plain chest radiography, fiberoptic bronchoscopy, and CT scanning if there is clinical suspicion of the disease despite a normal chest radiograph. Treatment includes anti-TB drugs, such as isoniazid, rifampin, pyrazinamide, ethambutol, and streptomycin. Table 2–19 provides a review of the side effects of anti-TB drugs.

## Table 2–19 Antituberculosis Drug Side Effects

| DRUG | SIDE EFFECT | TEST TO MONITOR DRUG | DRUG INTERACTIONS |
|---|---|---|---|
| Isoniazid | Peripheral neuropathy<br>Hepatitis<br>Rash<br>Mild CNS affects | AST<br>ALT<br>Neurological examination | Phenytoin<br>Disulfiram |
| Rifampin | Hepatitis<br>Fever, rash<br>Flu-like illness<br>GI upset<br>Bleeding problems<br>Renal failure<br>Urine discoloration (orange)<br>Contact lens discoloration | CBC<br>Platelets<br>AST<br>ALT | Inhibits affects of OCP (oral contraceptive pills), quinine, corticosteroids, warfarin, methadone, digoxin, and oral hypoglycemic<br>Aminosalicylic acid interferes with absorption of rifampin |
| Pyrazinamide | Hyperuricemia<br>Hepatotoxicity<br>Rash, GI upset<br>Joint aches | Uric acid<br>AST<br>ALT | Rare |
| Ethambutol | Optic neuritis (reverses when stopped)<br>Rash | Red–green color discrimination<br>Visual acuity | Rare |
| Streptomycin | 8th nerve damage<br>Nephrotoxicity<br>Use with caution in elderly and renal diseases | Audiogram<br>BUN, creatinine | Neuromuscular blocking agents may be potentiated |

Adapted from Nurse Practitioner Prescribing Reference, Winter 2008–2009. New York: Haymarket Media Publications, 2009.

## Diarrhea

Diarrhea can be caused by acute or chronic illness. Its acute sources include infections (viral, bacterial, or protozoal), stress, food intolerances, antibiotics, magnesium antacids, laxative abuse, and intestinal obstructions. Chronic diarrhea may be related to chronic bowel disease, malabsorption syndrome, GI surgery, endocrine disorders, IBS, Crohn's disease, lactose intolerance, or ulcerative colitis.

## Assessment

Assessment of the patient with diarrhea begins with the patient's history. Obtain a complete GI history including surgeries, medical diagnoses, and medications taken. Check for complaints of pain, cramping, weakness, or nausea. Obtain a 24-hour diet recall and ask the patient to identify any food allergies and recent increases in stress and to provide a travel history.

The physical evaluation of patients with diarrhea should include an assessment of skin turgor and of the mucous membranes, BP and vital signs, an abdominal assessment, an examination of the patient's skin for rashes.

Use the Rome III criteria for evaluating diarrhea. Table 2–20 shows common symptoms and causative agents for infectious acute diarrhea. Table 2–21 shows chronic diseases that are often associated with or which contribute to diarrhea.

### Table 2–20 Acute Diarrhea Related to Infectious Diseases

| DISEASE | PRESENTING SYMPTOMS | ORGANISM/TREATMENT |
|---|---|---|
| Q Fever | Diarrhea with high fever, chills, severe headache, malaise, chest pain, vomiting, sore throat, clay stools<br>Severe: hepatitis, pneumonia, thrombocytopenia (transient)<br>Seen in workers with sheep, cattle | *Coxiella burnetii*<br>Spread: Inhalation, ingestion, or insect bites<br>Treatment: Doxycycline or quinolones for 21 days |
| Rotavirus | Fever, nausea, vomiting, followed by diarrhea<br>Lasts 3–9 days | Rotavirus<br>Treatment: Rehydration |
| *Clostridium difficile* | Soft, unformed stools to watery diarrhea, foul smell, may be grossly bloody, abdominal pain, tenderness, fever | *C. difficile*<br>Treatment: Metronidazole or vancomycin |
| Cholera | Abrupt watery diarrhea, vomiting, thirst, weakness, muscle cramps, dehydration, oliguria, tachycardia<br>Without treatment: Death within hours<br>Can lose up to 1000 mL/hr | *Vibrio cholerae*<br>Treatment: Rehydration |

*Continued*

## Table 2–20  Acute Diarrhea Related to Infectious Diseases—cont'd

| DISEASE | PRESENTING SYMPTOMS | ORGANISM/TREATMENT |
|---|---|---|
| Anthrax (GI) | Severe bloody diarrhea: late sign | *Bacillus anthracis*<br>Treatment: Ciprofloxacin and either doxycycline or quinolone for 60 days |
| *Escherichia coli* | Watery or bloody diarrhea, nausea, vomiting, fever, abdominal cramps | *E. coli*<br>Traveler's diarrhea<br>Treatment: Rehydration |
| Acute viral, bacterial, or protozoal | Sudden-onset watery diarrhea, abdominal pain, cramps, nausea, vomiting, fever | Treatment: Rehydration |
| Pseudomembranous enterocolitis | Copious watery, green, foul-smelling, bloody diarrhea, colicky, distention, fever, dehydration<br>Follows antibiotic administration | *C. difficile*<br>Treatment: Metronidazole or vancomycin |
| Listeriosis | Diarrhea with fever, abdominal pain, myalgia, nausea, vomiting<br>Pregnancy, neonates and immunocompromised | Check stool for ova, parasites CBC, ESR, and C-reactive protein<br>Treatment: Rehydration |

Adapted from Desai, S. Clinician's Guide to Diagnosis. Cleveland, OH: Lexi-Comp Inc., 2001

## Table 2–21  Chronic Diseases Causing Diarrhea

| DISEASE | PRESENTING SYMPTOMS |
|---|---|
| Carcinoid syndrome | Severe diarrhea with face/neck flushing<br>Usual cause: Stress, ingestion of hot food or alcohol |
| Crohn's disease | Diarrhea with abdominal pain, nausea, possible fever, chills, weakness, anorexia, weight loss, perianal fistulas |
| Intestinal obstruction | Diarrhea, abdominal pain, tenderness, guarding, nausea, possible distention |
| Irritable bowel syndrome (IBS) | Diarrhea alternating with constipation or normal bowel function, may have abdominal pain, tenderness, distention, dyspepsia, nausea |

| Table 2–21 | Chronic Diseases Causing Diarrhea—cont'd |
|---|---|
| **DISEASE** | **PRESENTING SYMPTOMS** |
| Ischemic bowel disease | Bloody diarrhea with abdominal pain |
| Lactose intolerance | Diarrhea within several hours of milk ingestion, with cramps, abdominal pain |
| Ulcerative colitis | Recurrent bloody severe diarrhea with pus or mucus; tenesmus, urgency, low abdominal cramping, hyperactive bowel sounds, late findings: weight loss, anemia |

Adapted from Portable Signs and Symptoms. Philadelphia: Lippincott Williams & Wilkins, 2008.

# Dizziness

Dizziness is a common condition marked by a sensation of imbalance or faintness. It may be mild or severe and is generally aggravated by rapidly standing up and relieved by lying down.

## Differential Diagnoses

### Anemia

In anemia, dizziness is aggravated by movement or exertion. Other symptoms include pallor, dyspnea, fatigue, tachycardia, and a bounding pulse.

### Emphysema

In emphysema, dizziness is exacerbated by exertion.

### Generalized Anxiety Disorder

GAD presents with continuous dizziness; the patient may also have anxiety, insomnia, poor concentration, and muscle aches.

### Hyperventilation

Short episodes of dizziness follow hyperventilation.

### Hypovolemia

The patient with hypovolemia will present with dizziness, dry mucus membranes, decreased blood pressure, and tachycardia.

**COACH CONSULT**

Other causes of dizziness include cardiac arrhythmias, hypertension, concussion, transient ischemic attack, and medications such as anxiolytic agents, central nervous system (CNS) depressants, opioids, decongestants, antihistamines, and antihypertensive and vasodilator drugs.

# Dyspepsia

Patients who present with complaints of dyspepsia may also report accompanying symptoms of belching, heartburn, fullness, early satiety, nausea, vomiting, and anorexia.

## Differential Diagnoses

### Medication-Induced Dyspepsia

Medications that can cause dyspepsia include antibiotics, such as ampicillin and erythromycin; digoxin; iron supplements; potassium supplements; and theophylline.

### Gastroesophageal Reflux Disease

GERD presents as heartburn moving from the xiphoid region to the oropharynx. Its symptoms are precipitated by bending, straining during defecation, running, lifting, and the ingesting of foods such as chocolate, onions, coffee, peppermint, spicy foods, citrus products, and tomato products. Diagnostic procedures for GERD include an upper GI series and endoscopy, especially if bleeding is present.

### Irritable Bowel Syndrome

Dyspepsia is seen in 80% of patients with IBS.

### Biliary Tract Disease

Dyspepsia is present in biliary tract diseases such as cholelithiasis and dysfunction of the sphincter of Oddi. Diagnostic procedures for these conditions include a small-bowel study.

### Disorders of Carbohydrate Metabolism

Lactase deficiency presents with abdominal pain, bloating, flatulence, and diarrhea after the ingestion of lactose-containing products. Ingestion of fructose and sorbitol ingestion can cause bloating, abdominal pain, flatulence, and diarrhea, which generally resolve with the elimination of fructose and sorbitol from the diet.

## Table 2–22 Options for Eradicating *Helicobacter Pylori*

| ACID SUPPRESSANT | ANTIBIOTIC 1 | ANTIBIOTIC 2 | DURATION OF TREATMENT |
|---|---|---|---|
| Rabeprazole (Aciphex) 20 mg bid | Amoxicillin 1000 mg bid | Clarithromycin 500 mg bid | 7 days with a.m. and p.m. meals |
| Esomeprazole (Nexium) 40 mg daily | Amoxicillin 1000 mg bid | Clarithromycin 500 mg bid | 10 days |
| Lansoprazole (Prevacid) 30 mg bid | Amoxicillin 1000 mg bid | Clarithromycin 500 mg bid | 10–14 days Sold as PrevPac |
| Lansoprazole (Prevacid) 30 mg tid | Amoxicillin 1000 mg bid | — | 14 days |
| Omeprazole (Prilosec) (Zegerid) 20 mg bid | Amoxicillin 1000 mg bid | Clarithromycin 500 mg bid | 10 days. If ulcer present, continue omeprazole 20 mg qd x 18 days |
| Omeprazole (Prilosec) (Zegerid) 40 mg qd | Clarithromycin 500 mg tid | — | 14 days. If ulcer present, continue omeprazole 20 mg qd x 14 days |
| H2 receptor blocker (Axid, Pepcid, Tagamet, Zantac) | Metronidazole 250 mg AND | Tetracycline 500 mg with two 262.4 mg bismuth subsalicylate chewable tablets qid | Sold as combination pack. Take each dose with full glass of water x 14 days |
| Omeprazole (Prilosec) (Zegerid) 20 mg bid | Metronidazole 125 mg, tetracycline 125 mg, bismuth subcitrate 140 mg in a single capsule. Take three capsules qid | | Take each dose with full glass of water x 14 days |
| Nizatidine (Axid) 300 mg hs | Any of the above combinations | | Take with two antibiotics for 2 weeks. May take Axid for 4–8 wk |

*Continued*

| Table 2–22 Options for Eradicating *Helicobacter Pylori*—cont'd | | | |
|---|---|---|---|
| ACID SUPPRESSANT | ANTIBIOTIC 1 | ANTIBIOTIC 2 | DURATION OF TREATMENT |
| Famotidine (Pepcid) 40 mg hs | Any of the above combinations | | Take with 2 antibiotics for 2 weeks. May take Pepcid for 4–8 weeks |
| Cimetidine (Tagamet) 800 mg hs | Any of the above combinations | | Take with two antibiotics for 2 weeks. May take Tagamet for total of 4–8 weeks |
| Ranitidine (Zantac) 300 mg hs | Any of the above combinations | | Take with 2 antibiotics for 2 weeks. May take Zantac for total 4–8 weeks |

Adapted from Nurse Practitioner Prescribing Reference Winter 2008–2009. New York: Haymarket Media Publications, 2009.

# Dysphagia

Dysphagia, or difficulty in swallowing, may be seen in up to 10% of adults older than 50 years of age. Similar problems that should be considered in a work-up for dysphagia include odynophagia, or pain on swallowing, and globus, or a constant sensation of a lump or tightness in the throat. In some cases, dysphagia and odynophagia may be present simultaneously.

## Assessment

When assessing for dysphagia, pay attention to the following signs and symptoms:

- Aspiration
- Choking during swallowing
- Coughing during swallowing
- Difficulty initiating a swallow
- Drooling of food or saliva
- Food sticking in the throat

When patients complain of food sticking in the throat, the problem may be esophageal dysphagia. The condition is typically gradual in onset.

Potential causes of esophageal dysphagia include:

- Achalasia or a motility disorder; check for symptoms and a history of these
- Cigarette smoking, alcohol use, or Barrett's mucosa

The patient may also report substernal chest pain radiating to the back and regurgitation of food that worsens at night. Endoscopy reveals a dilated esophageal body with retained esophageal contents.

In some cases postural changes relieve dysphagia, such as with raising of the arms over the head, straightening of the back, or standing erect.

## Diagnostic Testing

If the NP suspects esophageal dysphagia, two diagnostic options are available:

- Barium esophagography, which reveals structural lesions of the esophagus and esophageal motility, and can show esophageal rings and webs that may be missed on endoscopy
- Endoscopy, which is the preferred procedure if any of the following situations exist:
  - Significant weight loss
  - Possible esophageal carcinoma
  - Persistent heartburn
  - A clinical presentation suggesting peptic stricture
  - Dysphagia of acute onset

Other diagnostic tests in patients with esophageal dysphagia include a plain chest radiograph to detect gastric air bubbles and esophageal air fluid levels, a barium swallow to identify esophageal abnormalities, and manometry to visualize relaxation of the lower esophageal sphincter (LES) and to identify problems with peristalsis.

## Differential Diagnoses

### *Scleroderma*

Patients with scleroderma may also have telangiectasia, subcutaneous calcifications, or sclerodactyly. Scleroderma is characterized by abnormalities of smooth-muscle function in the lower esophagus

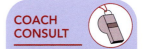

**COACH CONSULT**

Medications that may precipitate symptoms of oropharyngeal dysphagia include:

- Angiotensin-converting enzyme (ACE) inhibitors
- α-Adrenergic blockers
- Angiotensin II receptor blockers
- Antiarrhythmics
- Anticholinergics
- Antihistamines
- Antipsychotics
- Diuretics
- Opiates
- Benzodiazepines
- Neuroleptics
- Corticosteroids
- Hydroxymethylglutaryl-coenzyme A (HMG-CoA) reductase inhibitors

**COACH CONSULT**

Dysphagia may be a secondary response to neuromuscular conditions such as myasthenia gravis, hyperthyroidism, motor neuron diseases, or Parkinson's disease.

and esophageal sphincter. A barium esophagogram may reveal a dilated esophagus. A manometric examination will show peristalsis of the LES.

### Mediastinal Masses

Patients who have mediastinal masses may also present with unilateral wheezing.

### Aortic Aneurysm

Diagnostic procedures used to check for an aortic aneurysm include ultrasonography, CT scan, MRI, and aortography.

### Esophageal Carcinoma

Patients with esophageal carcinoma may have progressive dysphagia occurring over a period of months and a history of melena. Diagnostic procedures for esophageal carcinoma include:

- Barium swallow
- Esophagoscopy with biopsy
- CT scan for staging purposes
- Endoscopic ultrasound examination

Other differential diagnoses associated with dysphagia include:

- Esophageal spasms
- Lymphadenopathy
- Esophageal diverticula
- Esophageal rings or webs (Schatzki's ring)

## Dysuria

Pain or burning with urination is a more common presentation in female than in male patients, but it does also occur in men. Typically, dysuria is the result of inflammation or irritation of the urinary tract. This discussion of dysuria is divided into two sections: one for male and the other for female complaints of dysuria.

### Dysuria in Males

The most common causes of dysuria in male patients are acute pyelonephritis, cystitis, epididymitis, prostatitis, and urethritis. Symptoms associated with each of these conditions are listed below.

### Acute Pyelonephritis

**Assessment**

Assessment of a patient with acute pyelonephritis may include evaluation for back pain, fever, flank tenderness, nausea, vomiting, and CVAT. Acute pyelonephritis may be preceded by 1 to 2 days of dysuria, urinary frequency, or urinary urgency.

## Diagnostic Testing

Diagnostic testing for acute pyelonephritis includes:

- Urinalysis and urine and blood cultures for all men with acute pyelonephritis
- A CT scan if the condition is unresponsive to treatment
- Ultrasound examination to detect possible abscess

## Treatment

Treatment for acute pyelonephritis can consist of any of the following:

- Ampicillin: 1 g q6h + gentamycin 1 mg/kg q8h IV for 21 days
- Ciprofloxacin: 750 mg PO q12h for 21 days; or
- Trimethoprim/sulfamethoxazole (Bactrim DS): one tablet PO q12h for 21 days

## *Cystitis*

### Assessment

Assessment of a patient with cystitis should reveal urinary frequency, urgency, suprapubic pain, and hematuria.

### Diagnostic Testing

If a urethral discharge is present, consider urethritis as the diagnosis and obtain culture of the discharge fluid for gonorrhea and chlamydia. If these cultures are positive, consider serological tests for syphilis as well. Urinalysis in patients with cystitis reveals pyuria, bacteriuria, and hematuria.

### Treatment

Treatment for cystitis includes:

- Cephalexin (Keflex): 250 to 500 mg q6h for 1 to 3 days; or
- Ciprofloxacin (Cipro): 250 to 500 mg q12h for 1 to 3 days; or
- Norfloxacin (Noroxin): 400 mg q12h for 1 to 3 days; or
- Ofloxacin (Floxin): 200 mg q12h for 3 days; or
- Trimethoprim/sulfamethoxazole (Bactrim DS): two tablets as a single dose

## *Epididymitis*

### Assessment

Assessment of a patient with epididymitis should reveal scrotal pain, a urethral discharge, and tender swelling of the epididymis. These symptoms often present after heavy lifting, sexual intercourse, or trauma. Epididymitis is most common in men aged 20 to 35 years who have sexually transmitted diseases (STDs) caused by *Neisseria gonorrhea* or *Chlamydia trachomatis.* Older men with epididymitis typically have benign prostatic hyperplasia.

To differentiate epididymitis from testicular torsion, remember that epididymitis is marked by:

- Abnormal elevation of the affected testicle, with a palpable twist of the spermatic cord
- An abnormal axis of the affected testicle with the patient in the upright position
- Abnormal position of the epididymis within the scrotum
- An appearance of great patient discomfort

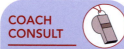

**COACH CONSULT**

Diagnostic procedures for testicular torsion include :
- Ultrasound examination with a color Doppler scan
- A radionuclide flow study to visualize diminished flow on the symptomatic side

### Diagnostic Testing

Diagnostic testing for epididymitis includes urinalysis, urine culture, and the testing of any discharge for sexually transmitted diseases (STDs). A CBC will show leukocytosis with a shift to the left. A scrotal ultrasound examination may aid in the diagnosis of a large hydrocele.

### Treatment

Treatment for epididymitis involves bedrest with scrotal elevation. If the epididymitis is related to an STD, the patient should be treated with Ceftriaxone at 250 mg IM as s single dose + doxycycline 100 mg q12h for 10 days. If the infection is not STD related, the patient should be given Ciprofloxacin at 250 to 500 mg PO q12h for 1 to 3 month or trimethoprim/sulfamethoxazole (Bactrim DS), with one tablet PO bid for 1 to 3 months.

## Prostatitis

Prostatitis presents with signs and symptoms of back pain, fever, a urethral discharge, scrotal pain, tenderness of the prostate on palpation, malaise, arthralgia, irritation, and problems in voiding. The patient may also have urinary frequency, urgency, and retention.

**COACH CONSULT**

*Escherichia coli* is the most common pathogen identified in prostatitis; other pathogens that may be seen include *Proteus, Klebsiella, Pseudomonas, Serratia, Enterobacter,* and *Providencia.*

### Assessment

Examination of the prostate in a patient with prostatitis may reveal it to be very tender, boggy, and edematous.

### Diagnostic Testing

Diagnostic testing for prostatitis includes urinalysis and urine and blood cultures.

### Treatment

The treatment of prostatitis is the same as that for acute pyelonephritis.

### Urethritis

Urethritis presents as a urethral discharge. Its diagnosis is made through urethral culture, and its treatment is with appropriate antibiotic drugs selected on the basis of culture results.

## Dysuria in Female Patients

Common causes of dysuria in female patients include cystitis, urethritis, vaginitis, and pyelonephritis. Bacterial infections are the predominant cause of dysuria in female patients. Noninfectious causes of dysuria include:

- Bladder calculus
- Bladder cancer
- Drug-induced cystitis
- Eosinophilic cystitis
- Hemorrhagic cystitis
- Interstitial cystitis
- Psychogenic dysuria
- Radiation-induced cystitis
- Ureteral calculus
- Urethral cancer
- Urethral diverticulum
- Urethral stricture

Clues in the physical examination that indicate the etiology of female dysuria caused by urinary tract infections (UTIs) are given in Table 2–23.

### Complicated Cystitis

Women with complicated cystitis should definitely have a urine culture to permit the selection of an appropriate antibiotic for its treatment. Patients with the following should be evaluated for complicated cystitis:

- Diabetes mellitus
- A history of frequent infections
- A history of resistant organisms
- Immunocompromise
- Indwelling catheters
- Known structural or functional urological abnormalities
- Pregnancy

**COACH CONSULT**

If you suspect prostatic abscess, order a transrectal ultrasound examination or CT scan, especially in patients with comorbid diabetes or those in immunocompromised states.

**COACH CONSULT**

Female patients who present with uncomplicated urinary UTIs may be treated empirically with appropriate antibiotics. Pretreatment cultures have not provided evidence to support the use of these antibiotics in uncomplicated cystitis.

| Table 2–23 **Dysuria in Female Patients** | |
|---|---|
| **PHYSICAL EXAMINATION FINDING** | **CONDITION SUGGESTED** |
| Suprapubic tenderness | Cystitis |
| Fever | Acute pyelonephritis |
| Costovertebral angle tenderness | Acute pyelonephritis |
| Vaginal discharge | Vaginitis Genital herpes |
| Satellite vaginal pustules | Vaginitis, vaginal candidiasis |
| Grouped painful vesicles Tender inguinal lymphadenopathy | Genital herpes |

Adapted from Desai, S. Clinician's Guide to Diagnosis. Cleveland, OH: Lexi-Comp Inc., 2002.

- Recent antibiotic treatment
- Recent hospitalization
- A recurrent or reinfective UTI

If an uncomplicated urinary tract infection is treated and the patient nevertheless presents after 2 weeks with symptoms, reinfection has occurred. Factors that require patient education for preventing future infections include:

- Avoiding a full bladder
- Maintaining a high fluid intake on a daily basis
- Emptying the bladder after intercourse
- Considering changing of contraception methods if using a diaphragm or spermicide for contraception
- Wiping from anterior to posterior after voiding

# Ear Pain

Earaches generally stem from diseases or conditions in the inner or middle ear, typically related to infection, trauma, or obstruction.

## Differential Diagnoses
### *Barotrauma*
Barotrauma presents with poor eustachian tube function, problems with the equalization of pressure in the middle and outer ear during activities

such as flying, diving, or changes in altitude. It may also appreciate ecchymosis or bleeding of the tympanic membrane (TM).

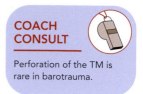
Prevention of barotrauma can be accomplished by frequent swallowing or yawning to autoinflate the middle ear. Systemic decongestants taken before travel may also be helpful. Topical decongestant nasal sprays, such as 1% phenylephrine, should be administered 1 hour before an activity that might cause barotrauma. Underwater divers are at risk for rupture of the TM because of the severe negative pressures they experience. Persons with persistent middle ear pressure may want to consider taking decongestants or undergoing myringotomy or, if frequent flyers, the insertion of ventilation tubes.

### Abscess
An abscess usually presents with ipsilateral headache, a low-grade fever, fatigue, and malaise.

### Cerumen Impaction
Cerumen impaction may present with partial hearing loss, itching, and dizziness. Treatment includes instilling a cerumen-softening agent for 3 to 5 days and irrigating with water warmed to body temperature or a solution of half water and half hydrogen peroxide.

### Mastoiditis
Mastoiditis often follows several weeks of unresolved otitis media (OM). It presents as a dull aching behind the mastoid process, with a low-grade fever. The TM will be dull, edematous, and possibly perforated with a purulent discharge. Radiography reveals coalescence of mastoid air cells. Treatment is accomplished with IV antibiotics or myringotomy, with culture of the drainage fluid.

### Herpes Zoster Oticus
Herpes zoster oticus presents as a burning or stabbing pain in ear; there may be vesicles in the ear canal or concha, and the patient may have hearing loss or dizziness. Treatment consists of giving antiviral medications.

### Meniere's Disease
Meniere's disease presents with ear pain associated with severe vertigo, tinnitus, and hearing loss. The classic syndrome consists of

episodic vertigo lasting from 20 minutes to hours, fluctuating low-frequency sensorineural hearing loss, tinnitus, and a sensation of aural pressure. Treatment includes a low-salt diet and diuretics (acetazolamide). In refractory cases, intratympanic administration of corticosteroids, vestibular ablation, and labyrinthectomy may be considered.

### Otitis Externa

Otitis externa presents as ear pain aggravated with movement of the tragus, an erythematous canal, and possibly a purulent discharge. Common causative organisms include gram-negative rods (*Pseudomonas, Proteus*) or fungi (*Aspergillus*). Treatment involves gently removing any purulent discharge by drainage, using a wick if there is significant edema so as to keep the ear canal open. Other treatment considerations include:

- Management of pain with NSAIDs and topical corticosteroids
- Acidic otic antibiotic drops with or without corticosteroids
- Aminoglycosides or fluoroquinolones
- Neomycin sulfate
- Polymyxin B sulfate with hydrocortisone

### Otitis Media, Acute

**ALERT**

An increased incidence of penicillin-resistant *S. pneumoniae* has been encountered in the treatment of OM.

Acute serous OM presents as a sense of fullness in the ear, hearing loss, otalgia, fever, and aural pressure, with decreased motility of the TM. Acute supparative OM presents with throbbing ear pain that progresses in intensity, a low-grade fever, and hearing loss. The most common causative pathogens of acute OM are *Streptococcus pneumoniae, Haemophilus influenzae, S. pyogenes, and Moraxella catarrhalis.* Treatment involves giving antibiotics, such as amoxicillin or erythromycin, cefaclor, or Augmentin, and nasal decongestants. Cases of recurrent OM are treated with long-term antibiotic administration.

## Edema

Edema can result from disorders in many body systems, including the cardiovascular, renal, endocrine, and hepatic systems; as well as after acute burns. Key pathophysiological factors in edema include excessive sodium ingestion or retention and conditions marked by hypoalbuminuria. Premenopausal women may experience cyclic edema related to increased aldosterone secretion.

Edema localized to a specific part of the body has particular implications. For example:

- Edema of the arm: Potential causes include arm trauma, burns, snakebites, superior vena cava syndrome, thrombophlebitis, and mastectomy. The edema may be bilateral or unilateral and of gradual or abrupt onset
- Edema of the face: May be localized or generalized on the face. Potential causes include trauma, allergy, malnutrition, and drugs. Edema around the eyes may be caused by chalazion, conjunctivitis, dacryoadenitis, dacryocystitis, nephritic syndrome, orbital cellulitis, pre-eclampsia, rhinitis, sinusitis, superior vena cava syndrome, trachoma, and trichinosis
- Edema of the leg: May be unilateral or bilateral and pitting or nonpitting; causes include burns, cellulitis, snake bites, heart failure, trauma, osteomyelitis, thrombophlebitis, and venous insufficiency

## Differential Diagnoses

### Heart Failure

Diagnostic procedures for heart failure with edema include plain chest radiography to detect cardiomegaly, echocardiography to detect dilated cardiac chambers, MRI to detect abnormalities in stroke volume and cardiomyopathy, and electron-beam CT scanning for calcification in the coronary artery.

### Myxedema (Hypothyroid)

Myxedema presents with weakness, fatigue, cold intolerance, constipation, weight changes, depression, menorrhagia, hoarseness, dry skin, bradycardia, and diminished deep tendon reflexes. Laboratory findings include a low or low-normal level of free thyroxine (FT4), elevated level of TSH, and ANAs not indicative of lupus. Other diagnostic procedures include assays for cholesterol, triglycerides, lipoprotein, liver enzymes, CK, and a CBC. The patient may also present with hyponatremia, hypoglycemia, and anemia. Imaging studies include CT scanning or MRI to detect goiter and MRI of the head to detect pituitary gland enlargement. Treatment involves giving levothyroxine before morning meals, with a follow-up in 1 to 2 weeks to recheck thyroid hormone levels and assess the effectiveness of medication.

### Pericardial Effusion

Pericardial effusion presents with dyspnea and cough and, in the case of a large effusion, a pericardial friction rub. Pain may be absent or present.

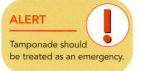
Patients with tamponade will have tachycardia, tachypnea, a narrow pulse pressure, and pulsus paradoxus. Imaging studies used to diagnose pericardial effusion include plain chest radiography to visualize an enlarged cardiac silhouette, echocardiography to detect accentuations in left ventricular (LV) filling, an ECG revealing nonspecific T-wave changes and a low voltage of the QRS complex, a CT scan to identify localized effusions, and MRI to identify the character of effusion fluid as either blood or serous fluid. The management of pericardial effusion involves close monitoring of small effusions by careful observation of jugular venous pressures (JVP) and by serial echocardiogram diagnostics to monitor the patient's status.

### Pericarditis

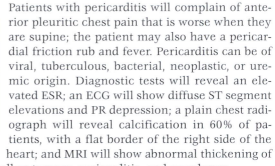

**COACH CONSULT**

Other potential causes of edema include:
• Angioneurotic edema
• Burns
• Medications
• Malnutrition
• Renal failure

Patients with pericarditis will complain of anterior pleuritic chest pain that is worse when they are supine; the patient may also have a pericardial friction rub and fever. Pericarditis can be of viral, tuberculous, bacterial, neoplastic, or uremic origin. Diagnostic tests will reveal an elevated ESR; an ECG will show diffuse ST segment elevations and PR depression; a plain chest radiograph will reveal calcification in 60% of patients, with a flat border of the right side of the heart; and MRI will show abnormal thickening of the pericardium, as well as tumors, pericarditis, and neoplasms.

Treatment for viral pericarditis is symptomatic, with monitoring of the CBC and cardiac enzymes, administration of acetylsalicylic acid (ASA; aspirin) at 650 mg q4h or NSAIDs, and corticosteroids. Treatment for TB-related pericarditis consists of anti-TB drugs. Dialysis is used to treat uremic pericarditis.

## Facial Pain

When a patient presents with complaints of facial pain, localize the pain if possible, determine whether the pain is sensitive to touch or movement (chewing, moving the head up or down), and identify any associated symptoms (headaches, recent trauma, anxiety, depression, fever, ear pain, disturbances of vision, eye pain, nasal discharge, and toothache). Table 2–24 presents acute and chronic causes of facial pain complaints.

## Table 2–24 Acute and Chronic Causes of Facial Pain

| DIAGNOSIS | HISTORY | PHYSICAL EXAMINATION |
|---|---|---|
| **ACUTE PROBLEMS** | | |
| Acute sinusitis | Headache, nasal congestion, nasal discharge, pain increases when head is lowered | Fever, sinus tenderness, erythema and edema may overlie the area, purulent nasal discharge, decreased or absent transillumination |
| Acute open-angle glaucoma | Painful red eye, headache, nausea, vomiting. May be precipitated by mydriatics, darkness, or stress. Blurred vision, halo around lights | Mildly dilated unreactive pupil. Inflamed eye, steamy cornea, shallow anterior chamber |
| Dental abscess | Toothache | Poor dental hygiene, tooth tender to direct percussion |
| Herpes zoster | Continuous unilateral facial pain, with vesicular rash | Unilateral vesicular eruption confined to one or more dermatomes |
| Bell's palsy | | |
| **CHRONIC PROBLEMS** | | |
| Tic douloureux | Brief "jabs" of unilateral severe pain. Precipitated by cold, hot, or pressure over "trigger" areas | Pressure over certain areas of the face may induce an attack of pain |
| Temporomandibular joint pain (TMJ) | Pain on chewing. May have history of rheumatoid arthritis | Crepitation, tenderness over TMJ area |
| Chronic or acute otitis media | Earache, decreased hearing | Perforated, inflamed, or thickened tympanic membrane |
| Migraine headache | | |

Adapted from Wasson, J. The Common Symptom Guide, ed. 5. New York: McGraw-Hill, 2002.

# Fatigue

Patients with fatigue will report symptoms of extreme tiredness, low energy levels, exhaustion, and a strong desire to rest. Fatigue is expected after extreme physical exertion for a short period and can also be evident after a period of emotional stress or sleep deprivation. Typically, such fatigue is short-lived and explainable when it accompanies a history of the patient's current or recent life situation. Fatigue that persists can be a nonspecific symptom of a psychological or physiological disorder, such as severe infection or a decline in function of the cardiac, endocrine, or neurological systems.

## Differential Diagnoses

### Acquired Immune Deficiency Syndrome

Patients with AIDS will typically present with fever, night sweats, weight loss, diarrhea, and a cough.

### Adrenocorticoid Insufficiency

Adrenocorticoid insufficiency, also known as adrenal crisis, initially presents after stress and later increases in severity. Other signs and symptoms include weakness and weight loss, GI upset, anorexia, nausea, diarrhea, abdominal pain, and dehydration. Laboratory studies reveal a high eosinophil count (EOS), hyponatremia, hypokalemia, and hypoglycemia. Cultures should be taken of the patient's blood, sputum, and urine. The gold-standard test for adrenocorticoid insufficiency is the cosyntropin stimulation test, which involves administering adrenocorticotropic hormone (ACTH) in a dose of 0.25 mg parenterally, waiting 30 minutes and 60 minutes, and checking the patient's serum cortisol levels. Normally a rise to at least 20 mcg/dL is expected. Treatment for adrenocorticoid insufficiency consists of giving hydrocortisone at 100 to 300 mg IV + saline, along with treating underlying situations such as bacterial infections and abnormalities in glucose metabolism.

### Anemia

Anemia presents with pallor, tachycardia, dyspnea, and pica. It is essential to determine whether the anemia is microcytic, normocytic, or macrocytic. (See Chapter 3 for more information on identifying the different types of anemia.)

#### Iron Deficiency Anemia

Iron deficiency anemia, which is a microcytic anemia, is marked by fatigue, tachycardia, palpitations, and tachypnea. In severe cases the patient may present with a smooth tongue, brittle nails, and cheilosis. Diagnostic tests include a CBC and assays for serum iron, serum ferritin, and total iron-binding capacity (TIBC). Treatment consists of oral iron replacement with ferrous sulfate at 325 mg tid. With this, the patient's laboratory test values should improve by 50% within 3 weeks and 100% in 2 months. The patient may also be given parenteral iron replacement upon referral to a hematologist.

## Anemia of Chronic Disease

In anemia of chronic disease, the patient will have normal or increased iron stores. This type of anemia is a chronic disease state marked by a decreased serum iron level, decreased TIBC, and normal ferritin level.

## Thalassemia

The patient with thalassemia presents with profound microcytic anemia and a family history of this disease. Microscopic study of the patient's red cell morphology will show acanthocytes and target cells. In beta-thalassemia, hemoglobin A2 and F are increased; in alpha-thalassemia, the mean corpuscular volume (MCV) will be 60 to 75 fL. Treatment is not required in mild cases of thalassemia, but in more serious cases of hemoglobin H disease the patient may be given folate supplements and be told to avoid iron and sulfonamides. In severe cases of thalassemia transfusion and folate supplementation are necessary.

## Sideroblastic Anemia

Patients with sideroblastic anemia present with general symptoms of anemia. Their bone marrow will show marked erythroid hyperplasia, ineffective erythropoiesis, increased iron stores, and ringed sideroblasts. Laboratory testing will demonstrate an elevated serum iron level and transferrin saturation. Severe cases require transfusion.

## Vitamin B12 Deficiency

Vitamin B12 deficiency is a type of macrocytic anemia. Its symptoms include peripheral nerve paresthesias, pallor, icterus, decreased vibratory and positional sensation, and a red tongue. Laboratory tests will show macrocytic anemia with a low serum level of vitamin B12; in severe cases of vitamin B12 deficiency the WBC may be elevated WBC and the platelet count decreased. Treatment involves vitamin B12 replacement at 100 mg IM weekly for 4 weeks and then at monthly intervals for life.

## Folic Acid Deficiency

Folic acid deficiency is a type of macrocytic anemia with symptoms similar to those of vitamin B12

> **ALERT**
>
> It is clinically possible for a patient to have a mixed presentation of anemias, including vitamin B12 deficiency and iron deficiency anemia, or anemia of chronic disease. Carefully consider all anemias in diagnostic work-ups.

deficiency, but without neurological deficits. Laboratory results will show macrocytic anemia, with normal vitamin B12 levels and low folate levels. Treatment consists of giving folic acid at 1 mg daily. This should totally correct the condition within 2 months.

## Anxiety

Patients with anxiety may also present with apprehension, restlessness, insomnia, and trembling. For more information on anxiety, see pages 56 to 69.

## Carbon Monoxide Poisoning

Patients with carbon monoxide poisoning will present with headache, dyspnea, and confusion, as well as flushed skin. Other symptoms include abdominal pain, nausea, syncope, hypotension, coma, seizures, and dizziness. Carbon monoxide poisoning is more common in the winter months than at other times of the year because of greater use of heaters. Treatment consists of giving 100% oxygen on high flow with a reservoir mask.

## Chronic Fatigue Syndrome

Chronic fatigue syndrome (CFS) presents as an incapacitating fatigue. The patient may also have a sore throat, myalgia, cognitive disorders, weight loss, and sleep disorders. The clinical diagnosis of CFS is made when four or more of the following have been present for 6 months:

- Impaired memory or concentration
- Sore throat
- Tender cervical or axillary lymph nodes
- Muscle pain
- Multiple joint pain
- Headaches of new onset
- Nonrefreshing sleep
- Postexertion malaise

Diagnostic tests used to rule out medical abnormalities as causes of the fatigue in suspected CFS include the CBC and ESR, and assays for alanine aminotransferase (ALT), total protein, albumin, globulin, alkaline phosphatase, calcium, phosphorus, glucose, BUN, electrolytes, creatinine, and TSH. The goal of treatment in CFS is to correct any underlying medical problems. The patient may also be started on resistance training and aerobic exercise and given ventilation with continuous positive airway pressure (CPAP) for sleep management.

## Chronic Obstructive Pulmonary Disease

Patients with chronic obstructive pulmonary disease (COPD) present with progressive fatigue and dyspnea. Other symptoms include a cough, shortness of breath, and dyspnea on exertion, and the patient may have a history of cigarette smoking. The typical age of onset of COPD is between 50 and 60 years.

Physical examination reveals rhonchi, diminished breath sounds, and prolonged expiration. Diagnostic testing includes arterial blood gas measurements initially and periodically thereafter; pulmonary function tests demonstrate airflow limitations and a decreased forced expiratory volume in 1 second ($FEV_1$). Treatment of COPD is guided by the severity of the disease state, following the guidelines of the American Thoracic Society, but may include smoking cessation; oxygen therapy; inhaled bronchodilators; corticosteroids; theophylline; pulmonary rehabilitation; and, in patients with acute infections, antibiotics.

### Depression

Symptoms associated with depression include headache, anorexia, constipation, insomnia, irritability, a decreased ability to concentrate, feelings of worthlessness, and thoughts of suicide. For more on depression, see pages 56 to 69.

### Diabetes Type 2

With type 2 diabetes, fatigue may be insidious or abrupt. Associated symptoms include blurred vision, weight loss, polyuria, and polydipsia.

### Hypercortisolism (Cushing's Syndrome)

Patients with hypercortisolism, also known as Cushing's syndrome, may have one or more of the typical symptoms of truncal obesity with slender extremities, a buffalo hump, moon face, purple striae on the skin, acne, and hirsutism. Other symptoms include psychological changes, thirst, polyuria, renal calculi, and impaired wound healing. Laboratory test results show leukocytosis with granulocytosis and lymphopenia. Other tests to consider include a salivary cortisol test and 24-hour urine assay for cortisol levels. Treatment options include transsphenoidal resection of pituitary adenoma and hydrocortisone or prednisone replacement therapy.

### Hypothyroid Diseases

Patients with hypothyroid diseases may present with lethargy, cold intolerance, forgetfulness, weight gain, constipation, and metrorrhagia.

### Infection

Symptoms of infection vary with its source but may include a low-grade fever and weight loss.

### Lyme Disease

Patients with Lyme disease may present with malaise, intermittent fever, chills, a red rash, and aching muscles and joints.

### Malnutrition
Patients with malnutrition will present with apathy; lethargy; weight loss; muscle wasting; edema; and dry, flaky skin and will be easily fatigued.

### Myasthenia Gravis
Patients with myasthenia gravis will be easily fatigued and display muscle weakness. The symptoms will worsen with exertion.

### Renal Failure
Patients with renal failure present with sudden fatigue, drowsiness, lethargy, and marked changes in all body systems.

### Systemic Lupus Erythematosus
Patients with systemic lupus erythematosus (SLE) present with malaise, a generalized aching sensation, headache, irritability, and a low-grade fever.

### Valvular Heart Disease
Patients with valvular heart disease present with dyspnea, a cough, hemoptysis, and a cardiac murmur. Plain chest radiography reveals enlargement of the heart and valvular calcifications. Echocardiography demonstrates enlargement of the cardiac chambers, thickening of the heart wall, and an increased size of the valvular orifice. With Doppler ultrasonography, the degree of regurgitation can be determined.

## Headache

Headache is one of the most common complaints for which patients seek medical attention. Headache is defined as pain in the head. This includes pain in the scalp and face. A headache is caused by the activation of pain-sensitive structures in or around the brain, skull, face, sinuses, or teeth. Migraine underlies most of the common headaches seen in clinical practice, including sinus headache. Common triggers for migraine headaches are identified in Table 2–25.

### Assessment

Begin your assessment of the patient with headache by taking the patient's history. Make sure to inquire about the age at which the headache had its beginning and its location; duration; frequency; severity; nature of onset (sudden or gradual); quality (throbbing, constant intermittent, pressure-like); exacerbating and remitting factors, such as the position of head when headache occurs or worsens; the time of day or

**ALERT**

Headache of new onset in a person of age 50 years or older should be considered a secondary disorder until proven otherwise.

## Table 2–25 Potential Trigger Factors for Migraine Headaches

| ENVIRONMENTAL | PHYSICAL | FOOD RELATED |
|---|---|---|
| High humidity<br>Sunbathing<br>Heat<br>Physical exertion or fatigue<br>High altitudes<br>Airplane trips<br>Pungent odors from perfumes, smoke, or solvents<br>Weather changes<br>Intense light, glare, flickering lights<br>Intense noise | Emotional tension<br>Lack of sleep<br>Oversleeping<br>Menstruation<br>Birth control pills, estrogen<br>Pregnancy and postpartum<br>Overuse of pain medications<br>Head injury | Dairy<br>Yogurt, aged cheese, sour cream<br>Beverages<br>Coffee, colas, caffeine in tea or chocolate, alcohol, wine<br>Meat/fish<br>Canned, salted, dried meats<br>Pickled meats and fish<br>Nitrate- and nitrite-containing meats or fish<br>Fruits/vegetables<br>Avocados, bananas, citrus fruit, figs, onions, papayas, raspberries, red plums<br>Beans/grains<br>Broad beans, fava beans, lima beans, lentils, soy beans, wheat<br>Other<br>Chocolate, vanilla, licorice, molasses, yeast extracts, nuts, peanut butter, soy sauce, soup cubes, monosodium glutamate (MSG), ice cream, metabisulfate in wine and vinegar, aspartame |

Adapted from Ferri, F. Ferri's 2009 Clinical Advisor, St. Louis: Mosby Elsevier, 2009.

night of onset; the quality of the patient's sleep; triggering factors such as light, sounds, physical activity, odors, and chewing; the headache pattern (relationship to the menstrual cycle); responses to treatment; and whether previous or recurrent headaches were similar or different.

The review of systems should seek symptoms suggesting a cause, including:

- Vomiting: Migraine, increased intracranial pressure
- Fever: Infection (e.g., encephalitis, meningitis, sinusitis)
- Redness of the eye, visual symptoms (halos, blurring): Acute narrow-angle glaucoma
- Visual-field deficits, diplopia, or blurring vision: Ocular migraine, mass lesion of the brain, idiopathic intracranial hypertension
- Lacrimation and facial flushing: Cluster headache (CH)
- Rhinorrhea: Sinusitis
- Pulsatile tinnitus: Idiopathic intracranial hypertension
- Preceding aura: Migraine

- Focal neurological deficit: Encephalitis, meningitis, intracerebral hemorrhage, subdural hematoma, tumor or other mass lesion
- Seizures: Encephalitis, tumor or other mass lesion
- Syncope at headache onset: Subarachnoid hemorrhage
- Myalgias, vision changes (people > 55 years of age): Giant-cell arteritis

Review-of-symptom questions in patients with headache should include risk factors for headache. Ask about the patient's exposure to drugs or substances (caffeine) and toxins, recent invasive procedures (lumbar puncture), immunosuppressive disorders, or intravenous drug use to evaluate for risk of infection. Ask about hypertension to assess for risk of brain hemorrhage; about cancer for risk of brain metastases; and about dementia, trauma, coagulopathy, or use of anticoagulants or ethanol to assess for risk of subdural hematoma. Because migraine headache may be undiagnosed in the patient's family members, the family history should include questions about anyone in the family with a history of headaches.

Physical examination of the patient with headache includes an assessment of vital signs and body temperature. The patient's general appearance (calm or restless) should also be assessed, and the following steps should be taken:

**ALERT**

Historical risk factors for headaches of serious cause are sudden onset, new onset in the elderly, association with focal neurological signs and symptoms, or association with fever, rash, stiff neck, or arthritis.

- Perform a full neurological examination, focusing on the head and neck; the findings should be normal in primary headache syndromes (migraine, tension), except perhaps during a complicated migraine. A stiff neck; head tilt; decreased alertness; abnormal eye movements; asymmetric deep tendon reflexes; asymmetric motor weakness; and a sensory deficit, ataxia, and gait disturbance may signal a stroke, hemorrhage, tumor, or demyelination
- Assess the scalp for swelling and tenderness. Palpate the ipsilateral temporal artery. Also palpate both temporomandibular joints for tenderness and crepitance with the patient's jaw open and closed
- Inspect the eye and periorbital area for lacrimation, flushing, and conjunctival injection. Assess the pupillary size and light responses, extraocular movements, and visual fields. Check the fundi for spontaneous venous pulsations and papilledema. Measure visual acuity if the patient has vision-related symptoms

or eye abnormalities. If the conjunctiva is red, examine the anterior chamber and cornea with a slit lamp if possible; also measure intraocular pressure

- Inspect the nares for purulence. Inspect the oropharynx for swellings, and percuss the teeth for tenderness
- Assess the neck for range of motion; flex it to detect discomfort, stiffness, or both, indicating meningismus. Palpate the cervical spine for tenderness
- Assess the patient's weight. Obesity may indicate pseudotumor or sleep apnea syndrome
- Resting tachycardia may indicate anemia
- Assess for skin changes consistent with a neurocutaneous syndrome. Individuals with neurofibromatosis commonly experience migraine and are also at risk for developing an intracranial mass
- Auscultate for bruits in the supraclavicular areas, neck, and temporal and occipital areas. Observe for signs of arteritis, vascular malformation, or abnormal blood flow through a tumor
- Examine for sinus tenderness, limitation of jaw excursion, or occipital trigger points
- A funduscopic examination may require pharmacological dilatation or ophthalmological consultation. Benign drusen may blur the disc margins, giving the (false) appearance of papilledema. Look for obscuration of blood vessels as they cross the disc boundary, radially oriented splinter hemorrhages, and loss of the light-reflective sheen of the retina approaching the disc margin. The presence of venous pulsations, best seen at the origin or branch points of the wider, darker veins within the disc margins, definitively excludes intracranial hypertension (except in patients with glaucoma)

Indications of danger in patients with headache are:

- Symptoms or signs of neurological abnormality, such as altered mental status, weakness, diplopia, papilledema, and focal neurological deficits
- Immunosuppression or cancer
- Meningismus

> **ALERT**
>
> Unilateral eye pain should be considered an ophthalmological emergency. Unilateral pupillary dilation of new onset should trigger consideration of early brain herniation, possibly due to a mass lesion on the third cranial nerve.

- Onset of headache after age 50 years
- Thunderclap headache, a severe headache that peaks within a few seconds
- Symptoms of giant-cell arteritis, such as visual disturbances, jaw claudication, fever, weight loss, temporal artery tenderness, or proximal myalgias
- Systemic symptoms, such as fever or weight loss
- Progressively worsening headache
- Red eye and halos around lights

Red flags for an underlying disorder in the patient with headache are:

- A headache that the patient describes as the "worst headache ever"
- The patient's first severe headache
- A headache that worsens over days or weeks
- Abnormal findings on a neurological examination
- Fever or unexplained systemic signs of an abnormality
- Vomiting that precedes a headache
- Pain induced by bending, lifting, or coughing
- Night-time awakening with headache pain
- Onset after age 55 years
- Pain with local tenderness, such as in the region of the temporal artery

## Diagnostic Testing

MRI is the gold-standard radiographic study for identifying the cause of headache. CT scanning or MRI should be done in patients with any of the following findings:

- Thunderclap headache
- New, abnormal findings on a neurological examination, such as papilledema, hemiparesis, ataxia, asymmetric reflexes, abnormal eye movements, alteration of consciousness or mental status, or nuchal rigidity
- Signs of sepsis, including a rash and shock
- Severe hypertension, with a systolic BP above 220 mm Hg or a diastolic BP of 120 mm Hg or more on consecutive readings
- An acute first episode of severe headache
- Headaches or vomiting in the morning
- Headache that becomes worse in the supine position
- Presence of a ventriculoperitoneal shunt

## Migraine Headache

A migraine headache may be unilateral; throbbing; and aggravated by light, noise, odors, or movement of the body. Migraine headaches vary in intensity from moderate to severe. There may be associated features including nausea and vomiting.

A prodrome or early warning occurs consistently at up to 24 hours before headache in at least 40% of migraineurs. Prodromal features include hunger, thirst, euphoria, mania, depression, drowsiness, psychomotor slowing, or irritability. An aura occurs immediately before or during the early phase of a migraine headache and may include visual scotomata (dark spots), photopsias (bright spots), fortification spectra (jagged bright lines), numbness, tingling, weakness, confusion, or aphasia. Triggers of migraine headache include environmental stimuli such as intense light, sounds, or odors; certain foods (those that contain nitrates, sulfites, monosodium glutamate, or alcohol); irregular sleep or nutrition; exercise; stress; and hormonal fluctuations.

### Screening Assessment

No specific diagnostic test exists for migraine. Screening tools for migraine and disability assessments of patients with migraine headaches are widely available to help with rapid diagnosis of the condition and selection of treatment. One of the simplest tools asks the patient the following three questions:

- Are you nauseated or sick to your stomach when you have a headache?
- Has a headache limited your activities for a day or more in the last 3 months?
- Does light bother you when you have a headache?

Two of three positive responses has a positive predictive value of 93% for a diagnosis of migraine; three of three positive responses predicts migraine in 98% of cases. The diagnosis may not be this simple in patients seen by otolaryngologists, and the question of sinus headache is often raised.

### Migraine With and Without Aura

Migraine aura occurs consistently in 15% to 25% of migraineurs. The aura is a localizable and fully reversible neurological deficit preceding head pain and results from progressive neuronal dysfunction spreading across the cerebral cortex.

### Treatment of Migraine Headache

Treatment of migraine headache includes:

- Educating and reassuring the patient; emphasizing the absence of sinus, muscle, or spine disease; and recognizing the episodic nature of migraine and the genetic and environmental factors responsible for it
- Reviewing expectations of therapy: Medicines help to ease migraine headaches from 60% to 70% of the time

- Having the patient keep a headache diary to identify possible triggering factors
- Addressing comorbid depression, anxiety, substance abuse, and other medical conditions that may influence migraines
- Outlining a clear treatment plan
- Reviewing nonpharmacological approaches to managing migraine, including the avoidance of triggering factors for it
- Reviewing pharmacological treatment.
- For the acute treatment of migraine:
  - The first line drug is ibuprofen: 10 mg/kg. Antiemetics for nausea and vomiting enhance the effectiveness of this and other analgesics. Drugs containing isometheptene (Midrin) and butalbital (Fiorinal) may aggravate migraine headaches. Triptans drugs are not currently approved by the U.S. Food and Drug Administration for use in children
  - Almotriptan (Axert): 6.25 and 12.5 mg; may be repeated once after 2 hours
  - Eletriptan(Relpax): 20 and 40 mg tablets; may be repeated once after 2 hours
  - Frovatriptan(Frova): 2.5 mg tablet; may be repeated once after 2 hours
  - Naratriptan (Amerge):1 mg and 2.5 mg tablets; may be repeated once after 4 hours
  - Rizatriptan (Maxalt): 5 and 10 mg tablets and melts; may be repeated after 2 hours
  - Sumatriptan (Imitrex): 50 and 100 mg tablets; 5 mg and 20 mg nasal spray; 4 mg and 6 mg/0.5 mL injections; may be repeated once after 2 hours
  - Zolmitriptan(Zomig): 2.5 and 5 mg tablets and melts or dissolvable oral medication; 5 mg per nasal spray; may be repeated once after 2 hours

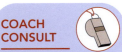

**COACH CONSULT**

Common side effects of triptans include chest tightness, throat or head pressure, tingling, nausea, and flushing. Start with lower doses and increase as needed. Be aware of drug interactions. Use triptans with caution in women of childbearing age. Attempt to taper the dose and discontinue use when migraine headaches are well controlled.

Rebound headaches can occur with the overuse of any class of medications used for headaches, including aspirin, acetaminophen, other NSAIDs, caffeine-containing preparations, ergotamine, and even triptan medications. As the frequency of headache increases, patients take more and larger doses of medications that become progressively less effective. Severe, incapacitating headaches require further neurological evaluation.

## *Prophylaxis of Migraine Headache*

The strategy for prophylaxis of migraine headache is to start medication at a low dose and to then increase the dose weekly or biweekly toward a target maximum dose until headaches relent or side effects supervene. Use of beta blockers (propranolol and nadolol) is discouraged in the setting of asthma, depression, or diabetes. TCAs (amitriptyline, nortriptyline) may benefit individuals with insomnia or depression. Anticonvulsants (topiramate, valproic acid) may benefit individuals with epilepsy. Cyproheptadine (Periactin), a combination antihistamine/antiserotonin agent, is often used to treat migraine in 10- to 12-year-old children. Other drugs for preventing migraine headaches are:

- Propranolol (Inderal) 10 mg; maximum dose 0.6 to 2 mg/kg/day; also available as long-acting capsules in 60, 80, and 120 mg strengths
- Timolol (Blocadren): 5 mg tablet
- Divalproex Na (Depakote): 125 mg tablet
- Methysergide (Sansert): 2 mg tablet

Table 2–26 lists pharmacological preparations used in the management of headache.

| Table 2–26 **Migraine Headache Management** | | |
|---|---|---|
| **DRUG CATEGORY** | **EXAMPLES** | **DOSAGE** |
| Simple analgesics | Acetaminophen Aspirin Caffeine Excedrin Migraine | Two tablets or caplets q6h (maximum: 8 tablets or capsules/24 hours) |
| Nonsteroidal anti-inflammatory drugs | Naproxen (Aleve, Anaprox) | 220–550 mg bid |
| | Ibuprofen (Advil, Motrin, Nuprin) | 400 mg q3–4h |
| | Tolfenamic acid | 200 mg PO, may repeat once in 1–2 hours |
| 5-Hydroxytryptamine agonists | Ergotamine (Ergomar) | 2 mg SL at onset, then q30 min (maximum: 3 tablets/day) |
| | Ergotamine 1 mg, caffeine 100 mg (Ercaf, Wigraine) | 1–2 tablets at onset, then one tablet q30min (maximum: 6 tablets/day) |

*Continued*

## Table 2–26 Migraine Headache Management—cont'd

| DRUG CATEGORY | EXAMPLES | DOSAGE |
|---|---|---|
| | Naratriptan (Amerge) | 2.5 mg tab at onset, may repeat once after 4 hours |
| | Rizatriptan (Maxalt) | 5–10 mg at onset, repeat after 2 hours (max 30 mg/day) |
| | Sumatriptan (Imitrex) | 50–100 mg tab at onset, may repeat after 2 hours (max 200 mg/d) |
| | Frovatriptan (Frova) | 2.5 mg at onset, repeat after 2 hours (maximum: 5 mg/day) |
| | Almotriptan (Axert) | 12.5 mg at onset, may repeat after 2 hours (maximum: 25 mg/day) |
| | Eletriptan (Relpax) | 40 or 80 mg |
| | Zolmitriptan (Zomig) | 2.5 mg at onset, may repeat after 2 hours (maximum: 10 mg/day) |
| Nasal sprays | Migranal Nasal Spray Imitrex Nasal Spray Zomig | 1 spray (0.5 mg) 5–10 mg (5 mg/spray) 5 mg spray |
| Parenteral | DHE 45 Imitrex injection | 1 mg IV, IM, SC at onset and 1 hour 6 mg SC at onset, may repeat once after 1 hour |

Adapted from Nurse Practitioner Prescribing Reference, Winter 2008–2009. New York: Haymarket Media Publications, 2009.

## Tension-Type Headache

Episodic tension-type headache is the most common head-pain syndrome. It is characterized by bilateral, nonthrobbing, aching pain of gradual onset over the frontal and temporal regions, often spreading to involve the occipital, posterior cervical, and trapezius musculature. The pain worsens as the day goes on. Associated symptoms such as nausea and vomiting are rare, and patients usually can continue activities of daily living during a headache. The headaches are not seasonal and do not awaken the patient from sleep. Adults rarely seek medical care for occasional tension headaches.

## Cluster Headache

CH is an uncommon disorder. The strictly unilateral, blinding, and short-duration attacks of abrupt onset that mark CH raise questions about potentially devastating consequences, including subarachnoid hemorrhage. Among the primary headache disorders, the pain of CH is assumed to be the most severe, and the accompanying autonomic features may confuse the diagnosis with pathology in the orbital or periorbital areas or sinuses. Cluster headaches may awaken the patient from sleep and may last from 15 minutes to 3 hours in length. The sleep loss related to the occurrence of cluster headaches and the seasonal or circannual occurrence of CHs suggest their association with a botanical allergy. Patients with cluster headaches may experience spontaneous remission followed by similar episodes of headaches within 4 to 8 weeks later, with recurrences several times a year. Precipitating factors for cluster headaches may include excessive alcohol intake, high emotional stress levels, or food allergy triggers. Secondary causes of CH can include cranial, cervical, or vascular disorders. The carotid artery, cavernous sinus, and various brain structures, including the periaqueductal gray matter, appear to participate in generation and modulation of the pain associated with CH.

CH occurs in 0.2 to 0.6% of the American population, with a male-to-female ratio of 4:1 to 12:1. Recent studies have suggested that although the gender ratio of CH may be changing, its overall prevalence has remained stable for the last two or three decades. Genetic studies suggest an autosomal dominant transmission of CH with a low frequency of the susceptibility allele.

CH has been recognized as a distinctive clinical entity since as early as the 1700s. During active periods, most commonly in the spring and autumn, clusters of individual headaches lasting between 30 and 180 minutes occur daily, with episodes lasting weeks or months. The majority of patients with CH have episodic, recurrent attacks of unilateral, temporal, or periorbital pain associated with autonomic features including ptosis, miosis, lacrimation, rhinorrhea, and ipsilateral nasal stuffiness. In a chronic form of this disorder, unrelenting and daily attacks of typical CHs persist without interruption.

Episodic CH is defined by gaps in time between painful periods. Chronic CH is unremitting. Episodes occur once or twice per year in 75% of patients, with a typical episode lasting approximately 2 months. Attacks typically last between 72 and 159 minutes, with a frequency of attack ranging from two per week to five per day, and 73% of patients have a predictable onset of attacks at night. Among patients with episodic CH, 43% describe a seasonal onset, and patients with chronic CH also describe seasonal exacerbations.

## Differential Diagnoses

### *Encephalitis*
Encephalitis presents as fever, an altered mental status, seizures, and focal neurological deficits.

### *Giant-Cell Arteritis*
Giant-cell arteritis generally occurs in patients 55 years of age and older. It presents with unilateral, throbbing pain. Patients will report pain when combing their hair, visual disturbances, claudicating pain in the jaw, fever, weight loss, sweats, temporal artery tenderness, and proximal myalgias.

### *Idiopathic Intracranial Hypertension*
In idiopathic intracranial hypertension, the patient complains of migraine-like headache as well as diplopia, pulsatile tinnitus, and loss of peripheral vision. Papilledema can be noted on assessment.

### *Meningitis*
Meningitis presents as fever, meningismus, and an alteration in mental status of rapid onset.

### *Sinusitis-Related Headaches*
Patients with sinus-related headaches may present with positional, facial, or tooth pain,. They may have purulent rhinorrhea and fever and may note tenderness with palpation of the frontal, ethmoid, or maxillary sinuses.

### *Subarachnoid Hemorrhage*
The hallmark of a subarachnoid hemorrhage is a "thunderclap headache" that has a peak intensity within a few seconds after it begins. The patient may also experience vomiting, syncope, obtundation, and meningismus.

### *Subdural Hematoma*
Patients with a subdural hematoma may present with drowsiness, altered mental status, hemiparesis, loss of spontaneous venous pulsations, and papilledema. Risk factors for this condition include older age, coagulation therapy, dementia, and ethanol abuse.

### *Tumor*
Patients with tumors have variable presentations of symptoms, including altered mental status, seizures, vomiting, diplopia, loss of spontaneous pulsations, focal neurological deficits, and papilledema.

## Hearing Loss

There are four primary classifications of hearing loss: conductive, sensorineural, mixed, and functional. Most commonly, hearing loss results from presbycusis, which is a sensorineural dysfunction occurring with advancing age. Other causes of hearing loss include trauma, infection, allergy, tumors, ototoxic drugs, and certain hereditary disorders.

## Assessment

Determine whether the hearing loss is of gradual onset or sudden onset; is mild or severe; is caused by aging, tumor, or trauma; and is marked by complete deafness. The Weber and Rinne tests are excellent diagnostic tests for hearing losses. Table 2–27 provides an overview of the findings with both of these tests.

## Differential Diagnoses

### *Acoustic Neuroma*

Acoustic neuroma presents as a progressive sensorineural hearing loss. The patient may also have tinnitus, vertigo, and facial paralysis. MRI is the preferred diagnostic test for acoustic neuroma because of its thin sections with high resolution, which is required for diagnosis of the condition. CT scanning can be used if there is no conductive hearing loss, though it will require thin sections with bone windows.

### *Adenoid Hypertrophy*

Adenoid hypertrophy leads to obstruction of the eustachian tube, causing gradual hearing loss. Patients with adenoid hypertrophy are mouth breathers and may report a sensation of fullness of the ear on the affected side of the head.

### *Aural Polyps*

Aural polyps can cause hearing loss if they occlude the ear canal.

### *Cholesteatoma*

Chronic OM with peeling layers of scaly or keratinized epithelium can lead to nerve damage in the middle ear and deafness. Cholesteatoma is marked by an expanding area of keratinization of the squamous epithelium of the middle ear or mastoid process and may be congenital or acquired.

### Table 2–27 Changes in Weber and Rinne Tests With Hearing Losses

| TEST | NORMAL FINDINGS | CONDUCTIVE HEARING LOSS | SENSORINEURAL HEARING LOSS |
|------|-----------------|-------------------------|----------------------------|
| Weber test | Sound heard equally bilaterally, does not lateralize | Sound lateralizes to affected ear | Sound lateralizes to the unaffected ear |
| Rinne test | Air conduction greater than bone conduction (AC>BC) | Abnormal in the affected ear (AC<BC) | Normal in the affected ear |

Adapted from Portable Signs and Symptoms. Philadelphia: Lippincott Williams & Wilkins, 2008.

**COACH CONSULT**

The following ototoxic drugs can cause hearing loss:
- Vancomycin
- Cisplatin
- Aminoglycosides
- Loop diuretics
- Bumetanide
- Erythromycin
- Salicylates
- Ethacrynic acid

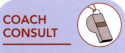

**COACH CONSULT**

Other causes of hearing loss include a tumor of the external ear, head trauma, and nasopharyngeal cancer.

Visual examination of the ear reveals a squamous epithelium-lined sac, filled with desquamated keratin; the ear canal may be filled with mucopus and granulation tissue, and there may be painless otorrhea. The patient may also report vertigo and possibly facial pressure. The condition is treated surgically.

### Cyst

Sebaceous or dermoid cysts can cause progressive hearing loss.

### Meniere's Disease

Symptoms of Meniere's disease include severe vertigo and a feeling of fullness in the ear.

### Otitis Externa (Swimmer's Ear)

Patients with otitis externa, also known as swimmer's ear, may experience tinnitus, pruritus, and severe ear pain. Ask the patient about recent water exposure or mechanical trauma. Physical examination and pneumatic otoscopy will demonstrate mobility of the TM. Management includes removal of debris and topical administration of otic drops.

### Otitis Media

OM is marked by infection followed by rupture of the TM with bloody or purulent drainage. Diagnostic procedures for OM include clinical examination with the finding of impaired mobility of the TM on pneumatic otoscopy, tympanometry, and culture of drainage fluid from the ear. Treatment involves giving the antibiotic amoxicillin and nasal decongestants.

### Otosclerosis

Patients with otosclerosis sometimes report that their hearing is better in noisy environments.

### Skull Fracture or Temporal Bone Fracture

With skull or temporal bone fracture, the patient may report ringing tinnitus and blood may be visualized behind the TM. The diagnosis is through plain films of the skull; CT scanning may be used to pick up lucent fracture lines and secondary signs of fracture, such as fluid in mastoid cells.

### Perforation of the Tympanic Membrane

Along with hearing loss, the patient with perforation of the TM may report ear pain, tinnitus, vertigo, and a sensation of fullness in the ear.

Table 2–28 provides an overview of acute and chronic causes of hearing loss.

| Table 2–28 **Causes of Acute and Chronic Hearing Loss** | | |
|---|---|---|
| **DIAGNOSIS** | **HISTORY** | **PHYSICAL EXAMINATION** |
| **CHRONIC HEARING LOSS** | | |
| Conductive hearing loss | Loss of hearing at all frequencies | Unilateral disease Rinne test shows air conduction less than bone conduction. Weber test lateralizes to involved ear. Whisper test abnormal if loss exceeds 40 db |
| Otosclerosis | Advanced age | Ear examination otherwise normal |
| Cerumen impaction or foreign body | Gradual or sudden hearing loss | Ear examination reveals wax or foreign body, hearing returns when removed |
| Chronic otitis externa, serious otitis | Decreased hearing in young child, foul ear discharge | Decreased motility of TM, discharge, TM perforation, cholesteatoma may be present |
| Nerve-deficit-type hearing loss | High-frequency loss noted, difficulty listening on telephone or in public groups | Unilateral disease: Both air and bone conduction are decreased, Weber test shows hearing lateralized to affected ear, Whisper test abnormal if loss exceeds 40 db |
| Presbycusis | Advanced age | Ear examination otherwise normal |
| Chronic noise-related losses, head trauma, mumps | History of these factors | Usually normal ear examination. With severe head trauma may have ear discharge or temporal bone tenderness |
| Acoustic neuroma | Decreased hearing, tinnitus | Decreased hearing, abnormal sensation of face, finger-to-nose test, or movement of facial musculature on the involved side |
| Ototoxic medications | Prolonged treatment with high-dose ethacrynic acid, furosemide, "mycin" antibiotics, quinine. Tinnitus is common | Examination is otherwise normal |
| Congenital | Deafness (usually bilateral) since birth. May have family history of deafness, delayed speech | Usually normal |

*Continued*

| Table 2–28 **Causes of Acute and Chronic Hearing Loss—cont'd** | | |
|---|---|---|
| DIAGNOSIS | HISTORY | PHYSICAL EXAMINATION |
| **ACUTE HEARING LOSS** | | |
| Acute hearing loss | Associated with ear pain or discharge<br>Associated with dizziness, movement or rotation of head, trauma | — |

Adapted from Wasson, J. The Common Symptom Guide, ed. 5. New York: McGraw-Hill, 2002.

# Hematemesis

Hematemesis, which results from bleeding in the GI tract, is a critical symptom that may signal a serious disease state, depending on the amount of bleeding, color of the blood that is egested, source of bleeding, and intensity of the blood loss over a period of time. Massive hematemesis, measuring 500 mL of blood or more, may be life threatening.

In addition to manifesting itself as hematemesis, GI bleeding may present as blood in the stools from either upper or lower GI sources of bleeding. Table 2–29 presents an overview of potential causes and symptoms of upper and lower GI bleeding. Box 2–2 looks at issues surrounding blood in the stools of newborns.

**COACH CONSULT**

Two rare causes of hematemesis are malaria and yellow fever. Malaria may present with chills, fever, headache, muscle pain, and splenomegaly. Yellow fever may be accompanied by jaundice, bradycardia, and fever of sudden onset.

## Assessment

Assessment of the patient with hematemesis begins with taking the patient's history. Critical questions to ask in the history are about alcohol use; a history of ulcers or liver disease; a history of coagulation disorders; and about current medications, especially aspirin, anticoagulants, and NSAIDs.

## Differential Diagnoses

### Anthrax

*Bacillus anthracis*, the cause of anthrax, is acquired from contaminated meat. Symptoms of anthrax include loss of appetite, nausea, vomiting, and fever, and may progress to hematemesis, abdominal pain, and bloody diarrhea.

## Table 2–29 Upper and Lower Gastrointestinal Causes of Rectal Bleeding

| DIAGNOSIS | HISTORY | PHYSICAL EXAMINATION |
|---|---|---|
| Upper gastrointestinal bleeding | Black tarry stools | |
| Peptic ulcer | Epigastric pain, history of aspirin or anti-inflammatory medications, pain relieved by antacids or food | Epigastric tenderness |
| Gastritis | Epigastric pain, excessive alcohol intake often precedes pain onset or bleeding | Possible epigastric tenderness |
| Esophageal varices | Chronic alcoholism or liver disease, may have nausea/vomiting | Spider angiomas, icterus, ascites, splenomegaly |
| **LOWER GASTROINTESTINAL CAUSES FOR RECTAL OR GASTROINTESTINAL BLEEDING** | | |
| Hemorrhoids/anal fissures | Blood-streaked stools, may have rectal pain | Hemorrhoids on rectal examination |
| Diverticular disease | Bright red blood, minimal discomfort | Usually normal |
| Ulcerative colitis; Salmonella or Campylobacter gastroenteritis Tropical: Schistosomiasis and worm infestation | Abdominal discomfort, diarrhea, loose stools, pus in bowel movement | Diffuse lower abdominal tenderness or fever |
| Intestinal tumors or polyps | Asymptomatic, weight loss, pain, change in bowel patterns, | Occasional palpable mass, weight loss |
| Gastrointestinal bleeding secondary to generalized bleeding disorders | Melena or red blood, prolonged and excessive bleeding from scratches or lacerations. May be taking anticoagulants | Skin assessment for petechiae or bruising |

Adapted from Wasson, J. The Common Symptom Guide, ed. 5. New York: McGraw-Hill, 2009.

In newborns, blood in the stool can indicate the following:
- Hemorrhagic diseases of newborns: Evidence of bruising or a bleeding disorder, bright red blood, or melena; relatively common in newborns not given vitamin K at birth
- Swallowing of blood: The physical examination will be normal; the source of blood is often the mother's nipple; may also be left on newborn from delivery
- Anal fissures/polyps: Usually indicated by bright red blood streaks in stool; fissures or polyps may be palpable on rectal examination
- Constipation: During bouts of constipation the stool may be streaked with bright red blood
- Volvulus intussusception: A rare disorder that presents as abdominal pain, vomiting, and decreased frequency of bowel movements. A plain abdominal film may be made to observe for a crescent sign and abdominal soft-tissue masses. Contrast enema may reveal a coiled spring appearance of the bowel, which is diagnostic of the condition. Ultrasound examination is used to identify a doughnut appearance of the bowel on a transverse scan
- Meckel's diverticulum: A rare condition in which there is no pain. A radionuclide scan will show increased isotope accumulation in the RLQ

Adapted from Osborn, L., DeWitt, T., First, L. and Zenel, J. *Pediatrics.* Elsevier-Mosby, St. Louis, 2005, pp 639–645.

### Esophageal Cancer

The patient with esophageal cancer may report chest pain that radiates down the back, substernal fullness, dysphagia, hiccups, melena, and halitosis.

### Esophageal Rupture

The patient with a rupture of the esophagus may present with severe pain in the neck, chest, and scapula.

### Esophageal Varices

Esophageal varices will present as massive GI bleeding followed by symptoms of shock. Endoscopy should be performed in patients with episodes of acute GI bleeding. A barium swallow may identify varices and shunting between the jugular vein and hepatic portal system.

### Gastric Cancer

Painless GI bleeding showing bright red or dark brown blood is a late sign of gastric cancer. The patient may also report anorexia, nausea, and chronic dyspepsia. Diagnostic procedures that should be done in such cases include an upper GI series, endoscopy, and CT scan for cancer staging.

### Gastritis, Acute
Acute gastritis may or may not be accompanied by melena, nausea, fever, malaise, and mild epigastric pain. The patient may also have a history of alcohol abuse.
### Mallory-Weiss syndrome
Mallory-Weiss syndrome generally presents as severe vomiting, retching, and straining at stool passage. Endoscopy will allow visualization of lacerations or fissures.
### Peptic Ulcer
The patient with peptic ulcer disease will present with melena, chills, fever, and dehydration. Diagnostic procedures for this condition include an upper GI series and endoscopy. Once a diagnosis is made, it is not necessary to repeat diagnostic procedures for recurrent episodes before beginning symptomatic treatment.

# Hematuria

Hematuria is generally associated with disorders of the kidneys and urinary tract, but may also result from GI, prostate, vaginal, or coagulation disorders. In addition, it may result from fever and hypercatabolic states or strenuous exercise.

## Differential Diagnosis
### Bladder Cancer
The patient with bladder cancer may report pain in the bladder, rectum, flank, or pelvis.
### Bladder Trauma
The patient with bladder trauma will generally present with lower abdominal pain, strong urinary urgency, scrotal swelling, and signs of shock.
### Calculi
Patients with renal calculi may present with UTI as a co-morbid condition and typically also experience severe flank pain and colicky pain that travels from the flank to the pelvis as calculi pass through the urinary tract.
### Coagulation Disorders
Macroscopic hematuria is an initial sign of thrombocytopenia and disseminated intravascular coagulation (DIC).
### Acute Cortical Necrosis
Acute cortical necrosis may present with acute flank pain, anuria, leukocytosis, and fever.

### Cystitis
Cystitis presents with urinary urgency, frequency, and dysuria. The patient may also have a fever.

### Diverticulitis
If the bladder is involved by diverticulitis, the patient may have symptoms of frequency, dysuria, and urgency.

### Glomerulonephritis
Glomerulonephritis may present as proteinuria, fever, fatigue, flank pain, an elevated BP, and pulmonary congestion.

### Nephritis
When seen in chronic interstitial nephritis, hematuria may be accompanied by polyuria and an increased BP. Ultrasound examination is used in making the diagnosis of nephritis.

### Obstructive Nephropathy
Patients with obstructive nephropathy report colicky flank pain and abdominal pain. Ultrasound examination is used in making the diagnosis of this condition.

### Polycystic Kidney Disease
Polycystic kidney disease is generally not seen until after the age of 40 years; it may present with an increased BP, flank pain, and signs of UTI. Diagnostic procedures include an ultrasound examination or CT scan to visualize large cysts. In children, ultrasound examination improves the visualization of echogenic kidneys and dilated renal tubules.

### Prostatitis
Prostatitis may present as urinary frequency, urgency, and dysuria.

### Pyelonephritis
Symptoms commonly associated with pyelonephritis include urinary urgency, burning on urination, chills, fever, flank pain, fatigue, and anorexia.

### Renal Cancer
Patients with renal cancer may report colicky pain and may pass blood clots. A CT scan differentiates hemorrhagic cysts from contrast-enhanced tumors. Ultrasound examination will identify a tumor or solid mass. MRI works as well as CT scanning, especially for patients who are sensitive to IV contrast media.

### Renal Infarction
Symptoms associated with renal infarction include CVAT, anorexia, nausea, and vomiting.

### Renal Trauma
Findings commonly reported in renal trauma are oliguria, flank pain, and hypoactive bowel sounds.

### Renal Tuberculosis
Renal tuberculosis may present as proteinuria, abdominal or flank pain, and urinary frequency.

### Schistosomiasis
Patients with schistosomiasis present with intermittent hematuria at the end of voiding. Bladder or abdominal pain and palpable abdominal masses may also be present.

### Sickle Cell Anemia
Patients in sickle cell crisis may present with fatigue, unexplained dyspnea, joint swelling, and increased susceptibility to infections.

### Systemic Lupus Erythematosus
SLE may present as hematuria, fever, anorexia, weight loss, nausea, vomiting, constipation, a rash, and polyarthralgia.

### Vasculitis
Patients with vasculitis may exhibit malaise, myalgia, polyarthralgia, fever, an elevated BP, and pallor, and possibly anuria.

# Hoarseness

Hoarseness can result from infection, inflammatory lesions or exudates of the larynx, laryngeal edema, and disruption of the vocal cords.

## Assessment
Assessment of the patient with hoarseness should include questions about:
- A history of overuse of the voice
- Dryness of the mouth, sore throat, shortness of breath, or difficulty in swallowing
- A history of rheumatoid arthritis, cancer, or aortic aneurysm
- A history of alcohol and tobacco use

## Differential Diagnoses
### Gastroesophageal Reflux
Retrograde flow of gastroesophageal reflux material spills this material into the hypopharynx, irritating the larynx and causing hoarseness.

### Hypothyroidism
Hoarseness is an early sign of hypothyroidism. Other signs include fatigue, cold intolerance, weight gain, and menorrhagia.

### Laryngeal Cancer
Patients with laryngeal cancer often have a long history of cigarette smoking.

### Laryngeal Leukoplakia
Patients with laryngeal leukoplakia usually have a history of tobacco smoking.

### Laryngitis
Patients with hoarseness can present with acute laryngitis.

### Rheumatoid Arthritis
Hoarseness is a precursor of laryngeal involvement in rheumatoid arthritis (RA).

### Thoracic Aortic Aneurysm
The most common symptom of a thoracic aortic aneurysm is severe, penetrating pain.

### Tracheal Trauma
Tracheal trauma may cause hoarseness, hemoptysis, and dysphagia.

## Insomnia

Insomnia is the inability to fall asleep or to remain asleep. The condition may be transient or chronic.

### Assessment
Patients complaining of insomnia should have a thorough sleep history recorded. The history should include the following questions :

- When did the insomnia begin? What circumstances were associated with the onset of insomnia?
- Have there been changes in the patient's medications, particularly in sedative-type agents?
- Is the patient currently taking any type of central nervous system (CNS) stimulant, such as an amphetamine, pseudoephedrine, theophylline derivative, cocaine, or a caffeine-containing drug?
- What is the patient's daily caffeine intake?
- Does the patient have any disease processes that could aggravate sleep cycles, such as endocrine or neurological diseases?
- Does the patient experience sleep apnea, or snore?
- Has the patient had any recent stress or psychological issues, such as anxiety?

### Differential Diagnoses
Potential causes of insomnia include:

- Alcohol withdrawal
- GAD
- Mood disorders
- Nocturnal myoclonus (restless leg syndrome)
- Sleep apnea

- Thyrotoxicosis
- Disorders of circadian rhythm
- Delayed-sleep-phase syndrome
- Difficulty in staying awake in the evening, or waking too early
- Problems related to shift work
- Difficulty in getting enough sleep during available sleep times

## Treatment
Behavioral therapy for general sleep hygiene includes
- Awakening at the same time every morning
- Going to bed at the same time every evening
- Avoiding caffeine intake from 4 to 6 hours before bedtime
- Avoiding nicotine use near  bedtime
- Avoiding alcohol use to facilitate sleep onset and avoid awakenings later in the night
- Avoiding heavy meals too close to bedtime
- Exercising regularly in the late afternoon
- Avoiding vigorous exercise late in the evening
- Minimizing noise, light, and excessive temperatures during sleep time
- Moving an alarm clock away from the bed if it is a distraction

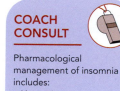

**COACH CONSULT**

Pharmacological management of insomnia includes:
- Hypnotics
- Antidepressants
- Antihistamines
- Anticholinergics
- Benzodiazepines

# Jaundice

There are three pathophysiologic mechanisms for the development of jaundice: prehepatic, hepatic, and posthepatic. Prehepatic jaundice typically occurs after a blood transfusion reaction or after a sickle cell crisis in which there is massive hemolysis. Hepatic jaundice results from the  inability of the liver to conjugate or secrete bilirubin. Posthepatic jaundice is identified in patients with pancreatic or biliary disorders.

**ALERT**

Obstruction of the biliary duct produces the Charcot triad of jaundice, pain in the RUQ, and fever with chills.

## Differential Diagnoses
### *Cholecystitis/Cholelithiasis*
Patients with cholecystitis or cholelithiasis report pain, nausea, vomiting, fever, diaphoresis, and a positive Murphy's sign. With cholelithiasis, the patient may also have symptoms of restlessness and tachycardia.

### Cirrhosis
Early findings in cirrhosis include weakness, ascites, leg edema, nausea and vomiting, diarrhea, anorexia, and weight loss.

### Dubin-Johnson Syndrome
Dubin-Johnson syndrome is a rare inherited liver disease whose classic symptom is jaundice that fluctuates in relation to stress. Other symptoms can include hepatic enlargement, upper abdominal pain, nausea, and vomiting.

### Heart Failure
Hepatomegaly may occur subsequent to heart failure. Other symptoms in such cases include ascites (a late sign), fatigue, dyspnea, orthopnea, tachypnea, arrhythmias, and tachycardia.

### Hepatic Abscess
Patients with a hepatic abscess present with fever, chills, and sweating. Other symptoms may include pain in the RUQ, nausea, vomiting, anorexia, hepatomegaly, an elevated right hemidiaphragm, and ascites. The diagnosis of hepatic abscess is made by a CT scan or ultrasound examination of the liver.

### Hepatitis
Early signs and symptoms of hepatitis include dark urine and clay-colored stools, fatigue, nausea and vomiting, malaise, arthralgia, myalgia, headache, anorexia, photophobia, pharyngitis, cough, and a low-grade fever.

### Pancreatitis, Acute
The primary symptom of acute pancreatitis is severe epigastric pain that radiates to the back. The diagnosis is made through CT scanning to locate focal extrahepatic inflammation or extrahepatic inflammation that is difficult to identify; ultrasound examination may reveal cholelithiasis.

### Sickle Cell Anemia
Sickle cell anemia causes jaundice from the hemolysis of red blood cells. Other symptoms can include susceptibility to infections, leg ulcers, swollen and painful joints, fever, and chills. In cases of severe hemolysis in sickle cell anemia, symptoms of hematuria, dyspnea, and tachycardia may be present.

**COACH CONSULT**

Other causes of jaundice include cancer and cholangitis.

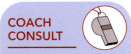

**COACH CONSULT**

Medications that negatively affect the liver include acetaminophen (Tylenol), isoniazid (INH), hormonal contraceptives, sulfonamides, erythromycin, niacin, androgenic steroids, phenothiazines, ethanol, methyldopa, rifampin, and phenytoin.

# Lymphadenopathy

Enlarged lymph nodes may result from the generation of lymphocytes within nodes or infiltration by lymphocytes into nodes. Lymphadenopathy can be generalized or localized. Generalized lymphadenopathy is marked by:

- An inflammatory process: Bacterial or viral
- Connective tissue disease
- Endocrine disorders
- Neoplasm

Localized lymphadenopathy is marked by infection and trauma. Table 2–30 identifies the the causes of this condition.

## Differential Diagnoses

### *Acquired Immunodeficiency Syndrome*

Patients with AIDS present with fatigue, night sweats, diarrhea, weight loss, and cough.

| Table 2–30 Localized Lymphadenopathy | |
|---|---|
| REGIONAL LYMPHADENOPATHY | POSSIBLE CAUSES |
| Auricular | Erysipelas<br>Herpes zoster ophthalmicus<br>Infection<br>Rubella<br>Squamous cell carcinoma<br>Hordeolum<br>Chalazion<br>Tularemia |
| Axillary | Breast cancer<br>Infection<br>Lymphoma<br>Mastitis |
| Cervical | Cat-scratch fever<br>Facial cancer<br>Oral cancer<br>Mononucleosis<br>Mucocutaneous lymph node syndrome<br>Rubella<br>Thyrotoxicosis<br>Tonsillitis<br>Tuberculosis<br>Varicella |

*Continued*

| Table 2–30  Localized Lymphadenopathy—cont'd | |
| --- | --- |
| REGIONAL LYMPHADENOPATHY | POSSIBLE CAUSES |
| Inguinal and femoral | Carcinoma<br>Chancroid<br>Infection<br>Lymphogranuloma venereum<br>Syphilis |
| Occipital | Infection<br>Roseola<br>Scalp infection<br>Seborrheic dermatitis<br>Tick bite<br>Tinea capitis |
| Popliteal | Infection |
| Submaxillary and submental | Cystic fibrosis<br>Dental infection<br>Gingivitis<br>Glossitis<br>Infection |
| Supraclavicular | Infection<br>Neoplastic disease |

Adapted from Portable Signs and Symptoms. Philadelphia: Lippincott Williams & Wilkins, 2008.

### Cutaneous Anthrax
Cutaneous anthrax presents as a lesion that progressively evolves into a painless ulcer with a necrotic center. Other symptoms include malaise, headache, and fever.

### Brucellosis
Brucellosis generally affects the cervical and axillary lymph nodes. It has an insidious onset, with headache, fatigue, weight loss, anorexia, and arthralgia.

### Cytomegalovirus Infection
Cytomegalovirus infection may present as fever, malaise, rash, and hepatosplenomegaly.

### Hodgkin's Disease
Hodgkin's disease may initially present as localized lymphadenopathy, but this progresses to generalized lymphadenopathy. Early signs may include fatigue, weakness, night sweats, weight loss, fever, and malaise.

### Leukemia

The patient with leukemia presents with generalized lymphadenopathy accompanied by fatigue, malaise, pallor, and a low-grade fever. The patient may also have a prolonged prothrombin time (PT). As the chronic disease progresses, it produces severe fatigue, hepatosplenomegaly, and weight loss.

### Lyme Disease

Lyme disease is a tick-borne infection that initially presents as a skin lesion. As the infection progresses, the patient experiences constant malaise, fatigue, headache, fever, chills, and body aches.

### Mononucleosis, Infectious

The patient with infectious mononucleosis presents with painful lymphadenopathy in the cervical, axillary, and inguinal nodes. The patient may experience symptoms of headache, malaise, and fatigue before lymph node enlargement; however, the classic triad of symptoms at presentation is lymphadenopathy, a sore throat, and an elevated temperature. Other symptoms may include hepatosplenomegaly, stomatitis, and pharyngitis.

### Mycosis Fungoides

Mycosis fungoides is a form of lymphoma accompanied by ulcerated brown tumors of the skin that are painful and pruritic.

### Non-Hodgkin's Lymphoma

Non-Hodgkin's lymphoma presents as a painless lymphadenopathy that may progress to generalized lymphadenopathy. Additional symptoms include dyspnea, cough, fever, night sweats, fatigue, malaise, and weight loss.

### Rheumatoid Arthritis

Lymph node involvement is an early sign of RA. Other symptoms include fatigue, malaise, a low-grade fever, weight loss, arthralgia, and myalgia. Common later symptoms are joint tenderness, swelling, and morning stiffness. Plain radiographs in patients with RA will identify periarticular demineralization, narrowing of joint spaces, and marginal erosions of bones in the hands and feet.

### Sarcoidosis

The patient with sarcoidosis presents with generalized hilar and right parenchymal lymphadenopathy. Other symptoms include arthralgia, fatigue, weight loss, and pulmonary symptoms. Plain chest radiography demonstrates bilateral and right lymphadenopathy as well as pulmonary infiltrates. A high-resolution CT scan will reveal pulmonary changes and affected lymph nodes.

### Sjögren's Syndrome

Sjögren's syndrome, a condition marked by RA, keratoconjunctivitis sicca, and xerostomia, involves the parotid and submaxillary lymph nodes.

Symptoms include dry mucus membranes, photosensitivity, poor vision, nasal crusting, epistaxis, and eye fatigue.

### Syphilis, Secondary
Secondary syphilis presents as a generalized lymphadenopathy along with a rash on the arms, trunk, palms, soles, face, and scalp. A palmar rash is a significant diagnostic sign of this condition.

### Systemic Lupus Erythematosus
The patient with SLE presents with generalized lymph node involvement. Signs and symptoms include a butterfly rash on the face, photosensitivity, Raynaud's phenomena, joint pain, and stiffness. The patient may also have systemic symptoms such as cough, anorexia, and weight loss.

### Tuberculous Lymphadenitis
The patient with tuberculous lymphadenitis presents with fluctuant (soft, rather than firm) lymph nodes that may occur locally or generally. Other symptoms include fever, chills, weakness, and fatigue.

### Waldenstrom's Macroglobulinemia
Waldenstrom's macroglobulinemia presents as lymphadenopathy accompanied by retinal hemorrhage, pallor, and heart failure.

## Menstrual Irregularities

The irregularities in vaginal bleeding included in this section are amenorrhea, dysmenorrhea, and abnormal vaginal bleeding. The essential history in patients with these disorders includes the date of the last menstrual period, possibility of pregnancy, timing of bleeding in relationship to menses, and amount of bleeding (number of soaked perineal pads in one day). Additional relevant information in the history includes data on the use of birth control pills; presence of an intrauterine device; and use of medications such as warfarin (Coumadin), thyroid medications, and steroids.

### Amenorrhea
Amenorrhea is the absence of menstruation. It occurs in two forms: primary and secondary. In primary amenorrhea menses have not been established by the age of 16 years. Causes of this form of amenorrhea include delayed puberty, systemic diseases such as diabetes mellitus and anorexia nervosa, thyroid disorders, and congential problems such as gonadal abnormalities and dysgenesis, and uterine hypoplasia.

Secondary amenorrhea, in which menses cease, can be caused by pregnancy, pituitary insufficiency, ovarian disorder, and endocrine disorders.

## Dysmenorrhea

Dysmenorrhea is pain associated with menstruation. Primary dysmenorrhea is indicated by pain without an organic pathology. The pain in this condition begins shortly after menarche and lasts from 8 to 72 hours. NSAIDs and paracetamol may be beneficial; topically applied heat and transcutaneous electrical nerve stimulation (TENS) may also be used to treat the condition.

Secondary dysmenorrhea is indicated by pain related to an underlying pathological condition, such as endometriosis. The patient with endometriosis may also have have dyspareunia, noncyclical pelvic pain, and subnormal fertility. The diagnosis is made by laparoscopy, removal of endometriotic deposits, and ultrasound examination. Treatment is with hormonal pharmaceuticals after surgery and oral contraceptives, danazol, gestrinone, gonadorelin analogues, and medroxyprogesterone acetate.

Ovarian cysts are another possible cause of secondary dysmenorrhea. They are diagnosed by pelvic or vaginal ultrasound examination.

## Abnormal Vaginal Bleeding

Abnormal vaginal bleeding, if sustained and heavy, can lead to iron deficiency anemia. It may be related to disorders of prostaglandin metabolism, use of an IUD, fibroids, or adenomyosis. The bleeding is managed with NSAIDs, tranexamic acid, and danazol, which will reduce blood loss Complicated cases may require hysterectomy for resolution.

Causes of abnormal vaginal bleeding include:

- Menarche
- Menopause
- Early pregnancy or spontaneous abortion
- Tumors of the cervix or uterus
- IUDs that cause intermenstrual bleeding or increase menstrual flow
- Disease processes, such as endocrine, ovarian, infectious, metabolic, or emotional disorders

**COACH CONSULT**

Abnormal vaginal bleeding may be a normal finding within the first 12 months of menarche and in early menopause.

# Nausea

Nausea is a common finding in a number of GI disorders, as well as during the first trimester of pregnancy.

## Differential Diagnoses

### *Adrenal Insufficiency*

Patients with adrenal insufficiency may present with vomiting, anorexia, and diarrhea.

### *Appendicitis*

Patients with appendicitis present with brief nausea together with abdominal discomfort and stabbing, colicky pain. Findings on physical examination of patients with acute appendicitis include a psoas sign (pain with extension of the right thigh), obturator sign (pain with internal rotation of the flexed right thigh), Rovsing's sign (pain in the RLQ upon the application of pressure to the left lower quadrant [LLQ]), and rebound tenderness. Diagnostic procedures include:

- Plain abdominal radiograph: This will pick up a calcified appendix
- CT scan: The gold standard procedure to identify a dilated appendix and appendiceal inflammation and abscesses
- Ultrasound examination: For use in children and during pregnancy
- WBC count: In appendicitis, this will be 10,000 to 20,000/µL

### *Cholecystitis*

Cholecystitis presents as pain in the RUQ that may radiate to the back and shoulders and is worse after meals. The patient may also have epigastric burning, jaundice, clay-colored stools, and Murphy's sign. Diagnostic procedures for suspected cholecystitis include ultrasound examination of the RUQ, cholescintigraphy, MRI, magnetic resonance cholangiopancreatography (MRCP) when ultrasound examination is not diagnostic; plain abdominal radiography to show radiopaque gallstones; and a WBC of 12,000 to 15,000. Also, the patient may have elevated serum levels of bilirubin, ALT, aspartate aminotransferase (AST), lactate dehydrogenase (LDH), alkaline phosphatase, and amylase.

### *Diverticulitis*

The patient with diverticulitis may report intermittent diarrhea, abdominal pain, and constipation. The presentation includes a low-grade fever and a palpable, tender, firm, fixed mass in the lower abdomen.

### *Gastritis*

In gastritis, nausea is worse after the consumption of alcohol, caffeine, aspirin, or spicy foods. The patient may vomit mucus or blood and experience belching, fever, and malaise.

### *Gastroenteritis*

Besides having nausea, the patient with gastroenteritis may have vomiting, diarrhea, and abdominal cramping. Common organisms causative of infectious gastroenteritis and the time frames for incubation of the disease with each are:

- *E. coli*: 24 to 72 hours
- Campylobacter: 2 to 5 days
- Staphylococcus: 1 to 6 hours
- Shigella: 8 to 24 hours
- Salmonella: 8 to 24 hours
- *Clostridium botulinum*: 12 to 36 hours
- Giardia: 7 to 21 days

Diagnostic procedures for gastroenteritis include plain abdominal radiography to identify gastric-outlet and small-bowel obstruction and a CT scan to reveal inflammation. Treatment includes hydration, a diet progressing from soups to complex carbohydrates and consisting of minimal foods of high sugar and fat content, and cautious use of antimobility drugs because they may prolong the illness. Antibiotics should be considered when:

> **COACH CONSULT**
>
> If infection spreads from the intestines, treatment may include ampicillin, gentamycin, trimethoprim/sulfamethoxazole (Bactrim), or ciprofloxacin.

- An organism is isolated and symptoms remain unresolved
- Leukocytosis or dysentery is present
- The patient is passing more than eight stools per day
- Traveler's diarrhea can be managed with bismuth subsalicylate

If the patient was recently treated with an antibiotic, consider *Clostridium difficile* as a possible pathogen; if a culture is positive for *C. difficile*, treat with metronidazole. In immunocompromised patients, treatment depends on the infecting organism, as follows:

> **ALERT**
>
> Avoid the use of bismuth-containing preparations in patients who are pregnant or allergic to aspirin; also avoid concurrent use of bismuth-containing preparations and anticoagulants, probenecid, or methotrexate.

- Salmonella: Cefotaxime or ceftriaxone for 10 to 14 days
- Shigella: Trimethoprim/sulfamethoxazole (Bactrim DS) or cefixime for 5 days
- Yersinia: Bactrim DS, aminoglycosides, cefotaxime, or tetracycline (for patients over 8 years of age)

## Heart Failure

The patient with heart failure may present with nausea and vomiting, particularly with right-sided heart failure.

## *Hepatitis*

Along with nausea, symptoms of hepatitis include vomiting, fatigue, myalgia, anorexia, cough, photophobia, pharyngitis, and fever. Other symptoms may be weight loss, headache, aversion to smoking and alcohol, pruritus, clay colored stool, dark urine, and pain in the RUQ. Patients with hepatitis B may also present with a nonspecific macular rash and arthralgia early in the disease course. Diagnostic procedures and results indicative of hepatitis include:

- WBC: Low to normal
- Urinalysis: May show proteinuria or bilirubinuria
- AST and ALT: Elevated; these values rise prior to the onset of jaundice, but fall after jaundice occurs
- LDH, bilirubin, alkaline phosphatase, and PT: Normal or slightly elevated
- Serologic tests according to type of hepatitis:
- Active hepatitis A: Anti-hepatitis A virus (HAV) antibody, immunoglobulin M (IgM)
- Recovered hepatitis A: Anti-HAV antibody, IgG
- Active hepatitis B: Hepatitis B surface antigen (HBsAg), hepatitis Be antigen (HBeAg), anti-hepatitis B core (HBc) antibody, IgM
- Chronic hepatitis B: HBsAg, anti-HBc antibody, IgM, IgG
- Recovered hepatitis B: Anti-HBc antibody, anti-HBsAg antibody
- Acute hepatitis C: Anti-hepatitis C virus (HCV) antibody, HCV ribonucleic acid (RNA)
- Chronic hepatitis C: Anti-HCV antibody, HCV RNA
- Hepatitis D: Anti-hepatitis D virus (HDV) antibody, IgM, HDV RNA
- Hepatitis E: None

Treatment for hepatitis is supportive and involves:

- Rest
- Fluid intake of 3,000 to 4,000 mL/day
- Vitamin K when the PT >15 sec
- Lamivudine (Epivir)-HBV for hepatitis B
- Interferon and ribavirin for hepatitis C
- Immunization again hepatitis B virus infection

## *Hyperemesis Gravidarum*

Hyperemesis gravidarum presents with profound vomiting and nausea in the first trimester of pregnancy.

## *Intestinal Obstruction*

Nausea is common in small bowel obstruction. Vomiting may be bilious or fecal, and the patient may also have colicky abdominal pain. Diagnostic procedures include the following:

- Biliary tract: CT scan or ultrasound examination and endoscopy
- Bowel: Plain abdominal film, barium enema, and CT scan

## Meniere's Disease
Patients with Meniere's disease exhibit sudden, brief episodes of nausea, together with vomiting, vertigo, tinnitus, diaphoresis, and nystagmus. Patients may also report ear fullness or hearing loss.

## Mesenteric Venous Thrombosis
Observe the patient with suspected mesenteric venous thrombosis for nausea, vomiting, diarrhea, abdominal distention, hematemesis, and melena.

## Metabolic Acidosis
The patient with metabolic acidosis also presents with vomiting, anorexia, diarrhea, and Kussmaul's breathing.

## Migraine Headache
The patient with a migraine headache will present with a severe headache accompanied with nausea, vomiting, photophobia, and phonophobia.

## Motion Sickness
The patient with motion sickness will present with nausea and vomiting brought about by motion. The patient may also have headache, dizziness, fatigue, diaphoresis, hypersalivation, and dyspnea.

## Myocardial Infarction
The patient with an MI will present with severe substernal pain that may or may not be accompanied by nausea, vomiting, or both.

## Pancreatitis
Nausea and vomiting are early signs of pancreatitis. There may also be severe epigastric pain with possible radiation to the back.

## Peptic Ulcer
In cases of peptic ulcer, nausea and vomiting may follow an acute attack of burning epigastric pain. The pain is relieved with eating if the ulcer is duodenal and is exaggerated with eating in cases of gastric ulcer. Peptic ulcer may be triggered by an empty stomach or ingestion of alcohol, caffeine, or aspirin. More than 90% of adult cases of peptic ulcer are related to *H. pylori* infection; other causes include NSAIDs and glucocorticoids. Diagnostic testing is not needed in uncomplicated cases, but in complicated cases of peptic ulcer a CBC may reflect anemia, and serology or a urea breath test may reflect *H. pylori*. Evaluation by endoscopy is performed after 8 to 12 weeks of treatment.

The treatment of peptic ulcer involves antisecretory drugs such as H2 receptor antagonists and proton-pump inhibitors, mucosa-protective agents such as sucralfate (1 g qid), bismuth subsalicylate, misoprostol (four times daily with food), and antacids. Treatment to eradicate *H. pylori* is considered combination therapy, in that two antibiotics are combined with either a proton-pump inhibitor or bismuth.

### Peritonitis
Peritonitis presents with nausea and vomiting along with acute abdominal pain.

### Pre-Eclampsia
Pre-eclampsia presents, usually in the last trimester, with nausea and vomiting along with rapid weight gain, oliguria, and a severe frontal headache. The triad of signs and symptoms of pre-eclampsia is hypertension, proteinuria, and edema.

## Palpitations

Palpitations, or an awareness of one's own heart beating, may be described as pounding, jumping, turning, fluttering, flopping, or skipped beats. These aberrations in heartbeat may vary in rate, rhythm, onset, and pattern of occurrence. Pathologic palpitations may result from cardiac or metabolic disorders, whereas nonpathologic palpitations are generally related to prosthetic valve emplacement, emotional or physical stress, or ingestion of stimulants such as caffeine or nicotine.

### Differential Diagnoses
### Acute Anxiety
The patient with acute anxiety may present with diaphoresis, flushing, hyperventilation, or trembling.

### Cardiac Arrhythmias
Cardiac arrhythmias may be accompanied by nausea, dizziness, weakness, or fatigue. Changes in heart rate and rhythm may be evident. Drugs that precipitate cardiac arrhythmias or increase cardiac output include:
- Cardiac glycosides
- Thyroid supplements
- Ganglionic blockers
- Beta-adrenergic blockers
- Calcium channel blockers
- Atropine
- Minoxidil
- Sympathomimetics (cocaine)

### Hypertension
The patient with hypertension may have persistent or transient palpitations along with headache, dizziness, tinnitus, and fatigue. The patient may also have epistaxis, arteriovenous (AV) nicking on ophthalmoscopic examination, and left ventricular hypertrophy. Proteinuria and hematuria may be seen. Primary and secondary hypertension are exacerbated

by smoking, stress, obesity, excessive alcohol intake, use of NSAIDs, use of nasal decongestants, and pregnancy. Chest radiograph may be performed to rule out coarctation of the aorta and cardiomegaly. Baseline studies in cases of hypertension include urinalysis; a CBC; and assays for bone morphogenetic protein (BMP), calcium, phosphorus, uric acid, cholesterol, and triglycerides. An ECG can reveal dysrhythmias, bundle-branch block, and left ventricular hypertrophy. Treatment of hypertension involves lifestyle modifications, smoking cessation, stress management, and relaxation.

### Hypocalcemia
Hypocalcemia may produce palpitations. Progressive changes in muscle behavior may also occur, from paresthesias to muscle tension and possibly muscle twitching.

### Mitral Prolapse
Mitral prolapse may present with sharp or stabbing precordial pain. The classic sign is a midsystolic click followed by an apical systolic murmur.

### Mitral Stenosis
Mitral stenosis presents with sustained palpitations, together with exertional dyspnea and fatigue. Assessment of the heart reveals a loud first heart sound or opening snap, as well as a diastolic murmur at the apex.

### Thyrotoxicosis
Patients with thyrotoxicosis present with sustained palpitations. They may also have weight loss, diaphoresis, tachycardia, dyspnea, and heat intolerance.

# Skin Problems

When determining the correct diagnosis for skin disorders, such as rashes or urticaria, the NP must consider whether skin lesions are primary lesions or secondary lesions. Among primary lesions are macules, papules, pustules, vesicles, cysts, nodules, tumors, and wheals. Secondary lesions result from the natural evolution of a primary lesion or as a result of scratching.

## Assessment
The assessment of skin lesions should begin with a determination of their type; configuration; precipitating events, such as outdoor exposures, contact with allergic substances, and medications; the presence of pruritus with the rash; and any underlying illnesses or associated symptoms.

Infectious lesions of the skin are categorized by their causation, including fungal, viral, bacterial, and infestational. Table 2–31 presents information to aid in the identification and treatment of skin rashes.

## Table 2–31  Skin Rashes: Identification and Treatment

| RASH/SKIN CONDITION | PHYSICAL FINDINGS/TREATMENT OPTIONS |
|---|---|
| Acne | Blackheads, whiteheads, pustules, and inflammatory papules over face, neck shoulders, chest, and back<br>Treatment: benzoyl peroxide, topical antibiotics (clindamycin, erythromycin), tretinoin<br>Oral antibiotics may be helpful (doxycycline, erythromycin, minocycline, and tetracycline) |
| **FUNGAL SKIN INFECTIONS** | |
| Diagnostic procedure for dermatophyte infections: Scrape border of lesion with #15 blade, add 1–2 drops of KOH solution, add coverslip, and examine under microscope; identify hyphae | |
| Tinea capitis (scalp) | Scaling red plaques with hair loss and broken hairs<br>Treatment: Griseofulvin (Grifulvin V) orally for up to 12 weeks, selenium sulfide shampoo twice a week for 2 weeks<br>With Grifulvin treatment, monitor liver enzymes, take with high-fat foods |
| Tinea corporis | Itching, scaling, inflamed plaques consisting of confluent vesicles and plaques, eventual central healing with peripheral spread of the lesion (like ringworm)<br>Treatment: Topical antifungal |
| Tinea cruris (groin) | Marginated, symmetrical, itching, red, scaling lesions with advancing, actively inflamed borders<br>Treatment: Topical antifungal |
| Tinea of hands and feet | Itching, vesicles on the palms and soles, scaling and fissuring between toes<br>Treatment: Topical or oral antifungal |
| Psoriasis (adult) | Well-circumscribed, silvery-coated plaques on scalp, knees, elbows, may also involve nails, groin, trunk; itching very common. Removal of scales will cause point bleeding<br>Treatment: Tazarotene, vitamin D topical, dithranol, keratolytics, topical corticosteroids<br>May also use PUVA, heliotherapy, and ultraviolet B |
| Seborrheic dermatitis | Poorly demarcated, greasy, scaly plaques on scalp, eyebrows, and nasolabial areas; may also involve back, ears, chest, and groin<br>Treatment: Antifungal with ketoconazole, selenium sulfide shampoo |

## Table 2–31  Skin Rashes: Identification and Treatment—cont'd

| RASH/SKIN CONDITION | PHYSICAL FINDINGS/TREATMENT OPTIONS |
|---|---|
| Tinea versicolor | Flat, barely palpable, superficial scaling plaques over neck, shoulders, and trunk<br>May look tan on light skin<br>Treatment: Topical selenium sulfide lotion daily for 1 week, leave on for 10 min before rinsing off, may repeat in 1 month; or Ketoconazole shampoo to skin daily for 3 days |
| Yeast infections (Candida) | Red, moist, grouped papules and pustules. Common in diabetics and children. Itching common. Common sites are high-moisture areas such as groin, base of nails. |
| **BACTERIAL SKIN INFECTIONS** | |
| Impetigo | Red papules and superficial vesicles that become confluent. Honey-colored crusts. Lesions often heal centrally while spreading. Common sites are head, neck, and diaper area. Contagious.<br>Treatment: For multiple lesions, give oral antibiotics (dicloxacillin or cephalexin for 10 days)<br>For small numbers of lesions, apply topical mupirocin ointment (Bactroban) |
| Boils | Tender superficial abscesses, commonly in hairy areas<br>Treatment: I&D (incision and drainage) if indicated; culture drainage. Oral antibiotics, topical antibiotics to lesion. For boils caused by methicillin-resistant *Staphylococcus aureus:* use Bactrim DS twice daily and rifampin as oral antibiotics. Consider treating finger- and toenails with topical antibiotics; also coat nares with topical antibiotics daily |
| Hives (urticaria) | Itching, migratory pink itchy wheals, may follow ingestion of drugs, shellfish, may be stress-related eruptions<br>Treatment: Symptomatic, antihistamines may be helpful |
| **INFESTATIONS** | |
| Scabies | Itchy papules and vesicles, generally in warm, moist body folds, such as between fingers, at the navel, behind the knees, and in the groin area. Lesions may have burrows (zigzag threadlike channels) with variable degrees of inflammation. Contagious<br>Treatment: Lindane lotion apply to body for 8–12 hours, then shower<br>Others: Crotamiton, permethrin |

*Continued*

## Table 2–31  Skin Rashes: Identification and Treatment—cont'd

| RASH/SKIN CONDITION | PHYSICAL FINDINGS/TREATMENT OPTIONS |
|---|---|
| **INFESTATIONS** | |
| Lice | Itching, papules, urticaria, and eventual secondary bloody crusts in hair-bearing areas. Hair with nits. Contagious<br>Treatment: Malathion lotion, permethrin lotion, apply twice, 7 days apart<br>Educate on household cleaning to eradicate lice |
| **COMMON PEDIATRIC RASHES** | |
| Pityriasis rosea | Oval, salmon-colored, superficial, scaling plaques along trunk, preceded by a large herald patch. Eruption is self limited, may last up to 6 weeks. |
| Papovavirus (Fifth disease) | Red cheeks, circumoral pallor, truncal rash, fever. |
| German measles | Fever, posterior cervical node enlargement for up to 7 days, followed by sudden red, finely papular rash on face that fades after 1 day then spreads to trunk and extremities |
| Measles | Cough, fever, conjunctivitis for 3 days, followed by generalized purple-red macular and papular rash starting at the head and spreading over the body in 3 days. May have Koplik spots (red spots with small white centers) on throat |
| Chickenpox | Umbilicated vesicles, mostly on the trunk, but also on extremities, face; vesicles crust within several days of onset. May have low fever |
| Molluscum contagiosum | Flesh-colored, dome-shaped papules with central umbilicated areas. Viral, spread by direct contact. Lesions usually 2–5 mm, generally no more than 20 lesions with an outbreak. Self limiting.<br>Treatment: Liquid nitrogen to genital lesions; other options include salicylic acid, podofilox gel bid x 3 days, Imiquimod cream 3 times a week for 2 weeks, or tretinoin gel hs for 2 weeks. |
| Atopic dermatitis | Itching, worse in evenings, erythematous papular lesions that become confluent; scaling, lichenification from repeated scratching, very dry skin<br>Involves flexural areas, foot, occasional exudative lesions<br>Treatment: Skin hydration, cleansing with mild soaps. Topical moisturizing lotions, creams, or ointments. May use topical steroid ointments and oral antihistamines for acute flare-ups. Use lowest potency steroid ointment that will control the symptoms |

Adapted from Wasson, J. The Common Symptom Guide, ed. 5. New York: McGraw-Hill, 2002.

## Diagnostic Testing
Laboratory diagnostic studies for pruritic conditions unrelated to primary skin lesions include assays of the:
- Hemoglobin and hematocrit
- Serum iron, TIBC, and ferritin
- Serum BUN and creatinine
- Alkaline phosphatase, bilirubin, AST, and ALT
- TSH, free thyroxine, and FT4
- Serum glucose
- Anti-HIV antibody titer
- Follicle stimulating hormone (FSH) level
- Stool for occult blood

## Treatment
Oral and topical agents are available for treating skin disorders that present with pruritus, including oral antihistamines and topical antipruritics.

### *Oral Antihistamines (Second Generation H1-receptor Blockers)*
- Fexofenadine (Allegra) in 60 mg capsules and tablets of 30, 60, and 180 mg
  - Children 6 to 11 years: 30 mg bid
  - Adults: 60 mg bid
- Loratadine (Claritin).
  - Children 2 to 5 years: 5 mg qd
  - Adults: 10 mg qd
- Desloratadine (Clarinex)
  - Adults and children over 12 years: 5 mg qd
- Cetirizine (Zyrtec)
  - Children 2 to 5 years: 2.5 mg qd
  - Children 6 to 11 years: 5–10 mg qd
  - Adults and children over 12: 5 to 10 mg qd

### *Oral Antihistamines First-Generation H1-Receptor Blockers*
- Hydroxyzine (Atarax) (an inexpensive medication; administer at bedtime; drowsiness is a common side effect)
  - Children 0.5 mg/kg/dose tid prn, available as syrup at 10 mg/5 mL
  - Adults: 25 to 50 mg dose tid

### *Topical Antipruritic Agents*
- Pramoxine (Sarna) Lotion, Prax Lotion, Itch-X Gel (all are available as OTC products
- Cetaphil with menthol and phenol
- Doxepin HCL cream (Zonalon) for adults only, qid, prn

## *Topical Steroids*

Topical steroids provide relief for many corticosteroid responsive skin diseases. The NP should remember that systemic absorption may occur, especially if such steroids are used over large skin areas, over broken or inflamed skin, on the face, or in occluded dressings. Use of the lowest potency product that proves efficacious is recommended. Table 2–32 provides an overview of topical steroid preparations by level of potency.

| Table 2–32 **Topical Steroid Preparations by Potency** | | |
|---|---|---|
| **LOW POTENCY** | | |
| Alclometasone dipropionate 0.05% *(Aclovate cream)* Fluocinolone acetonide 0.01% *(Synalar solution)* Hydrocortisone base or acetate 0.5% *(Cortisporin cream)* | Hydrocortisone base or acetate 1% *(Cortisporin ointment Hytone cream/ointment, U-cort cream, Vytone cream)* | Hydrocortisone base or acetate 2.5% *(Anusol HC cream Hytone cream, ointment)* Triamcinolone acetonide 0.025% *(Aristocort A cream, Kenalog cream, lotion)* |
| **INTERMEDIATE POTENCY** | | |
| Betamethasone valerate 0.12% *(Luxiq foam)* Clocortolone pivalate 0.1% *(Cloderm lotion)* Desonide 0.05% *(Desonate gel DesOwen cream, lotion, ointment; Verdeso foam)* Desoximetasone 0.05% *(Topicort LP emollient cream)* Fluocinolone acetonide 0.01% *(Derma-Smoothe/ FS oil Capex shampoo* | Fluocinolone acetonide 0.025% *(Synalar cream, ointment)* Flurandrenoline 0.025% *(Cordran SP cream, ointment)* Flurandrenolide 0.05% *(Cordran SP cream, lotion)* Fluticasone propionate 0.05% *(Cutivate ointment)* Fluticasone propionate 0.05% *(Cutivate cream, lotion)* Hydrocortisone probutate 0.1% *(Pandel cream)* | Hydrocortisone butyrate 0.1% *(Locoid cream, ointment, solution)* Hydrocortisone valerate 0.2% *(Westcort cream, ointment)* Mometasone furoate 0.1% *(Elocon cream, lotion, ointment)* Prednicarbate 0.1% *(Dermatop emollient)* Triamcinolone acetonide 0.1% *(Aristocort A cream, ointment Kenalog cream, lotion)* Triamcinolone acetonide 0.2% *(Kenalog aerosol)* |

## Table 2–32 Topical Steroid Preparations by Potency—cont'd

### HIGH POTENCY

| | | |
|---|---|---|
| Amcinonide 0.1% (Cyclocort cream, lotion, ointment) Betamethasone dipropionate augmented 0.05% (Diprolene AF emollient cream; Diprolene lotion) Desoximetasone 0.05% (Topicort gel) | Desoximetasone 0.25% (Topicort emollient cream, ointment) Diflorasone diacetate 0.05% (Psorcon E emollient cream, ointment) Fluocinonide 0.05% (Lidex cream, gel, ointment, solution; Lidex E emollient cream) | Halcinonide 0.1% (Halog cream, ointment, solution) Triamcinolone acetonide 0.5% (Aristocort A cream; Kenalog cream) |

### VERY HIGH POTENCY

| | | |
|---|---|---|
| Betamethasone diproprionate augmented 0.05% (Diprolene ointment, gel) | Clobetasol propionate 0.05% (Clobex lotion, shampoo, spray; Cormax ointment, scalp application; Olux foam; Olux E foam) Temovate cream, gel, ointment, scalp application Temovate E emollient cream | Fluocinonide 0.1% (Vanos cream) Flurandrenoline 4 mcg/ cm$^2$ (Cordran tape) Halobetasol propionate 0.05% (Ultravate cream, ointment) |

Adapted from Nurse Practitioner Prescribing Reference Winter 2008–2009. New York: Haymarket Media Publications, 2009.

### Topical Antifungals
Topical antifungal agents are available for the management of dermatophytic skin eruptions. Table 2–33 is a presentation of topical antifungal agents with dosing guidelines included.

### Moisturizers
Conditions marked by dryness of the skin, such as atopic dermatitis, require daily lubrication of the skin to control the dryness. Bathing should always be followed by the application of emollients after patting the skin dry. Patients should be educated to use mild soaps such as Dove, Basis, or Eucerin for cleansing. Moisturizers are available as lotions, creams, and ointments.

The following are good examples of skin moisturizers, lotions, creams, and ointments:
- Moisturizing lotions
  - Petrolatum-based: Dermasil, Moisturel, Replenaderm

## Table 2–33 Topical Antifungals for Management of Tinea Corporis, Pedis, and Cruris

| ANTIFUNGAL AGENT | AVAILABLE AS | DOSING | DURATION OF TREATMENT | USE IN CHILDREN |
|---|---|---|---|---|
| Miconazole (Monistat Derm) | Cream 15 g, 1 oz, 3 oz | BID | Tinea corporis/cruris 2 weeks Tinea pedis 4 weeks | Yes |
| Terbinafine (Lamisil) | Solution, 30 mL Pump spray | Daily for Tinea corporis, cruris Twice daily for Tinea pedis | 1 week | Not recommended |
| Econozole (Spectazole) | Cream, 15, 30 g | Daily | Tinea corporis, cruris 2 weeks Tinea pedis 4 weeks | Yes |
| Ciclopirox (Loprox) | Cream 15, 30, 60 g Lotion 30, 60 mL | Twice daily | Up to 4 weeks | <10 not recommended |
| Ketoconazole (Nizoral) | Cream 15, 30, 60 g | Daily | Tinea corporis, tinea cruris 2 weeks Tinea pedis 6 weeks | Yes |
| Oxiconazole (Oxistat) | Cream 15, 30 g Lotion 30 ml | Daily or twice daily | Tinea pedis 4 weeks Tinea corporis, cruris 3 weeks | Not recommended |
| Sulconazole (Exelderm) | Cream 15, 30, 60 g Solution 30 ml | Twice daily for Tinea pedis Daily or twice daily for Tinea corporis and cruris | Tinea pedis 4 wks Tinea corporis, cruris 3 weeks | Not recommended |
| Butenafine (Mentax) | Cream 15, 30 g | Twice daily or daily for Tinea pedis Daily for Tinea corporis, cruris | Tinea pedis 1 week twice daily or 4 weeks daily Tinea corporis, cruris 2 weeks | Not recommended |

Adapted from Nurse Practitioner Prescribing Reference Winter 2008–2009. New York: Haymarket Media Publications, 2009.

- Mixtures of lanolin and petrolatum: Eucerin Lotion, Lubriderm Lotion, Nivea Lotion
- Without lanolin or petrolatum: Corn Husker's Lotion, Cetaphil Lotion
- Moisturizing creams
  - Petrolatum-based: Purpose Dry Skin Cream, Cetaphil Cream, Keri Cream
  - Mixtures of lanolin and petrolatum: Eucerin Cream
  - No lanolin or petrolatum: Neutrogena Norwegian Formula Hand Cream
- Moisturizing ointments
  - Petrolatum-based: Vaseline Pure Petrolatum Jelly
  - Mixtures of lanolin and petrolatum: Aquaphor Natural Healing Ointment

## Differential Diagnoses

### Diabetes Mellitus

The patient with diabetes mellitus will present with an elevated serum glucose level.

### Hyperthyroidism

The patient with hyperthyroidism will present with fatigue, heat intolerance, increased appetite, increased sweating, nervousness, palpitation, weight loss, fine tremor, hyperreflexia, ocular signs, Plummer's nails, pretibial myxedema, proptosis, a staring gaze, and warm, moist skin. The patient will have a decreased serum level of TSH and an elevated level of FT4.

> **COACH CONSULT**
>
> Pruritus can be the result of a primary skin disease or may be a clue to an underlying pathology. There are multiple causative factors for generalized pruritus.

### Hypothyroidism

The patient with hypothyroidism will have cold and dry skin, constipation, hair loss, a sensation of coldness, weakness, weight gain, hoarseness, a large tongue, periorbital puffiness, prolonged DTRs, and sparse hair. Diagnostic tests will reveal and elevated TSH and decreased FT4.

### Iron Deficiency Anemia

The patient with iron deficiency anemia will present with microcytic or normocytic anemia, a decreased serum iron concentration, low serum level of ferritin, elevated TIBC, and decreased transferrin saturation.

### Liver Disease

The patient with liver disease will present with an elevated alkaline phosphatase level.

### Neoplasms

The patient with Hodgkin's disease may present with fever, night sweats, weight loss, splenomegaly, and lymphadenopathy. The patient with non-Hodgkin's lymphoma may have fever, night sweats, weight loss, splenomegaly, and lymphadenopathy. Leukemia and solid tumors of the pancreas and stomach can also have effects on the skin.

### Polycythemia Vera

The patient with polycythemia vera may have a history of venous or arterial thrombosis, burning pain in the hands and feet, and splenomegaly. Laboratory tests will show elevated hemoglobin and hematocrit levels.

### Postmenopause

Skin problems in women who are postmenopausal may be accompanied by an elevated serum level of FSH.

### Primary Skin Conditions

Some primary skin conditions present as pruritus without or with only minimal manifestations on the skin. These include:

- Aquagenic pruritus: Itching that follows bathing or water exposure
- Fiberglass dermatitis: Caused by fiberglass particles that may be visible by microscopic examination of a skin scraping
- Xerosis: Excessive dryness of the skin in winter months
- Scabies: A contagious infestation of the skin by the itch mite

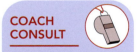
### Pregnancy

The pregnant patient may present with an elevated urine or serum level of hCG, or both.

### Psychologic Factors

The patient with a psychologic source of skin disturbance may complain of a sensation of bugs crawling on the skin.

### Uremia

The patient with uremia will present with an elevated BUN and creatinine.

## Sore Throat

Throat pain can include discomfort in the pharynx, nasopharynx, oropharynx, or hypopharynx. It typically results from infection, trauma, or allergy. Other causative factors can include a systemic disorder or cancer. Patients who are mouth breathers also experience throat pain, from increased dryness of the mucous membranes. Other throat irritants include vocal strain and exposure to alcohol, tobacco, or ammonia.

## Differential Diagnoses
### Agranulocytosis
In addition to a sore throat, patients with agranulocytosis will frequently have fever, chills, and a headache.
### Bronchitis
Besides having a sore throat, patients with bronchitis present with a cough, fever, chills, and muscle and back pain. Auscultation may reveal rhonchi, wheezing, and occasionally crackles.
### Chronic Fatigue Syndrome
Patients with CFS present with intense fatigue and may also present with a sore throat, myalgia, and cognitive decline.
### Common Cold
The patient with a common cold will typically present with a cough, sneezing, nasal congestion, rhinorrhea, headache, arthralgia, and myalgia.
### Contact Ulcers
Contact ulcers appear on the posterior vocal cords, causing pain aggravated by talking. The patient may also have ear pain.
### Foreign Body
A foreign body in the throat will present as localized throat pain.
### Gastroesophageal Reflux Disease
The patient with GERD will present with a chronic sore throat and hoarseness.
### Influenza
The patient with influenza may have fever, chills, headache, weakness, malaise, cough, and muscle weakness.
### Laryngeal Cancer
The primary symptom of laryngeal cancer is pain or burning in the throat when consuming citrus drinks. A classic sign of this malignancy is hoarseness lasting longer than 3 weeks.
### Mononucleosis
Mononucleosis commonly occurs in teenagers and young adults 15 to 24 years of age. It has an incubation period of 1 to 2 months and is generally self-limiting. The Epstein-Barr virus is the causative agent. Mononucleosis has the distinctive triad of symptoms consisting of a sore throat, cervical lymphadenopathy, and fluctuating temperature. However, it may also present with fever, chills, malaise, anorexia, and splenomegaly. Laboratory findings include a positive Monospot test and increased WBC count with relative lymphocytosis and neutropenia. Treatment of

mononucleosis includes supportive care, prednisone for severely enlarged tonsils, and avoidance of contact sports for 3 weeks to a period of months until splenomegaly is resolved.

## Necrotizing Ulcerative Gingivitis (Trench Mouth)

Necrotizing ulcerative gingivitis (trench mouth) presents as a sore throat of abrupt onset along with gingivitis and bleeding of the gums.

## Peritonsillar Abscess

Peritonsillar abscess presents as a severe throat pain, but the patient may also have dysphagia, drooling, halitosis, and fever.

## Pharyngitis

Pharyngitis may be bacterial, fungal, or viral. Bacterial pharyngitis begins abruptly with unilateral soreness of the throat. Fungal pharyngitis presents with a burning sensation accompanied by pharyngeal edema and erythema; additionally, the patient may have white plaque marks on the tonsils, pharynx, tongue, and oral mucosa. Viral pharyngitis presents with a diffuse sore throat, malaise, fever, and mild erythema and edema of the posterior pharynx. Laboratory tests for the cause of pharyngitis include a rapid streptococcal antigen test, Monospot test, and CBC with a differential count. Treatment of pharyngitis involves hydration, saline gargles, antibiotics (penicillin or erythromycin) to treat streptococcal infection, ceftriaxone for gonococcal infection, and acetaminophen (Tylenol) or aspirin for pain and fever.

## Sinusitis

Patients with sinusitis may present with a sore throat related to a post-nasal drip, which may result in halitosis; pain and pressure over the face, nose, cheeks, and molar teeth; a purulent nasal discharge; tenderness over the sinuses; and headache. Common bacterial of sinusitis causes include *Haemophilus influenzae, Streptococcus pneumoniae,* and various anaerobes. Diagnostic testing includes culture as needed, CT scans or sinus radiographs, and transillumination studies of the sinuses. Treatment of sinusitis involves hydration, decongestants, antihistamines, antibiotics for bacterial sinusitis, analgesics, and supportive care.

## Tongue Cancer

The patient with tongue cancer presents with localized throat pain; there may also be a raised white lesion or ulcer on the tongue.

## Tonsillar Cancer

Tonsillar cancer presents as a soreness of the throat that radiates to the ear. There may also be a superficial ulcer on the tonsil.

## Tonsillitis

Tonsillitis presents as mild to severe throat pain, with dysphagia and headache. Lingual tonsillitis presents with a red, swollen tongue covered in exudates. Treatment and laboratory testing for tonsillitis are the same as for pharyngitis.

### Uvulitis

The patient with uvulitis reports a sensation of something stuck in the throat. Signs and symptoms of uvulitis include uvular erythema and edema of the uvula. Clinically the patient may also present with dysphagia; gag easily; or complaint of sore throat, fever, and a muffled voice.

## Vaginal Discharge

A normal vaginal discharge is generally nonodorous, clear to white, and mucoid in appearance. Several pathologic vaginal conditions are differentiated on the basis of the vaginal discharge in each. Table 2–34 compares discharges in various vaginal disease conditions and the diagnosis and treatment procedures for each condition.

| Table 2–34 | Differential Diagnoses and Treatment for Diseases Causing Vaginal Discharge | | |
|---|---|---|---|
| **VAGINAL DISEASE CONDITION** | **DISCHARGE CHARACTERISTICS** | **DIAGNOSTIC TEST** | **TREATMENT PER CDC RECOMMENDATIONS** |
| Atrophic vaginitis | Thin, scant, watery discharge | Pap smear | — |
| Bacterial vaginosis | Thin, green or gray-white, foul smelling discharge | Vaginal pH >4.5 Positive whiff test Clue cells on wet prep DNA probe based test for *Gardnerella vaginalis* | Nonpregnant: metronidazole 500 mg bid x 7 days OR Metro gel daily x 5 days OR |
| | | | Clindamycin cream intravaginally x 7 days Pregnant: Metronidazole 250 tid x 7 days OR Clindamycin 300 mg orally bid x 7 days Avoid alcohol during and post treatment with metronidazole |

*Continued*

| Table 2–34 | Differential Diagnoses and Treatment For Diseases Causing Vaginal Discharge—cont'd | | |
|---|---|---|---|
| **VAGINAL DISEASE CONDITION** | **DISCHARGE CHARACTERISTICS** | **DIAGNOSTIC TEST** | **TREATMENT PER CDC RECOMMENDATIONS** |
| Candidiasis | White, curdlike, profuse discharge with yeasty sweet odor | Vaginal pH <4.5 Microscopic KOH with hyphae and budding yeast | Intravaginal agents OR Oral: Fluconazole 150 mg as a single dose *Note with repeated vaginal candidiasis consider testing for diabetes mellitus |
| Chancroid | Mucopurulent, foul smelling | | — |
| Chlamydia Reportable STD | Yellow mucopurulent, odorless | NAATs to identify *Chlamydia trachomatis* Wet prep to identify coexisting vaginal infections | Azithromycin 1 g orally in single dose OR Doxycycline 100 mg bid x 7 days Alternative: Erythromycin 500 mg QID x 7 days OR Ofloxacin 300 mg bid x 7 days OR Levofloxacin 500 mg daily x 7 days Note: Avoid intercourse until fully treated, get partners treated (past 60 days) Pregnancy: Treat with erythromycin 500 qid x 7 days OR Amoxicillin 500 mg tid x 7 days |

| VAGINAL DISEASE CONDITION | DISCHARGE CHARACTERISTICS | DIAGNOSTIC TEST | TREATMENT PER CDC RECOMMENDATIONS |
|---|---|---|---|
| Genital herpes | Copious mucoid d/c Incubation 2–14 days, recurrent life long viral infection First clinical episode: burning, itching, dysuria, pain, and tenderness in perineal area, may also have fever and lymphadenopathy Recurrent episodes: localized lesions, prodrome | HerpeSelect Unroof lesion and swab with Dacron tipped swab | Initial episode: Acyclovir 400 mg tid x 7–10 days OR Acyclovir 200 mg 5 times/day for 7–10 days OR Famciclovir 250 mg tid x 7 days OR Valacyclovir 1 g bid x 7–10 days Recurrent episode: Acyclovir 400 mg tid x 5 days OR Acyclovir 800 mg bid x 5 days OR Famciclovir 125 mg bid x 5 days OR Valacyclovir 500 mg bid x 3–5 days OR Valacyclovir 1.0 g qd x 5 days Evaluate and treat symptomatic sex partners |
| Genital warts | Can be asymptomatic or subclinical Visible genital warts | Clinical exam Use 3–5% acetic acid to visualize warts Pap smear to detect cervical dysplasia | Patient applied: Podofilox gel bid x 3 days Imiquimod cream daily for up to 16 weeks Provider administer: Cryotherapy Podophyllin resin TCA or BCA Sex partners: assess and treat visible warts |

*Continued*

## Table 2–34  Differential Diagnoses and Treatment for Diseases Causing Vaginal Discharge—cont'd

| VAGINAL DISEASE CONDITION | DISCHARGE CHARACTERISTICS | DIAGNOSTIC TEST | TREATMENT PER CDC RECOMMENDATIONS |
|---|---|---|---|
| Gonorrhea Reportable STD | Yellow or green, foul odor Incubation period 2–7 days Women: Urethra, endocervix, upper genital tract, pharynx, and rectum Men: Urethra, epididymis, prostate, rectum, and pharynx | Gram-stain smear NAATs to detect *N. gonorrhoeae* organism Women: Pelvic examination to check for adnexal tenderness, cervical motion tenderness Men: Examine for urethral discharge and rectal exam for tenderness or discharge | Cefixime 400 mg PO OR Ceftriaxone 125 mg IM as a single dose OR Ciprofloxacin 500 mg orally as a single dose OR Levofloxacin 250 mg as a single dose PLUS: If *Chlamydia* not ruled out: Azithromycin 1 g orally as a single dose OR Doxycycline 100 mg bid x 7 days Refer sex partners for treatment |
| Gynecologic cancer | Chronic, watery, bloody, or purulent discharge, may have odor | Pap smear | — |
| Trichomoniasis | Frothy, green and profuse, foul smell, vulvar irritation Incubation period 4–28 days | Vaginal pH >4.5 Microscopic examination reveals organisms with whiplike flagella Culture most sensitive | Metronidazole 2 g in one dose OR Metronidazole 500 mg bid x 7 days Avoid sex until after treated, treat partners, no alcohol while taking metronidazole |

| Table 2–34 | **Differential Diagnoses and Treatment for Diseases Causing Vaginal Discharge—cont'd** | | | |
|---|---|---|---|
| **VAGINAL DISEASE CONDITION** | **DISCHARGE CHARACTERISTICS** | **DIAGNOSTIC TEST** | **TREATMENT PER CDC RECOMMENDATIONS** |
| Syphilis Reportable STD | *Treponema pallidum* Primary: Ulcer/ chance at site Secondary: 6–8 weeks later with generalized arthralgia, malaise, fever, lymphadenopathy, rash Latent: Neurological symptoms | Darkfield microscopy RPR, VDRL Treponemal specific tests: TP-PA | Primary and secondary: Benzathine penicillin G 2.4 million units IM *always test for HIV |

BCA: bichloracetic acid; HIV: human immunodeficiency virus; NAAT: nucleic acid amplification test; TCA: trichloroacetic acid; VDRL: Venereal Disease Research Laboratory
From CDC.gov/STD Treatment Guidelines (2006).

# Vertigo

Vertigo is defined as an illusion of movement, often a revolving movement, that worsens with actual movement. Vertigo may be accompanied by nausea, vomiting, nystagmus, and tinnitus.

## Differential Diagnoses
### *Brainstem Ischemia*
Brainstem ischemia presents as a sudden, severe vertigo that is initially episodic but is later persistent.
### *Head Trauma*
The patient with head trauma presents with persistent vertigo following the causative injury. The patient may also have nystagmus and hearing loss.
### *Herpes Zoster*
The patient with herpes zoster presents with vertigo of sudden onset. Other symptoms include hearing loss, herpetic vesicles in the ear canal, and facial paralysis.

### Labyrinthitis
Labyrinthitis may occur with severe ear infection, and vertigo may occur as a single event or recur.

### Meniere's Disease
The patient with Meniere's disease presents with unpredictable episodes of vertigo and gait disturbance of abrupt onset.

### Multiple Sclerosis
MS presents as episodic vertigo as well as visual disturbances such as diplopia and blurring.

### Vestibular Neuritis
Vestibular neuritis presents as vertigo of abrupt onset that may last for several days. The patient may also have nausea, vomiting, and nystagmus.

## Vision Problems

Many eye conditions can contribute to optical symptoms such as vision loss, blurred vision, and visual floaters. Table 2–35 identifies known causes of these ocular symptoms.

### Differential Diagnoses
### Hordeolum (Stye)
Hordeolum (stye) is typically caused by *Staphylococcus aureus*. It may be external, pointing toward the skin surface of the eyelid, or internal, pointing toward the conjunctival side of the lid. Signs and symptoms include pain and erythema of the eyelid and a localized, tender mass in the eyelid. Treatment involves warm compresses and topical bacitracin or erythromycin ophthalmic ointment.

### Chalazion
A chalazion appears as a beady nodule on the upper eyelid. It is painless, but does present with edema of the eyelid, eyelid tenderness, sensitivity to light, and increased tearing. Management involves the application of warm compresses and surgical removal of the nodule.

### Blepharitis
Blepharitis is seborrheic dermatitis of the eyelid edge. It is marked by red, scaly, greasy flakes, with a thickened, crusted lid margin, itching, and tearing. Treatment involves the application of hot compresses, topical antibiotics such as bacitracin or erythromycin, and scrubbing of the eyelashes and lid margins with the eyes closed.

### Conjunctivitis
The patient with conjunctivitis presents with inflammation or infection of the conjunctiva, caused by allergy; chemical irritation; or infection with

## Table 2–35 Identified Causes of Visual Disturbances

| VISION LOSS | BLURRED VISION | VISUAL FLOATERS |
|---|---|---|
| Cataract | Brain tumor | Retinal detachment |
| Concussion | Cataract | Uveitis |
| Diabetic retinopathy | Concussion | Vitreous hemorrhage |
| Glaucoma | Corneal abrasions | |
| Macular degeneration | Concussion | |
| Ocular trauma | Corneal foreign object | |
| Optic atrophy | Diabetic retinopathy | |
| Optic atrophy | Dislocated lens | |
| Paget's disease | Eye tumor | |
| Pituitary tumor | Glaucoma | |
| Retinal artery occlusion | Hereditary corneal | |
| Retinal detachment | dystrophies | |
| Retinal vein occlusion | Hypertension | |
| Steven's–Johnson | Hyphema | |
| syndrome | Iritis | |
| Temporal arteritis | Retinal detachment | |
| Vitreous hemorrhage | Macular degeneration | |
| | Stroke | |
| | Temporal arteritis | |
| | Vitreous hemorrhage | |

Adapted from Munden, J. & Schaeffer, L. (Ed). Portable Signs and Symptoms. Philadelphia: Lippincott Williams & Wilkins, 2008.

bacterial, viral, or gonorrheal/chlamydial organisms. Signs and symptoms include itching, burning, tearing, redness of the eye or eyelid, possible blurred vision, swelling of the eyelid, and patient reports of the sensation of a foreign object in the eye. Bacterial conjunctivitis presents with a purulent discharge and is treated with ophthalmic levofloxacin, ofloxacin, ciprofloxacin, tobramycin, or gentamycin applied as eyedrops. Gonococcal or chlamydial conjunctivitis presents with a copious, purulent discharge. Treatment of the various types of conjunctivitis consists of:

- Gonococcal conjunctivitis: Ceftriaxone: 250 mg IM
- Chlamydial conjunctivitis: Erythromycin ophthalmic ointment
- Systemic gonorrhea or chlamydia: Oral tetracycline, erythromycin, clarithromycin, azithromycin, or doxycycline, according to the guidelines of the U.S. Centers for Disease Control and Prevention

The patient with allergic conjunctivitis presents with a stringy discharge accompanied by increased tearing and is treated with oral antihistamines. Viral conjunctivitis presents with a watery discharge and is treated symptomatically.

# Urinary Incontinence

Urinary incontinence can result from a bladder anomaly, neurological disorder, or loss of pelvic muscle strength. The classification of urinary incontinence is based on its cause, including neurogenic etiologies, stress, overflow, urgency, or total incontinence. Table 2–36 presents an overview of the classes of urinary incontinence.

## Differential Diagnoses
### *Benign Prostatic Hypertrophy*
Benign prostatic hypertrophy (BPH) presents as overflow incontinence related to urethral obstruction. Signs and symptoms of BPH include incomplete emptying of the bladder, a reduced urine stream, and inability to initiate a urine stream.
### *Bladder Cancer*
Bladder cancer presents as overflow incontinence from obstruction of urine flow by the tumor.
### *Diabetic Neuropathy*
Diabetic neuropathy presents as painless bladder distention and overflow incontinence. The patient may also have episodic diarrhea or constipation.

| Table 2–36 **Classification of Urinary Incontinence** | |
| --- | --- |
| **INCONTINENCE TYPE** | **DESCRIPTION** |
| Neurogenic | Damage to spinal nerves that control bladder relaxation and contraction |
| Stress | Intermittent incontinence following coughing, sneezing, laughing, or sudden movement |
| Overflow | Urinary retention from overfilling of bladder to the point that bladder muscles cannot contract strongly enough to expel urine |
| Urge | Inability to suppress a sudden urge to urinate |
| Total | Total inability of the bladder to retain urine |

Adapted from Munden, J. & Schaeffer, L. (Ed.). Portable Signs and Symptoms. Philadelphia: Lippincott Williams & Wilkins, 2008.

### Multiple Sclerosis
Common urologic symptoms of MS include urinary incontinence, urgency, and frequency. MRI will demonstrate demyelination plaques.
### Prostatitis
An enlarged prostate in prostatitis may obstruct urine flow. Other symptoms of prostatitis include urinary frequency and urgency, hematuria, dysuria, urethral discharge, distended bladder, and perineal pain.
### Spinal Cord Injury
In spinal cord injury, overflow incontinence follows rapid bladder distention. Diagnostic procedures for spinal cord injury include plain film radiography to identify a vertebral fracture line, and CT scanning to detect subtle abnormalities.
### Stroke
Stroke can be accompanied by transient or permanent urinary incontinence.
### Urethral Stricture
Urethral stricture may eventually lead to overflow incontinence.
### Urinary Tract Infection
Symptoms of UTI include dysuria, frequency, urgency, hematuria, cloudy urine, and possibly bladder spasms.

# Weight Gain and Loss

Changes in weight may have multiple causes. Weight losses of less than 10 pounds a month may be attributed to changes in diet, recent acute illness (especially when accompanied by nausea, vomiting, or diarrhea), diuretic therapy, fever, decreased nutrient metabolism, or increased energy consumption as seen with exuberant exercise. Minor gains in weight may be related to increased calorie consumption, fluid retention, and a decline in metabolic rates.

## Differential Diagnoses for Excessive Weight Gain
### Acromegaly
The patient with acromegaly presents with moderate weight gain, coarse facial features, enlarged hands and feet, back and joint pain, and heat intolerance.
### Hypercortisolism
Hypercortisolism presents as accumulations of fat, particularly on the trunk and back of the neck. The patient may also display cushingoid features.

**COACH CONSULT**

Medications that may cause weight gain include:
- Corticosteroids
- Phenothiazines
- TCAs
- Hormonal contraceptives
- Lithium

### Hyperinsulinism
Hyperinsulinism causes an increase in appetite that leads to weight gain. The patient may also have behavioral irritability, indigestion, weakness, diaphoresis, and tachycardia.
### Hypogonadism
Findings with hypogonadism include sparse facial and body hair and voice changes.
### Hypothalamic Dysfunction
Hypothalamic dysfunction presents as excessive appetite, an altered body temperature, and sleep disturbance.
### Hypothyroidism
Symptoms of hypothyroidism include cold intolerance; constipation; menorrhagia; dry, pale skin; and thick, brittle nails.
### Nephrotic Syndrome
Nephrotic syndrome presents as weight gain from edema, orthostatic hypotension, and abdominal distention.
### Pancreatic Islet Cell Tumor
The patient with a pancreatic islet cell tumor presents with excessive hunger, emotional lability, malaise, fatigue, diaphoresis, palpitations, tachycardia, and syncope.
### Pre-Eclampsia
Patients with pre-eclampsia may have nausea and vomiting, epigastric pain, an elevated BP, and blurred vision.
### Sheehan's Syndrome
Sheehan's syndrome is most common in women with severe obstetric hemorrhage.

## Differential Diagnoses for Excessive Weight Loss
### Adrenal Insufficiency
Adrenal insufficiency may present as anorexia, weakness, fatigue, irritability, syncope, abdominal pain, and diarrhea. Physical assessment may also reveal hyperpigmentation of the skin over joints and the belt line, palmar creases, lips, gums, tongue, and buccal mucosa.
### Anorexia
In addition to having weight loss, the patient with anorexia may present with muscle atrophy, dental caries, hypotension, cold intolerance, and amenorrhea.
### Crohn's Disease
The patient with Crohn's disease may experience abdominal cramping or pain, anorexia, diarrhea, and tachycardia and may manifest hyperactive bowel sounds and abdominal distention.

### Cryptosporidiosis
The patient with cryptosporidiosis presents with a protozoal infection that leads to watery diarrhea, abdominal cramping, flatulence, anorexia, nausea, vomiting, and myalgia.

### Esophagitis
Esophagitis presents as an avoidance of eating caused by esophageal pain upon swallowing. It may also present with hypersalivation, dysphagia, and tachypnea.

### Gastroenteritis
Gastroenteritis presents as weight loss secondary to dehydration and malabsorption.

### Leukemia
Leukemia presents as weight loss, weakness, dyspnea, tachycardia, palpitations, and abdominal or bone pain.

### Lymphoma
Lymphoma presents as gradual weight loss accompanied by fever, fatigue, and night sweats. The patient may also have hepatosplenomegaly and lymphadenopathy.

### Pulmonary Tuberculosis
Pulmonary tuberculosis presents as gradual weight loss, fatigue, weakness, anorexia, night sweats, and a low-grade fever.

### Thyrotoxicosis
The patient with thyrotoxicosis presents with increased metabolism that contributes to weight loss. Other findings include nervousness, heat intolerance, diarrhea, palpitations, tachycardia, diaphoresis, and fine tremors.

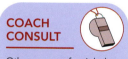

**COACH CONSULT**

Other causes of weight loss include:
- Cancer
- Depression
- Diabetes mellitus

# 3 Guidelines for Diagnostic Testing

# CHAPTER 3

# Guidelines for Diagnostic Testing

## Using Laboratory Diagnostics to Your Advantage

Some of the easiest and least expensive diagnostic tools at your fingertips are diagnostic laboratory studies, many of which can be performed in your own office.

### The Complete Blood Count

A complete blood count (CBC) with a differential count gives you a vast amount of information about your patient's chief complaints. Indications for a CBC include:

- Ruling out viral versus bacterial diseases in patients presenting with fever
- A patient presentation of fatigue, weight loss, or both
- Cases involving physiological stress, such as surgery
- Pallor or weakness in a patient
- A presentation of pica: The eating of ice, cornstarch, clay, dirt, or other nonfood items
- A presentation with any bleeding disorder or complaint
- A family history of hereditary hematological abnormalities
- For screening a patient in a general physical examination
- For screening a patient before surgery
- For monitoring a patient's hematologic status during pregnancy
- For monitoring of patients treated for hematological diseases

Normal values for a CBC are given in Table 3–1. Keep in mind that values in the CBC may vary slightly from one clinical laboratory to another and that local laboratory values should be used as a reference for normal ranges.

Abnormal values in a CBC may represent a multitude of hematological illnesses, depending on the particular component of the CBC that is above or below its normal value. Many of the values in the CBC provide helpful clinical information for the diagnosis of anemias, hydration status, and infectious diseases. Table 3–2 identifies some common causes of abnormal values in the differential component of the CBC.

| Table 3–1 **Normal Values of the Complete Blood Count** | |
|---|---|
| **LABORATORY PROCEDURE** | **RANGE OF NORMAL VALUES** |
| WBC | 4300–10,800/mm |
| RBC | 4.5–5.6 million/mm |
| Hgb<br>• Male<br>• Female | <br>14–18 g/100 mL<br>12–16 g/100 mL |
| Hct<br>• Male<br>• Female | <br>40%–54%<br>37%–48% |
| MCV | 88–98 |
| MCH | 27–32 |
| RDW | 11.6%–14.6% |
| Reticulocyte count | 0.5%–2.5% |
| Platelets | 150–450,000 |
| ESR<br>• Male<br>• Female | <br>1–13 mm (giant cell inflammation)<br>1–20 mm |

ESR: erythrocyte sedimentation rate; MCH: mean corpuscular hemoglobin concentration; RDW: red cell distribution width.

## Table 3–2 Meanings of Differential-Count Results in the Complete Blood Count

| DIFFERENTIAL COMPONENT | INCREASED IN | DECREASED IN |
|---|---|---|
| RBC | Bone marrow failure, anxiety, dehydration, high altitudes, polycythemia vera, COPD with hypoxia | Chemotherapy, dietary deficiencies, hemoglobinopathies, hemolytic anemia, hemorrhage, Hodgkin's disease, chronic inflammatory disease, leukemia, multiple myeloma, organ failure, overhydration, pregnancy, subacute endocarditis |
| Hgb | Burns, COPD, CHF, dehydration, high altitudes, polycythemia vera | Anemia, carcinoma, fluid retention, hemoglobinopathies, Hodgkin's disease, leukemia, pregnancy, nutritional deficits, splenomegaly |
| Hct | Erythrocytosis, shock, hemoconcentration, polycythemia vera | Anemia, blood loss, bone marrow hyperplasia, burns (severe), chronic diseases, hemolytic reactions |
| Reticulocyte count | Blood loss, hemolytic anemia, iron deficiency anemia, megaloblastic anemia | Alcoholism, anemia of chronic disease, aplastic anemia, bone marrow replacement, endocrine disease, renal disease, sideroblastic anemia |
| Platelets | Acute infections, postexercise, anemia, chronic heart disease, cirrhosis, chronic leukemia, malignancies, pancreatitis, polycythemia vera, essential thrombocythemia, rheumatic fever, rheumatoid arthritis, splenectomy, postoperative status, trauma, ulcerative colitis | Alcohol/drug toxicity, prolonged hypoxia, viral infections, megaloblastic anemias, iron deficiency anemia, lymphoma, severe hemorrhage, DIC, uremia, burns, malaria, radiation, splenomegaly |
| ESR | MI, anemia, cat scratch fever, cancer, heavy metal poison, Crohn's disease, endocarditis, pregnancy, nephritis, rheumatic fever, temporal arteritis, lymphoma, inflammation, infections | High RBC, high Hg; elevated blood glucose Normal in CHF, G6PD deficiency, hemoglobin C, polycythemia, sickle cell, spherocytosis |

DIC: disseminated intravascular coagulation; G6PD: glucose-6-phosphate dehydrogenase

The WBC provides particular clinical information for diagnosing infectious, viral, or autoimmune diseases. Table 3–3 presents common clinical diagnoses marked by increases or decreases in the WBC and its differential components.

Peripheral blood smears may also provide clues to the diagnoses of clinical diseases. In these smears, blood cells are identified microscopically by their shapes. Table 3–4 presents a summary of some findings in peripheral smears and their possible clinical significance.

## Serum Chemistry Studies

Serum chemistries, electrolytes, liver function studies, and lipid panels are all cost- effective, highly efficient studies for diagnosing and monitoring patients in your practice.

| Table 3–3 Interpretation of Differential Count Results in the White Blood Count | | |
|---|---|---|
| DIFFERENTIAL COMPONENT | INCREASED IN | DECREASED IN |
| WBC | Infancy, stress, menstruation, labor, infections, anemia, appendicitis, collagen d/o, Cushing's disease, leukemia | Diurnal rhythms, alcoholism, anemia, bone marrow depression, malaria, SLE, malnutrition, radiation, rheumatoid arthritis, viral infections |
| Neutrophils | Acute hemolysis, acute hemorrhage, infectious disease, inflammatory disease, malignancy, DKA, Cushing's, myelocytic leukemia, stress, tissue necrosis | Acromegaly, anaphylaxis, anorexia, vitamin B12 or folate deficiency, bone marrow depression, SLE, viral infections |
| Lymphocytes | Addison's disease, infections, lymphocytic leukemia, malnutrition, myeloma, ulcerative colitis | Antineoplastic drugs, aplastic anemia, burns, hemolytic disease newborns, high doses of adrenocorticosteroids, Hodgkin's disease, immunodeficiency diseases, pernicious anemia, pneumonia, radiation, rheumatic fever, transfusion reaction |
| Monocytes | Cancer, cirrhosis, hemolytic anemia, Hodgkin's disease, infections, lymphomas, monocytic leukemia, polycythemia vera, radiation, sarcoidosis, SLE, thrombocytopenic purpura, ulcerative colitis | — |

DKA: diabetic ketoacidosis; SLE: systemic lupus erythematosus;

## Table 3–4  Clinical Interpretations of the Peripheral Blood Smear

| PERIPHERAL SMEAR FINDING | DESCRIPTION | CLINICAL SIGNIFICANCE |
| --- | --- | --- |
| Poikilocytosis | A variety of abnormally shaped cells on smear | Sickle cell disease<br>Red cell membrane disorders |
| Spherocytosis | Spherical shaped cells | Acquired hemolytic anemia<br>Direct physical or chemical injury to cells, such as from heat |
| Elliptocytes | Elliptical | Iron deficiency anemia<br>Sickle cell anemia<br>Megaloblastic anemias<br>Myelofibrosis |
| Leptocytes | Thinner than normal | Obstructive jaundice<br>Postsplenectomy<br>Hemoglobin C disease<br>Hypochromic anemias |
| Schistocytes | Cell fragments | Megaloblastic anemias<br>Severe burns |
| Basophilic stippling | Fine or coarse basophilic staining | Increased production of RBCs<br>Lead poisoning<br>Megaloblastic anemias |
| Howell–Jolly bodies | Smooth, round, blue dots within red cells | Megaloblastic anemias |
| Cabot rings | Blue, threadlike rings | Erythropoiesis |
| Heinz bodies | Refractile inclusions | Postsplenectomy<br>Hereditary deficiency |
| Acanthocytosis | Thornlike projections | Alcoholic cirrhosis<br>Postsplenectomy |

An initial chemistry panel can permit an analysis of suspected abnormalities. Once the initial chemistry panel has been completed, the healthcare provider can monitor treatment with sequential laboratory tests for specific indices so as to maintain a cost-effective approach to care. If, for example, the only abnormal values in an initial chemistry panel that were abnormal were the blood urea nitrogen (BUN) and creatinine, it would not be necessary to repeat full chemistry panels on the patient's subsequent visits, but only to continue to monitor the BUN and creatinine as indicators of a response to treatment. Table 3–5 provides ranges of normal values for basic serum chemistry studies.

## Hemoglobin A$_{1C}$

Hemoglobin A$_{1C}$ (HbA$_{1C}$) reflects the average daily blood glucose concentration over the previous 90 days. If the HbA$_{1C}$ is 6.0, the patient's average daily glucose level during that 90-day period was 135 mg/dL. Each increase of 1.0 points in the HbA$_{1C}$ represents an increase of 35 mg in the serum glucose level. For example:

| HbA$_{1C}$ | Serum glucose level |
|---|---|
| 6.0 | 135 mg/dL |
| 7.0 | 170 mg/dL |
| 8.0 | 205 mg/dL |
| 9.0 | 240 mg/dL |
| 10.0 | 275 mg/dL |
| 11.0 | 310 mg/dL |
| 12.0 | 345 mg/dL |

## Liver Function Studies

Bilirubin provides one measure of hepatic function. To identify liver disease, both the total and direct bilirubin level are needed. Hepatocellular injury can be identified by the assay for aspartate aminotransferase (AST)

| Table 3–5 **Normal Values of Serum Chemistry Tests** | |
|---|---|
| TEST | NORMAL VALUE |
| Sodium | 135–145 mmol/L |
| Potassium | 3.5–5.0 mEq/L |
| Chloride | 100–106 mEq/L |
| Osmolality | 280–296 mmol/L |
| BUN | 8–25 mg/dL |
| Creatinine | 0.6–1.5 mg/dL |
| Glucose | 70–100 mg/dL |

or alanine aminotransferase (ALT); the AST is typically elevated in alcoholic and toxic injuries, while the ALT is more often elevated in viral injuries to the liver.

Values of lipid metabolism may vary with the methods used for its measurement. Studies performed in a controlled laboratory will yield the most valid results. Analyses done at health fairs and screenings should be evaluated more cautiously, since some variability is to be expected due to their quality control. It is also important to consider physiological variability in the patient. As much as an 8% variation can be found with multiple cholesterol screenings within a single 24-hour period. it is therefore imperative that treatment decisions about lipid management be based on at least two values recorded at least 1 week apart. When medical interventions are instituted for elevated lipid concentrations, retesting should be scheduled for 6 weeks later.

Interference with cholesterol panels can be attributed to a number of factors. Among them are use of oral contraceptives or estrogen and high serum levels of vitamin C.

Table 3–6 identifies normal ranges for common liver function studies.

| Table 3–6 **Laboratory Studies of Liver Function** | |
|---|---|
| **REFERENCE** | **NORMAL VALUE** |
| Total bilirubin | Up to 1.0 mg/dL |
| Direct bilirubin | Up to 0.4 mg/dL |
| Alkaline phosphatase | 40–130 IU/dL |
| AST/SGOT | 20–40 IU |
| ALT/SGPT | 10–35 IU |
| Amylase | 23–85 |
| Cholesterol | <200 mg/dL |
| Triglycerides | <150 mg/dL |
| HDL | 35–45 mg/dL |
| LDL | <130 mg/dL |

## Laboratory Studies of Thyroid Function

Thyroid hormones are responsible for a variety of physiological functions, including oxygen consumption, metabolism of proteins and carbohydrates, and electrolyte mobilization. Thyroid dysfunctions are generally classified as hyperthyroid, with excessive thyroid hormone production; hypothyroid, with deficient thyroid hormone production; and euthyroid, with normal thyroid hormone secretion. Normal values for thyroid hormones include:

- TSH: 0.4 to 10 mIU
- T3: 80 to 200 ng/mL
- T4: 5.8 to 11.0 ng/mL

## Testing for Coagulation Disorders

Disorders of blood coagulation are classified as hypocoagulative disorders, with failure to achieve adequate thrombus formation, or hypercoagulative disorders, with inappropriate thrombus formation. The American College of Chest Physicians and the National Heart Lung and Blood Institute recommend an International Normalized Ratio (INR) of 2.0 to 3.0 for:

- Preventing venous thrombosis
- Treating venous thrombosis
- Treating pulmonary embolism
- Preventing systemic embolism
- Implanted tissue heart valves
- Acute myocardial infarction (MI)
- Treating valvular heart disease
- Treating atrial fibrillation (AF)

Normal values for basic coagulation tests are:

- Prothrombin time (PT): 0 to 13 sec
- INR: Normal = 1.0
  - Thrombosis/embolism: 2.0 to 3.0 sec
  - Mechanical heart: 2.5 to 3.5 sec
- Partial thromboplastin time (PTT): 5 to 39 sec

Table 3–7 identifies dosage adjustment for the anticoagulant warfarin based on INR values.

Bear in mind that the metabolism of warfarin can be affected by illness, some medications, foods with a high vitamin K content, herbal remedies, and alcohol. Baseline values of INR should be obtained at the initiation of warfarin therapy and then determined on a daily basis until dosage adjustments have been made. Once the warfarin dosage has been stabilized, the patient's condition may be well controlled with INR testing for 4 to 8 weeks.

## Table 3–7  Dosage Adjustment Algorithm for Warfarin

| | | CURRENT DAILY DOSE | | | | |
|---|---|---|---|---|---|---|
| | | 2.0 | 5.0 | 7.5 | 10.0 | 12.5 |
| INR | WARFARIN DOSE ADJUSTMENT* | ADJUSTMENT IN DAILY DOSE | | | | |
| 1.0–2.0 | Increase x 2 days | 5.0 | 7.5 | 10.0 | 12.5 | 15.0 |
| 2.0–3.0 | No change | - | - | - | - | - |
| 3.0–6.0 | Decrease x 2 days | 1.25 | 2.5 | 5.0 | 7.5 | 10.0 |
| 6.0–10.0[1] | Decrease x 2 days | 0 | 1.25 | 2.5 | 5.0 | 7.5 |
| 10.0–18.0[2] | Decrease x 2 days | 0 | 0 | 0 | 0 | 2.5 |
| >18.0[2] | Discontinue warfarin, consider in patient management or reversal of anticoagulation | | | | | |

*Allow 2 days after dosage change for clotting factor equilibration. After increase or decrease in dosage for 2 days, go to new higher (or lower) dosage level (example: if 5.0 mg daily, alternate 5.0/7.5; if alternating 2.5/5.0, increase to 5.0 daily).
[1]Consider oral vitamin K at 2.5–5.0 mg.
[2]Oral vitamin K at 2.5–5.0 mg.

Remember that INR values will not be realized for up to 3 weeks after adjusting the dose of an anticoagulant. If the patient has an INR value other than the targeted value, consider more frequent monitoring.

## Prostate-Specific Antigen

The serum level of prostate-specific antigen (PSA) provides helpful information in monitoring and diagnosing prostate cancer. The normal level of PSA is <4.0 ng/mL. It is also important to monitor for upward trends in yearly PSA values, even if the values are not >4.0 ng/mL. A rise in the level of PSA from one year to the next could indicate abnormal prostate gland activity and should be investigated further.

## Cardiac Enzymes

Myocardial injury releases a number of enzymes, including creatine phosphokinase (CPK), lactate dehydrogenase (LDH), creatine kinase-MB (CK-MB), troponin, and AST. The timing of the enzyme release, peak serum level of the enzyme, and rate of clearance of the enzyme from the serum can be very helpful in the diagnosis of cardiac injury. Table 3–8 presents information on the timing factors in assaying serum levels of cardiac enzymes after myocardial injury.

## The Anemias

Anemias are classified as microcytic, macrocytic, or normocytic according to the size of the red blood cells (RBCs) in each, which is represented by the mean corpuscular volume (MCV). The most common microcytic anemias include iron-deficiency anemia, the thalassemias, and sideroblastic anemias; each presents with a low value of MCV. Macrocytic anemias are marked by high values of MCV levels and are typically seen in folic acid deficiency or vitamin B12 deficiency; they may also be seen in liver disease, hemolytic anemia, and anemia from blood loss.

A normal value of MCV in the presence of low values of hemoglobin (Hgb) and hematocrit (Hct) can represent hemolytic anemia, anemia from blood loss, anemia of chronic disease, acquired sideroblastic anemia, or early onset iron-deficiency anemia. When the MCV is below its normal range, the serum total iron-binding capacity (TIBC) and serum ferritin level will aid in the diagnosis of iron-deficiency anemia. Normal values for TIBC are 240 to 360 mcg/dL; normal values of serum ferritin are 20 to 250 ng/mL.

| Table 3–8 **Cardiac Enzyme Timetable** | | | | |
|---|---|---|---|---|
| **ENZYME** | **BEGINS** | **PEAKS** | **RETURNS TO BASELINE** | **NORMAL** |
| CPK/MB | 4–6 hours | 14–30 hours | 48–72 hours | <5% total CPK |
| LDH | 8–12 hours | 24–48 hours | 10 days | 45–90 U/L |
| Troponin | 3 hours | 8–12 hours | 5–14 days | <1.5 ng/mL |

The serum level of vitamin B12 and the serum folate level will aid in differentiating the various types of macrocytic anemia from one another. The normal ranges for serum vitamin B12 are 150 to 250 pg/mL; the normal ranges for folate are >3 ng/mL. Figure 3–1 depicts a decision tree for diagnosis and interpretation of the anemias.

## A Decision Tree for Diagnosis of Anemia

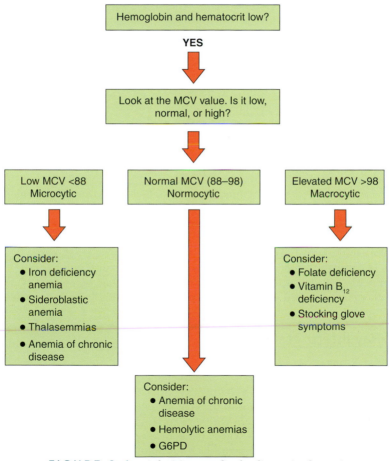

FIGURE 3-1: A decision tree for the diagnosis of anemia.

## COACH CONSULT

- If your patient presents with blood in the urine, you have to rule out a variety of illnesses, including stones in the ureters, urinary tract infection (UTI), prostate problems, and bladder neoplasms.

- Patients with a history of smoking have an increased risk of bladder neoplasms. It is imperative to get a follow up urinalysis to demonstrate that a patient is free of hematuria after a course of antibiotic treatment. If the hematuria continues beyond treatment of the UTI, refer the patient to a urologist for further evaluation of the hematuria.

## Urinalysis

A urinalysis can provide first clues to a disease process in an asymptomatic patient. For example, patients with diabetes mellitus may have elevated urine glucose levels identified before a diagnosis of diabetes has been made. The urinalysis can identify problems with hydration; infection; changes in physical activity; pathological conditions; and changes caused by foods or medications. Urine color, volume, turbidity, odor, and specific gravity (SG) can each help in diagnosing abnormalities. Thus, the normal urine SG is 1.003 to 1.025 g/mL. A low specific gravity would indicate a loss of the kidney's ability to concentrate the urine, such as is seen in diabetes insipidus, glomerulonephritis, pyelonephritis, and other tubular abnormalities of the kidney. A high specific gravity is often seen in patients with fever, vomiting, diarrhea, adrenal insufficiency, congestive heart failure (CHF), and hepatic diseases.

Other values identified in the urinalysis include the pH and levels of proteins, glucose, ketones, hemoglobin, and nitrites, and numbers of leukocytes. Table 3–9 names a number of potential causes of abnormal findings for these values in the urinalysis.

The urinalysis report can provide you with clues to differentiate a number of urological diseases based on the types of casts that are present in the specimen. Table 3-10 identifies disease processes likely to be responsible for specific casts identified in the urinalysis.

# X-Ray Interpretation

## Chest X-rays

Chest x-rays are among the most common diagnostic imaging tools used in clinical settings. When viewing any x-ray film, remember that the more dense the body material, the more x-radiation is absorbed, making the material appear more white on the film.

Conversely, air and fluids within the body absorb very little of the x-ray beam and thus appear darker on the x-ray film. On a gradient scale, the whitest x-ray images are obtained from lead, followed by bone and then by

## Table 3–9  Interpretation of Urinalysis Results

| URINALYSIS COMPONENT | INCREASED IN | DECREASED IN |
|---|---|---|
| pH | Ingestion of citrus fruits, metabolic or respiratory alkalosis, vegetarian diets | High-protein diets, ingestion of cranberries, metabolic or respiratory acidosis |
| Protein | Stress, exercise, diabetic nephropathy, glomerulonephritis, toxemia of pregnancy | NA |
| Glucose | Diabetes | NA |
| Ketones | Diabetes, fever, fasting, high-protein diets, starvation, vomiting | NA |
| Hemoglobin | Exercise, malignancy, menstruation, pyelonephritis, snake/spider bites, trauma, tuberculosis, UTI, urolithiasis | NA |
| Nitrites | Presence of nitrite-forming bacteria: Citrobacter, enterobacter, *Escherichia coli*, *Klebsiella*, *Proteus*, some *Staphylococcus* species | NA |
| Leukocytes | Bacterial infection, calculi formation, fungi or parasitic infection, glomerulonephritis, interstitial nephrititis | NA |

NA: not applicable.

body tissues or organs. Darker images portray fluids, and even darker images show air, such as air in the lungs.

Some basic rules for reading chest x-ray films will aid the NP in making the best possible diagnosis of what they show. These rules are to:

- Always use the same approach every time you look at a chest film, so that you do not miss something important on the films
- Verify the patient's right and left sides by looking at the stomach bubble and heart shape
- Count the ribs to be sure the patient made a good inspiratory effort before the x-ray film was taken (10 ribs posterior and 6 ribs anterior)

## Table 3–10 Urinary Casts and Their Significance

| CAST | PROBABLE DISEASE PROCESS |
|------|--------------------------|
| Red cell | Glomerulonephritis |
| White cell | Pyelonephritis<br>Interstitial nephritis |
| Hyaline | Diuretics<br>Heavy exercise<br>Fever<br>Concentrated urine |
| Renal tubular | Acute tubular necrosis<br>Interstitial nephritis |
| Broad, waxy | Chronic renal failure |
| Granular | Nonspecific |

- Check soft tissues for deformities, foreign bodies, or subcutaneous emphysema
- Look at the shape and line of the diaphragm
- Check the hilar and mediastinal areas for aorta size and shape and prominence of hilar vessels
- Look at the heart size, shape, and calcifications
- Check the lungs for infiltrates, masses, increased interstitial markings, and vascularity
- Check the lateral film to confirm any questionable masses or infiltrates, the anteroposterior (AP) diameter, and effusions

### Orthopedic X-Rays

Plain x-ray films are generally the first-line diagnostic approach to most orthopedic injuries. It is best to request two views of any bony structure so as to avoid missing small anomalies on the films. If in doubt about whether to order a plain x-ray film or more extensive diagnostic studies such as magnetic resonance imaging (MRI) or a computed tomographic (CT) scan, get the radiologist's opinion opinion in order to minimize patient costs and time.

Some general principles that apply in interpretation of orthopedic plain x-ray films are:

- Look at every film you order
- Have a systematic method of reading; always follow that method to avoid missing fine points
  - Observe the film both from a distance and close up
  - Observe the film generally and then focus on the site in question
  - Look at and through overlying structures
  - Look at all views
  - Use a hot lamp liberally
  - Compare the appearance of one side of the film to the opposite side if in doubt
  - Go back to the area of interest and repeat the examination if needed
- Always check the patient's demographic information (patient name, age, sex, and date of x-ray examination) on every film you read
- Evaluate the x-ray technique used in making the film: Is there over-/underpenetration? What is the patient's alignment?

Fracture lines on x-ray films may be obvious or subtle. X-ray films of normal bone reveal no interruption in the trabecula and show smooth joint spaces and an intact cortical line. With a fracture, the practitioner may observe:

- A lucent line
- Interruption of the cortical bone
- A dense line secondary to an overlap of fragments
- Clinical findings such as
  - Soft-tissue swelling
  - Joint effusion
  - Deformity
  - Dislocation
  - Loss of mobility
  - Tenderness with palpation

**COACH CONSULT**

Basic rules for interpretation of chest x-rays are that:
- The heart should be about one half of the chest width on a PA film
- With right ventricular enlargement, expect to see elevation of the cardiac apex
- With a diagnosis of CHF, Kerley B lines may appear on the x-ray; these increased vascular markings may be unilateral on the right side. If they are unilateral on the left side, the patient does not have CHF
- If the patient has chronic obstructive pulmonary disease (COPD), the lung fields will be darker and the x-ray film will show a flat hemidiaphragm
- Atelectasis appears as a white area signifying the absence of air

**COACH CONSULT**

The thymus, or "sail," is commonly seen on chest films of children. It usually recedes at some time between the ages of 8 and 12 years. It is most commonly noted on the right side of a child's chest x-ray film.

At 2 weeks after a fracture, bone callus formation can be visualized on x-ray films as new bone formation occurs. At 2 to 4 weeks after a fracture, the x-ray film will show a diminished fracture line with calcification. Complete bone remodeling requires 2 to 3 years for completion. Reasons for delayed bone healing include:

- Infection
- Poor blood supply to the bone
- Improper fixation of the fractured bone
- Destruction of bony fragments
- Tissue between the fragments and the corresponding bones

When viewing films of the forearm, observe for the fat pad sign to aid in interpretation of the findings. A small fat pad line is normally adjacent to the bone, but is displaced outward and away from the bone if a fracture is present. Visualization of this constitutes a positive fat pad sign.

## Computed Tomographic Scans

CT is a three-dimensional x-ray procedure that allows visualization of bone and calcifications within blood vessels, the bowel, and other body structures. The CT scan provides excellent spatial resolution and differentiation of benign from malignant tumors and permits the evaluation of vascular dysfunction and calcification, organ anomalies, and cysts. Some advantages of a CT scan include its relative rapidity in emergency situations, requiring less than 10 minutes to completion as compared to the 45-minutes required to complete an MRI. CT scans are excellent for detecting freshly coagulated blood and intracranial abnormalities such as bleeding or lesions, especially in emergency situations.

If necessary, contrast media may be used to further enhance abnormal tissues in a CT scan. These media are generally used to aid in the diagnosis of vascular, hemorrhagic, or bleeding disorders. In other disorders, non-contrast-enhanced CT scans are preferred. CT imaging is the mode of choice for evaluations of the inner ear and sinuses and for imaging other bony structures.

CT scans are contraindicated in:
- Patients with allergies to shellfish or iodine dyes
- Patients with claustrophobia
- Pregnant patients, unless the benefits of the examination outweigh its risks
- Elderly patients who are dehydrated
- Patients in renal failure
- Children of age 17 years and younger, unless the benefits outweigh risks related to radiation exposure

## Magnetic Resonance Imaging

MRI generates cross sectional images of the body in any plane. The MRI works by using water density and the magnetization of hydrogen ions to allow the camera to pick up any energy given off by the hydrogen ions. The brightness of the MRI image of a tissue is determined by the amount of fat and water content of the tissue. MRI is the best diagnostic tool for detecting and identifying tumors.

MRIs may be ordered with and without gadolinium contrast. For most purposes of family medicine and orthopedics, MRI should be ordered without contrast enhancement. If contrast enhancement is required, make certain that the patient does not have a history of renal failure, since gadolinium is cleared by the kidneys and exposure to it could have fatal effects on patients with a low creatinine clearance.

A distinct advantage of MRI for diagnostic use is that it provides high-contrast, high-resolution images of the nervous system and basilar brain structures. Its disadvantages include the greater time required to perform an MRI (45 minutes) than a CT scan (5 to 10 min). Cost factors must also be considered, as a CT scan is less expensive than an MRI. Table 3–11 provides assistance in choosing a CT scan or an MRI in specific clinical scenarios.

## Ultrasonography

Ultrasound examination permits the evaluation of body structures and the movements of internal organs and of blood flow within vessels. Listed below are examples of clinical situations in which ultrasound examination can provide excellent diagnostic assistance:
- Orthopedics: Helpful in diagnosing tendon tears, soft-tissue masses, and bleeding or fluid collection in muscle, bursae, spaces.

| | | | |
|---|---|---|
| **Table 3–11** | **Selection Criteria for Magnetic Resonance Imaging or Computed Tomographic Scan** | |
| **PATIENT SCENARIO** | **CT SCAN PREFERRED** | **MRI PREFERRED** |
| Head trauma | X | |
| Lower cost | X | |
| Subtle tumor or infarct of brain | | X |
| Brainstem injury | | X |
| Fresh brain hemorrhage | X | |
| Old brain hemorrhage | | X |
| Time-factor-emergent | X | |
| Skull fracture | X | |
| Calcified lesions | X | |
| Obese patient | X | |
| Pacemaker or metal fragments/prosthetics | X | |
| Anatomical detail needed | | X |

- Pregnancy: Permits the evaluation of fetal skeletal dysplasias and cysts, placental abnormalities, and the fetal urinary bladder and stomach
- Gynecology: Helpful in the evaluation of treatment responses of gynecological tumors, cysts, polyps, fibromas, and endometrial hyperplasia
- Abdominal: Helpful in identifying soft-tissue abnormalities

Table 3–12 compares the indications for diagnostic use of the CT scan, MRI, and ultrasound examination on each major body system.

## Electrocardiography

It is important to develop a standard system for reading a 12-lead electrocardiogram (ECG), with sequential steps used to avoid missing any important details. A 12-lead ECG will help you determine essential elements

## Table 3–12 Indications for Diagnostic Testing by Body System

| BODY SYSTEM | ULTRASONO-GRAPHY | CT SCAN | MRI |
|---|---|---|---|
| Ear, nose, throat | | Recalcitrant sinusitis | Suspected acoustic neuroma<br>Eye orbit with exophthalmos |
| Neurological | | Syncope, suspected lesions<br>Suspect hemorrhage<br>CVA<br>Carotid lesions<br>Cerebral aneurysm<br>Subarachnoid bleed<br>Acute head trauma | Seizures, suspected tumor<br>Headaches<br>AV malformation<br>Acute head trauma<br>Dementia<br>Suspected neoplasm<br>Spinal cord lesion |
| Respiratory | | Hemoptysis<br>Suspect PE<br>Lung abscess<br>Asbestosis<br>Bronchiectasis<br>Lung tumors<br>Mediastinal mass<br>Pleural effusion<br>Blunt trauma to chest | Mediastinal mass |
| Gastrointestinal | Abdominal pain<br>Abdominal ascites<br>Jaundice to rule out biliary obstruction<br>Abdominal mass in a child<br>Gallbladder pain<br>Pyloric stenosis<br>Small-bowel obstruction<br>Appendicitis | Abdominal pain<br>Fatty liver<br>Appendicitis<br>Antibiotic colitis<br>Epigastric mass<br>Diverticulosis<br>Liver abscess<br>Peritonitis<br>Intussusception<br>Pancreatitis | Abdominal aortic aneurysm |
| Genitourinary | Inguinal hernia<br>Scrotal hernia<br>Hydrocele<br>Varicocele<br>Undescended testicle, infant | Undescended testicles, older boy<br>Hematuria<br>Renal infarction<br>Renal trauma | Undescended testicles, adult |

*Continued*

## Table 3–12 Indications for Diagnostic Testing by Body System—cont'd

| BODY SYSTEM | ULTRASONO-GRAPHY | CT SCAN | MRI |
|---|---|---|---|
| Genitourinary (cont'd) | Hematuria Renal abscess Glomerulonephritis Pyelonephritis | Pheochromocytoma Pyelonephritis | |
| Reproductive | Ovarian cysts PID Breasts with questionable mammogram result Multiple pregnancy Placenta abruption | Ovarian cysts, tumors | |
| Musculoskeletal | Hips for developmental dysplasia | Ankle sprain taking longer than 6 weeks to heal Osteoarthritis of spine Spinal stenosis Sciatica | Herniated discs Rotator cuff tears Ligament injuries Spinal stenosis Sciatica Osteomyelitis Pelvic fracture Osgood–Schlatter disease |

AV: arteriovenous; CVA: cerebrovascular aneurysm; PID: pelvic inflammatory disease.

such as heart rate, rhythm, conduction issues in the atria and ventricles, axis determination, and a quick identification of areas of ischemia or heart-tissue damage. Interpretation of the 12-lead ECG is a skill that is easily learned, but also a skill that can be forgotten if not used regularly. It is important to take advantage of opportunities to refresh your interpretative skills in reading the 12-lead ECG, especially if you do not review 12-lead ECGs on a regular basis. A seven-step procedure for interpreting the 12-lead ECG is given in Box 3–1. Box 3–2 takes you through the steps for checking for atrial and ventricular hypertrophy with a 12-lead ECG. Figure 3–2 represents a normal 12-lead ECG.

## Box 3–1 Seven-Step Procedure for Interpreting the 12-Lead Electrocardiogram

**Step One:** What is the heart rate?

**Step Two:** What is the ECG rhythm? This can be determined with the rhythm strips on the lower half of the ECG report.

**Step Three:** What is the PRI?

If longer than 0.20 sec, consider AV block

If shorter than 0.20 sec, consider Lown–Ganong–Levine or Wolff–Parkinson–White (LGL/WPW) syndrome

**Step Four:** What is the width of the QRS complex?

A width > 0.12 sec indicates BBB, check leads $V_1$ to $V_6$

An ST and T-wave (STTW) or "check-mark" appearance in lead $V_1$ indicates right BBB; an STTW appearance in lead V6 indicates left BBB

**Step Five:** What is the mean ventricular axis?

Are both leads I and II more positive than negative? This is a normal axis. If not, go to Lead III

If Lead III is negative, read left axis deviation (LAD) = left anterior hemiblock (LAHB)

If Lead III is positive; read right axis deviation (RAD) = left posterior hemiblock (LPHB)

RAD with R > s in lead $V_1$ = right ventricular hypertrophy (RVH)

**Step Six:** Does the ECG show the changes of ischemia? Check all three lead groups.

Lead groups:

- I and aVL represent lateral heart tissue (left ventricle)
- II, III, and aVF represent the inferior part of the heart (changes in two of these three leads indicate that the inferior wall of the left ventricle is involved)
- $V_1$ to $V_6$ represent anterior heart activity

Are there any flat or inverted T waves? These indicate acute ischemia.

Are the ST segments within 1 mm of the baseline? This is an acute injury pattern.

Are there any pathological Q waves (wide or deep)? These indicate infarction.

- Check the V leads (R:S ratio). Is there normal progression of the R:S waves in leads $V_1$ through $V_6$? If there is not progression, this is indicative of an infarction.
- Q in positive lead indicates an infarct)

*Continued*

*Consider any of the foregoing changes in two or more leads of the same lead group as evidence of MI

Presence of a pathological Q wave alone with no acute S-T or T wave changes indicates an old injury or a healed transmural MI. ECG Changes seen in a Q wave MI

1. S-T segment elevates within the first hour following the MI
2. Q wave changes appear within the first 6 hours post MI
3. T wave inversion begins within the first 6 hours post MI
4. S-T segment normalizes within 7 days
5. T wave normalizes within 6 weeks of the MI
6. Q wave changes remain forever

**Step Seven:** What is the progression pattern for the anterior V1-6 leads?

$V_1$ = right ventricle

$V_2$, $V_3$, $V_4$ = anteroseptal leads

$V_5$ and $V_6$ = anterolateral leads

Check the R-wave progression (or the R:S ratio). The R wave progression pattern should begin with a dominant, high voltage S wave in $V_1$, which progressively diminishes in voltage until the $V_6$ lead. The R wave begins in the $V_1$ lead at its lowest voltage and progressively increases voltage through each of the V leads until it is the dominant lead in the $V_6$ lead. If there are significant changes in two or more contiguous leads of the V-leads, you can infer that the anterior wall of the left ventricle is involved.

---

Box 3–2 **Identifying Atrial and Ventricular Hypertrophy With a 12-Lead Electrocardiogram**

**ATRIAL HYPERTROPHY**

Check the P waves. Imagine that the first half of the P wave represents the right atrium and the second half the left atrium. If there is left atrial hypertrophy, the first half of the P wave will be larger than the second half, thus with a tall and peaked appearance.

• If the left atrium is hypertrophied, the second half of the P wave will be broad and notched

• Causes of right atrial enlargement: Chronic pulmonary disease, RVH, pulmonary valvular diseases, and congenital heart problems (pulmonary stenosis [PS], atrial septal defect [ASD], tetralogy of Fallot [TF])

• Causes of left atrial enlargement: Diseased mitral valve, CHF, valvular heart disease, hypertensive heart disease

## Box 3–2 Identifying Atrial and Ventricular Hypertrophy With a 12-Lead Electrocardiogram—cont'd

**VENTRICULAR HYPERTROPHY**

Ventricular strain patterns are noted in leads $V_1$ to $V_6$; hypertrophy causes changes in leads $V_1$ and $V_6$.

- Right ventricular hypertrophy: (1) QRS shift toward RAD; (2) positive deflection in RV lead ($V_1$); and (3) RV strain pattern in lead $V_1$ (sloping S-T segment). Causes: Congenital heart disease (PS, ASD, TF), long-term COPD, mitral stenosis, sometimes pulmonary embolism
- Left ventricular hypertrophy: Extreme voltage in leads $V_1$ and $V_6$
  - (1) Abnormally deep S waves in lead $V_1$ and very tall R waves in lead $V_6$ (total of deflections = 35 mm or more); (2) LV strain pattern in leads $V_5$ and $V_6$; and (3) an R wave in lead aVL that is 13 mm or taller. Causes are hypertensive heart disease and valvular heart disease.

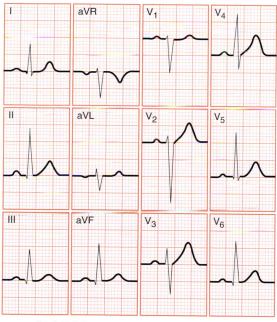

**FIGURE 3-2:** Normal 12-lead ECG.

## Electrocardiographic Basics
- One small square = 0.04 sec horizontally and 1 mm vertically
- One large square = 0.20 sec horizontally and 5 mm vertically
- PR interval (PRI) = 0.12 to 0.20 sec (within one large square); a longer time = atrioventricular (AV) block
- QRS interval = 0.04 to 0.10 sec (less than three small squares); an interval >3 small squares = bundle-branch block (BBB)
- ST interval = within 1 mm of baseline

Young, athletic males may have high-voltage ECG patterns but no left-ventricular (LV) strain pattern. High-voltage readings are related to the physiological nearness of the heart to the chest wall in these young athletes. Box 3–3 provides pearls for interpreting the ECG.

The 12-lead ECG provides clinical information that identifies specific regions of the heart muscle involved in an ischemic event or injury. The injury can be identified in a primary lead, but reciprocal changes may be evident in areas recorded by opposite leads. Table 3–13 demonstrates the use of lead interpretation for identifying specific areas of cardiac injury.

---

### Box 3–3 Pearls in Electrocardiographic Interpretation

The following pearls may aid the NP in the interpretation of the 12-lead ECG:
- Digitalis may produce a scooping of the ST wave because of a reduced repolarization time of the ventricles
- Quinidine prolongs ventricular repolarization and may flatten the T wave
- An elevated potassium level produces a tented T wave, and as the $K^+$ concentration rises, the PRI may get longer and the P waves get smaller or disappear, progressing to a widened QRS
- Effects of a decreased potassium level are ST-segment depression, a prominent U wave, and a small T wave
- Hypercalcemia will present as a short Q–T interval
- Hypocalcemia produces a long Q–T interval
- Pericarditis produces diffuse ischemic changes in all lead groups
- Pericardial effusion produces a low-voltage ECG
- Other causes of a low-voltage EKG are diffuse myocardial injury, infiltration of heart tissue (amyloidosis), obesity, COPD, CHF

Kernick, I. (2007) How to read that 12 lead EKG: A primer for electrocardiographic interpretation using the 12 lead EKG Course Workbook. Shreveport, LA: CHRISTUS Schumpert Health System. Used with permission.

## Table 3–13 Interpretive Summary of Findings in Electrocardiographic Leads

| WALL | LEAD | CHANGES IN ECG | ARTERY | RECIPROCAL |
|------|------|------|--------|------------|
| Inferior | II, III, aVF | Q, S–T, T | RCA | I, aVL |
| Lateral | I, aVL, V$_5$, V$_6$ | Q, S–T, T | Circumflex | V1, V3 |
| Anterior | V$_1$-V$_4$, I, aVL | Q, S–T, T | LCA | II, III, aVF |
| Posterior | V$_1$, V$_2$ | R>S, S–T, T↓ | RCA, Circumflex | II, III, aVF |
| Apical | V$_3$, V$_4$, V$_5$, V$_6$ | Q, S–T, T | LAD, RCA | II, III, aVF |
| Anterolateral | I, aVL, V$_5$, V$_6$ | Q, S–T, T | LAD, Circumflex | II, III, aVF |
| Anteroseptal | V$_1$, V$_2$, V$_3$, V$_4$ | Q, S–T, T No R in V$_1$ | LAD | II, III, aVF |

## Echocardiography

An echocardiogram can provide diagnostic information related to heart size and heart-wall thickness, the pumping strength of the heart, valve leakage and valvular abnormalities, degrees of vascular obstruction, and pressure gradients. Typically, patients who present with the following symptoms are candidates for an echocardiogram:

- Heart disease
- Murmurs
- Palpitations
- Hypertension
- Stroke
- Heart-valvular disease
- Suspected or known congenital heart diseases
- Cardiac tamponade
- Pericardial effusion

## Spirometry

Spirometry is a "gold standard" diagnostic tool for evaluating and monitoring asthma and COPD. This test provides an objective measure of the patient's ability to move air in and out of the lungs at a given point in time. Sequential spirometric measurements during office visits can allow the clinician to monitor progress in the treatment of asthma and COPD. Table 3–14 provides normal spirometric values.

## Indications and Contraindications

Indications for spirometry include:
- Detecting and monitoring pulmonary disease
- Chest pain, orthopnea
- Cough
- Wheezing, dyspnea
- Cyanosis
- Diminished breath sounds
- Finger clubbing
- Abnormal blood gas readings
- Pulmonary diseases
- History of smoking in patients age 45 years and older

Contraindications for spirometry testing include:
- Hemoptysis
- Nausea or vomiting
- Pneumothorax
- Recent abdominal, thoracic, or eye surgery
- Recent MI or unstable angina
- Thoracic aneurysm

A healthy person should achieve a forced expiratory volume in 1 sec ($FEV_1$) of 80% of the predicted value for the individual's age and sex. This declines with airway obstruction and increases when adequate treatment has been provided. The ratio of $FEV_1$ to forced ventilatory capacity

| Table 3–14 **Normal Values for In-Office Spirometry** | |
| --- | --- |
| TEST | NORMAL VALUES |
| $FEV_1$ | 80%–120% predicted |
| FVC | 80%–120% predicted |
| Absolute $FEV_1$/FVC | Within 5% of predicted |
| TLC | 80%–120% predicted |
| FRC | 75%–120% predicted |

(FEV$_1$/FVC) is particularly sensitive for the identification of mild or early-stage COPD.

The two most common patterns seen in spirometry are those of respiratory obstructive diseases and respiratory restrictive diseases. Patterns of obstructive disease are generally seen in patients who have difficulty exhaling adequately. Patterns of restrictive disease are typical in patients with limited lung capacity, such as those with cystic fibrosis, lung resections, severe scoliosis, and scarring of lung tissue. A three-step approach to interpreting spirometric readings is provided in Box 3–4.

When you evaluate the results of spirometric tests, first confirm the patient's identification information, then review the spirometric data for FEV$_1$ and FVC. If the numbers for FVC and FEV$_1$ exceed 80% of the predicted values, the results are interpreted as normal. Review the flow-versus-volume curve on the spirograph to ascertain the shape of the curve and the length of the curve line.

Normal spirometric flow chart results will exhibit:

- Smooth lines, resembling a sail that rises rapidly to a sharp peak and descends in a straight line or at a 45-degree angle
- An expiratory time >6 sec
- A rapid peaking of the peak expiratory flow (PEF) rate

**COACH CONSULT**

The absolute FEV$_1$/FVC ratio differentiates obstructive from restrictive spirometry patterns:

- In obstructive diseases, the FEV$_1$/FVC ratio is lower than the lowest level predicted. Examples of this would include asthma or COPD
- In restrictive diseases, the FEV$_1$/FVC is not lower than the predicted lowest level, but the FVC is lower than predicted

---

### Box 3–4 Interpreting In-Office Spirometry Results

**Step One:** Does the flow-volume curve demonstrate the patient's best effort? There should be a sharp peak and smooth descents on the flow–volume curve, with a flat plateau at the end of the time curve.

**Step Two:** Are the FVC and FEV$_1$ >80% predicted? Is the FEV$_1$/FVC ratio >70 to 80% of the predicted value? If the answer is yes, the spirometric results are normal.

**Step Three:** If the results are abnormal, determine whether the results indicate obstructive or restrictive airway disease.

- An FEV$_1$/FVC ratio <70% in adults or <80% in children indicates obstructive disease (asthma, COPD). An FEV$_1$ <80% confirms obstructive disease.
- If the FVC is <80% predicted and the FEV$_1$/FVC is >70% predicted, a restrictive disease pattern is identified. In this case the FEV$_1$ can be low or normal.

To determine whether an obstructive pattern is reversible, administer an inhaled short-acting- beta 2 agonist, preferably with a spacer or a nebulizer. Have the patient wait 20 to 30 min and repeat the spirometry test. An increase in the $FEV_1$ of 12% above the initial reading is indicative that the obstructive airway disease is reversible.

Figures 3–3 and 3–4 show the results of spirometric examinations of a 56-year-old woman with chronic bronchitis. The pattern is clearly that of an obstructive airway disease, with a reduced expiratory time; the FVC and the FEV are less than 80% of their predicted values.

## Tympanograms

A tympanogram is a useful in-office test for helping to differentiate between otitis media (OM) and other diseases of the ear canal. It is simple to perform and rapid. When you interpret a tympanogram, you must consider three features of the curve:

1. Compliance
2. Middle ear pressure
3. Shape of the curve

### Features of the Office Tympanogram

The features of the tympanogram allow the clinician to make an accurate diagnosis on the basis of its physical appearance. The peak of the tympanograph curve and its location on the chart reveal whether abnormalities are present. The three essential components of the tympanogram are compliance of the TM, middle ear pressure, and the shape of the peak.

- Compliance of the TM is determined by measuring the height of the peak of the curve. The peak is defined as:
  - High: >0.5 mL
  - Intermediate: >0.2 to <0.5 mL
  - Low: <0.2 mL
- Middle ear pressure: The TM is most compliant when the middle ear pressure is equal to the pressure in the external ear canal. The middle ear pressure classified as:
  - Normal: –100 to +50 daPa

**ALERT**

Tympanograms are not reliable in children 7 months of age or younger because of the highly compliant nature of the external ear canal.

**COACH CONSULT**

- Always correlate test results with clinical evidence from your physical examination of the ear canal and tympanic membrane
- Always remember to check for motility of the tympanic membrane (TM) by using the insufflator bulb attached to your otoscope

Patient ID: 000
Age: 56  Height: 62  Weight: 200
Sex: Female  Race Correction: 100
Test Date: 07/16/2008
Calibration Date: 08/16/2005
Software Revision: 2.01  HdT/V 2-7370/84
Notes: BTPS – 1.035
   Flow sensor used with filter
   Normals: Knudson, Knudson
   Interpretation Algorithm: ATS

Test Results — Best Test Report

| Test | Pred | Act 1 | %<br>Pred |
|---|---|---|---|
| FVC | 2.85 | 1.88 | 66% |
| FEV1 | 2.34 | 1.64 | 71% |
| FEV1/FVC | 82% | 87% | 107% |
| FEF25–75 | 2.59 | 2.07 | 80% |
| FEFMAX | 5.6 | 3.8 | 68% |
| FEV3 | 2.71 | 1.87 | 70% |
| MMET | 0.55 | 0.50 | 91% |
| ET | | 3.5 | |
| BESTFVC | 2.85 | 1.88 | 66% |
| BESTFEV1 | 2.34 | 1.64 | 71% |

Baseline Maneuvers
   Accepted:   3
   The maneuvers are reproducible
MODERATE RESTRICTION
Patient's Lung Age: 78
COPD Risk – Need smoking history

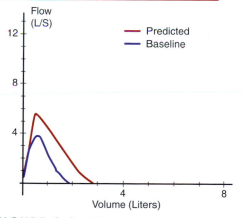

FIGURE 3-3: Office spirometry report, part one.

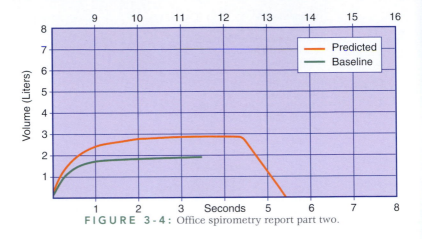

**FIGURE 3-4:** Office spirometry report part two.

- High negative: < –100 daPa
- High positive: > +50 daPa
- Peak shape: This may be sharp, rounded, or flat. The peak will be sharp in the absence of middle ear effusion and flat in the presence of effusion.

Figure 3–5 is an example of a normal tympanogram. Note how the curves for each ear are situated within the bars and the well-rounded peak, representing a normal examination.

## Interpreting Tympanogram Results

Several types and subtypes of diagnoses can be made by evaluating the results of a tympanogram. The types of diagnoses are differentiated by peak pressures and compliance data into the following categories:

- Type A Normal
  - Peak pressure curve between +50 and –150 daPA
  - Peak compliance between 0.2 and 1.8 mL $H_2O$
- Type A Shallow
  - Peak pressure normal, low compliance
  - Possible scarring of the TM (< 0.2mL $H_2O$)
- Type Ad
  - Very high peaks indicating increased middle ear pressures
- Type B (TM retracted, poor motility)
  - Peak absent or poorly defined (> –0.200 mL $H_2O$)

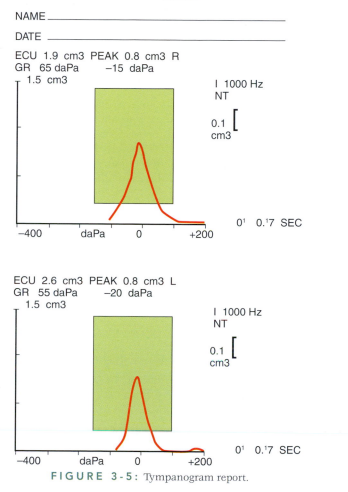

NAME _____

DATE _____

ECU 1.9 cm3 PEAK 0.8 cm3 R
GR 65 daPa        −15 daPa

1.5 cm3

I 1000 Hz
NT

0.1 [
cm3

0¹  0.¹7  SEC

−400        daPa        0        +200

ECU 2.6 cm3 PEAK 0.8 cm3 L
GR 55 daPa        −20 daPa

1.5 cm3

I 1000 Hz
NT

0.1 [
cm3

0¹  0.¹7  SEC

−400        daPa        0        +200

**F I G U R E   3 - 5 :** Tympanogram report.

- Compliance below normal
- May be otitis media
- Other causes: Occlusion of the ear canal with cerumen,
  perforation of the TM

- Type C
  - A clear peak is evident, but on the negative side of the chart (negative middle ear pressure), and compliance is normal
  - May indicate a eustachian tube dysfunction or a developing or resolving case of OM

## Monofilament Testing in Diabetic Neuropathy

The 10-g nylon monofilament evaluation of diabetic neuropathy involves a 10-point check of each foot. The patient must respond "yes" to pressure exerted when the monofilament is pressed just enough to bend it at each of the 10 sites on the foot. Ten points include the pads of toes 1, 3, and 5; three points occur across the pad of the foot; two points across the arch, one on the heel, and one point on the top of the foot between the first and second toes.

## Bone Densitometry

### T Scores and Z Scores

A T score is a comparison of the patient's bone density with that of a healthy 30-year-old of the same sex and ethnicity as the patient. Z scores utilize standard deviations to allow for differences in height, weight, and other variables. Z scores are reported for premenopausal women, men younger than age 50 years, and children.

The risk of a hip fracture is 1.5 to 2.5 times greater for every increase of 1 standard deviation (SD) in the hip T score. Hip T scores have fewer artifactual errors than do lumbar scores. The following T-score ranges indicate the degree of bone density:

- Normal: –1.0 or higher
- Osteopenia: < -1.0 to > –2.5
- Osteoporosis: –2.5 or lower

# 4 Skin and Wound Care

# CHAPTER 4

# Skin and Wound Care

A variety of wounds require medical interventions, from simple laceration repair to intensive wound care involving debridement, packing, and long-term wound care management. This chapter focuses on basic wound management, including wound assessment, wound cleansing, wound measurement, wound packing, wound dressings, and conservative wound debridement. Discussions of the management of skin wounds infected with methicillin-resistant *Staphylococcus aureus* (MRSA) and simple laceration repair are also included in the chapter.

## Basic Wound Care for Primary Care Settings

As with the treatment of any body system in health care, assessment is the initial step in wound care. Assessment and documentation of wounds throughout the healing process are critical to achieving positive outcomes in patient care. Initial wound assessment provides a baseline for monitoring the effectiveness of wound-care strategies and sequential follow-up is useful for assessing this effectiveness.

### Wound Assessment

Many wounds take considerable time and effort to heal. Initial and follow-up wound assessments are critical to effective healing. The NP should adopt a consistent pattern of wound assessment that considers all factors relevant to wound healing. When assessing a wound, include the following factors:

- Location of the wound, with reference to anatomical landmarks
- Accurate measurement of the wound size, including length, width, depth, and tunneling
- Appearance of the wound bed

- Appearance of skin surrounding the wound
- Any wound drainage, including amount, color, odor, and consistency
- Reports of pain or tenderness, which may indicate infection, tunneling, tissue destruction, or vascular insufficiency
- Skin temperature
- Wound classification, including:
  - Staging, as for decubitus pressure ulcers
  - Classification by depth as partial thickness or full thickness
  - Classification by color as red, yellow, or black
  - Distinction among arterial, diabetic, and venous ulcerations.

Table 4–1 provides differential descriptions of arterial, diabetic, and venous ulcerations. Figure 4–1 shows an arterial wound, and Figure 4–2 shows a venous ulceration.

## Table 4–1 Differentiating Arterial, Diabetic, and Venous Ulcers

| VARIABLE | ARTERIAL ULCERS | DIABETIC ULCERS | VENOUS ULCERS |
|---|---|---|---|
| Location | Between toes or tips of toes<br>Lateral malleolus<br>Trauma sites from footwear | Plantar aspect of foot<br>Over metatarsal head<br>Under heel | Medial lower leg and ankle<br>On malleolar area |
| Patient assessment | Thin, shiny skin<br>Hair loss<br>Thick toenails<br>Pallor on elevation<br>Cyanosis<br>Temperature decreased<br>Diminished or absent pulses | Diminished or absent foot sensation<br>Palpable pulses<br>Foot warm<br>May have foot deformities | Edema<br>Dry, thin, scaly skin<br>Dilated superficial veins<br>Hyperpigmentation<br>Possible dermatitis |
| Wound characteristics | Even wound margins<br>Necrosis<br>Deep, pale wound bed<br>Blanched or purpuric skin surrounding<br>Pain<br>Cellulitis<br>Minimal exudation | Deep wound bed<br>Wound margins even<br>Cellulitis<br>Granular tissue may be present<br>Small to moderate exudation | Wound margins irregular<br>Ruddy, granular tissue<br>Superficial wound<br>Some pain<br>Moderate to heavy exudation |

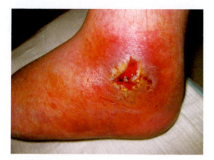

FIGURE 4-1: Arterial wound.

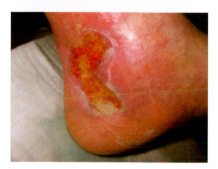

FIGURE 4-2: Venous wound.

## Wound Cleansing

Wound cleansing is essential for removing bacteria and debris from the wound bed before treating and dressing a wound. Gentle probing of a new wound is imperative to ascertain that all foreign objects have been removed before beginning wound treatment. Wounds should also be cleansed before each new change of dressing. Steps involved in wound cleansing are:

- Positioning the patient for comfort and privacy
- Setting up equipment and supplies for wound cleansing
- Having a means for disposing of soiled dressings and supplies
- With gloved hands, removing and discarding old dressings
- Changing gloves
- Inspecting the wound and noting the color, amount, and odor of any drainage
- Folding a sterile 4x4-in. piece of gauze and saturating it with wound cleansing solution (normal saline [NS])

- When cleansing a wound, moving from the least contaminated to the most contaminated areas in concentric circles, starting directly over the wound and moving outward in larger circles. Discard the soiled gauze and repeat the cleansing with a new sterile gauze, doing this as many times as needed until the entire wound is cleansed
- Measuring the perimeter of the wound with a disposable measuring device, and recording measurements from the widest section of the wound
- Measuring the depth of the wound at its deepest point
- Preparing to apply the appropriate topical dressings, and securing them with tape or netting. A comparison of appropriate dressings is provided in Table 4–2

Some wounds will require irrigation to cleanse the tissues and remove debris. This is especially true for open wounds in which foreign objects may have entered the wound bed. Commercial wound cleansers or NS can

### Table 4–2 Comparison of Wound Dressings

| DRESSING TYPE | INDICATIONS FOR USE | ADVANTAGES | DISADVANTAGES |
| --- | --- | --- | --- |
| Alginate | Wounds with moderate to heavy drainage Wounds with tunneling Infected wounds | Dressing turns to gel as it absorbs moisture Holds up to 20 times its own weight in fluid Can be cut to fit wound | May need irrigation to remove it from wound Requires a secondary dressing May dehydrate wound |
| Antimicrobial | Infected wounds Draining wounds Nonhealing wounds Minimally to heavily draining wounds | Forms: Transparent dressings, gauze, foams, absorptive fillers Reduces and prevents infection Works against a broad spectrum of organisms | May produce a hypersensitivity reaction May sting May contribute to development of resistance to antibiotics |
| Biological | Ulcers of varying thicknesses Skin grafting donor sites Burns | Temporary dressings, function like skin grafts Reduces healing time Prevents infection and fluid loss Eases discomfort | May cause allergic reactions May require a secondary dressing |

## Table 4–2 Comparison of Wound Dressings—cont'd

| DRESSING TYPE | INDICATIONS FOR USE | ADVANTAGES | DISADVANTAGES |
|---|---|---|---|
| Collagen dressings (made with bovine or equine collagen) | Chronic, nonhealing, granulated wound beds<br>Wounds with tunneling | Forms: Gel, granules, or sheet forms<br>Works well on chronic but clean wounds<br>Can be used on draining wounds | Possible allergic reactions<br>Require secondary dressings<br>Not for use on third-degree burns or wounds with dry beds |
| Composite | Primary or secondary dressing on draining wounds<br>IV or central line dressing | Multiple sizes/shapes | May dry the wound bed<br>Cannot be cut to fit<br>No for use on third-degree burns |
| Contact layer | Prevents other dressing from sticking to wound surface | Less pain with dressing changes<br>Cut to fit<br>Use with topical medications | Requires secondary dressing<br>Not for use on third-degree burns<br>Not for use with wound tunneling |
| Foam | Wounds with minimal drainage | Nonadherent<br>Use on infected wounds<br>Can be used with draining wounds | May require a secondary dressing<br>Not for nondraining wounds<br>May cause maceration if not changed regularly |
| Hydrocolloid | Wounds with minimal to moderate drainage | No sticking to wound<br>Keeps moisture<br>Change 2–3 times/week<br>Easy removal<br>Forms: Sheets, powder, gel | Not for use on burns or dry wounds<br>Can cause maceration |
| Hydrogel | Dry wounds<br>Minimally draining wounds<br>Wounds with necrosis or sloughing | Forms: Sheets, gel<br>Cooling to wound, eases pain | Requires a secondary dressing<br>Can macerate surrounding skin<br>Daily dressing changes |

be used for irrigation. Irrigation solution should be allowed to reach room temperature before being used in a wound. Never use wound irrigation solutions that have been open for more than 24 hours if they are kept in the patient's personal wound-care supplies. Supplies and equipment required for wound irrigation, and their uses, include:

- Wound irrigation solution
- Acetic acid, which is effective against *Pseudomonas aeruginosa* in superficial wounds
- Hydrogen peroxide, which has an effervescent action that provides mechanical cleansing and debridement
- Povidone iodine preparations, for use on intact skin or on small, clean wounds for broad-spectrum cleansing
- Sodium hypochlorite solutions, which is effective against *Staphylococcus* and *Streptococcus* species, controls odor, and dissolves necrotic tissue
- Sterile gloves
- Protective eyewear and a gown
- Wound-care materials following irrigation
- A 35-mL piston syringe with a 19-gauge needle or catheter

When cleansing a wound, gently instill a slow, steady stream of solution into it. Continue to irrigate until you have administered the prescribed amount of solution or the drainage from the wound is clear. After you have finished with the cleansing, dispose of all soiled dressings, catheters, and syringes.

## Wound Measurement

Sequential wound measurements provide objective measures of progress in wound healing. In addition to measuring the width, length, and depth of a wound, it is essential to determine the presence and extent of any wound tunneling. Tunneling, or undermining, is tissue destruction underlying the skin in the periphery of the wound. Tunneling may be more extensive in one part of the wound than in another part. It is important to monitor increases or decreases in tunneling with each dressing change. Tunneling can be measured by using the following steps:

- Put on sterile gloves
- Gently probe the wound bed and edges with a sterile cotton-tip applicator to identify tunneling
- Gently insert the cotton-tip applicator into the wound in the direction of the tunneling, advancing to the point where the tunneling ends

- Use the cotton-tip applicator to measure the point from the wound edge to the tip of the applicator after the applicator has been advanced to the full extent of the tunneling. Measure this distance with a centimeter ruler to identify the amount of tunneling present.

## Wound Packing

Wound packing is a form of mechanical debridement. Most infected wounds will require packing with appropriate packing materials to facilitate effective wound drainage and optimum wound healing. Wound packing materials can include gauze saturated with iodoform or another sterilizing agent or sterile gauze soaked with NS. Steps for wound packing are:

- Prepare wound packing and dressing supplies and equipment
- Wash hands and put on sterile gloves
- Remove old packing materials from the wound
- Cleanse the wound per protocol
- Soak sterile gauze in sterile NS and wring out until slightly moist
- With sterile forceps, loosely pack the gauze into the wound bed, covering the wound surface and edges
- Avoid overpacking the wound, to prevent excessive pressure on the wound bed
- Apply the appropriate topical dressing and use synthetic or non-woven gauze to secure the primary dressing

## Wound Dressings

Selection of wound dressings is critical to promoting effective wound healing. The amount of moisture or lack of moisture in a wound dictates the type of wound dressing required to maximize healing.

The purposes of wound dressings are to:

- Protect the wound from bacteria and trauma
- Control bleeding or edema, which may occur in the wound site
- Medicate the wound bed
- Absorb drainage from the wound bed
- Débride necrotic tissue
- Fill or pack the wound
- Protect the skin surrounding the wound

**COACH CONSULT**

The cardinal rule of wound dressings is to keep moist tissues moist and dry tissues dry.

Wound dressings are categorized by their moisture-related properties. More than 2,000 wound-care products are currently on the market, making wound-dressing decisions difficult. It is best to base the selection of wound-care products on the properties of the products within a category of product types, such as antimicrobial dressings or biological dressings. Table 4–2 compares the properties of wound dressings in different categories.

## Wound Debridement

Wound debridement removes unhealthy or necrotic tissue from the wound bed to enable the remaining tissues to heal effectively. The NP should consider wound debridement if the wound bed contains any necrotic tissue. Several types of wound debridement can be done, including:

- Autolytic debridement: Dissolves necrotic tissue by using the body's enzymes and defense mechanisms. There are many dressings designed to promote autolysis. Examples of products for autolytic debridement include Accuzyme® Papain Urea Débriding Ointment, which can be used to débride necrotic tissue from decubitus ulcers, diabetic ulcers, burns, postoperative wounds, and from pilonidal cysts, carbuncles, and other infected wound areas. Avoid contact of the ointment with the eyes. The ointment is applied in the following manner:
  - Cleanse the wound with NS. Do not use hydrogen peroxide; it may inactivate the papain product
  - Apply the ointment directly to the wound
  - Cover the wound with a dressing
  - Reapply the ointment one or two times daily
  - Flush the wound with NS to remove any accumulation of liquefied necrotic material before reapplying the débriding ointment
- Surgical debridement: Clears necrotic tissue surgically, leaving a clean wound bed. This debridement process requires a surgeon's expertise for removing necrotic tissue with a sharp instrument or a laser. This can be done at the bedside or in an operating room, depending on the extent of debridement indicated
- Mechanical debridement: Includes hydrotherapy, conservative sharp debridement, pulsatile lavage, and wet-to-dry dressings. To apply a wet-to-dry dressing, follow these steps:
  - Moisten gauze with a solution such as NS and wring it out until it is slightly moist
  - Fluff the gauze completely and place it over the wound bed
  - Remove the dressing when it is almost dry. Tissue debris and drainage will adhere to the gauze

# Wound Healing

Wound repair occurs by primary intention, secondary intention, and tertiary intention; each depends on a multitude of local and systemic factors. Healing by primary intention occurs in acute wounds that are closed with the skin edges being approximated. These wounds have a lower risk of infection, experience very little tissue loss, and heal with minimal scarring within 7 to 14 days. Wounds that heal by secondary intention tend to be more chronic, such as pressure ulcers. These wounds do involve tissue loss, have an increased risk of infection, and require more time for healing. Wounds that heal by tertiary intention are typically surgical wounds left open for 4 to 5 days to allow resolution of infection or edema and then closed with sutures or staples.

Some factors that can impede the progress of wound healing include:

- Sustained pressure on the wound site, affecting capillary blood flow
- A wound environment that lacks adequate moisture, which tends to cause formation of a scab or crust, impeding wound healing
- Edema at the wound site, which diminishes oxygen transport to the wound tissues
- Systemic or local infection delaying wound healing
- Necrosis, in the form of eschar or slough, which impedes healing
- Older age, which tends to be accompanied by slower wound healing owing to compromise of the immune system and diminished hydration
- Obesity, which impedes wound healing because of impaired circulation in adipose tissues
- Chronic disease states that delay wound healing
- Poor nutritional status
- A decreased blood supply, especially to lower extremities

Several complications are possible in wound healing. Any of them can impede the progress of healing. They are:

- Infection, if unchecked, possibly leading to osteomyelitis or sepsis
- Hemorrhage
- Dehiscence
- Evisceration
- Fistula

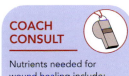

**COACH CONSULT**

Nutrients needed for wound healing include:
- Proteins
- Carbohydrates
- Fats
- Vitamins A, C, and K
- Pyridoxine, riboflavin, and thiamine
- Copper
- Iron
- Zinc

# Wounds Infected With Methicillin-Resistant *Staphylococcus aureus*

Infections with MRSA are becoming more common across the United States. The organism can be found on the skin of nearly 20% of healthy persons, yet over the past decade it has become an emerging agent of serious soft-tissue infections.

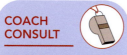

**COACH CONSULT**

Photographs of wounds taken sequentially throughout the healing process provide excellent documentation of the state and progress of healing. Consider taking such photographs with a digital camera that has grid lines.

MRSA can cause infections of the skin, soft tissues, bone, joints, blood, and heart. Skin and soft-tissue infections are the most commonly identified as harboring MRSA. These include:

- Cellulitis
- Impetigo
- Folliculitis
- Furunculosis
- Carbuncle
- Abscess
- Infected lacerations

The U.S. Centers for Disease Control and Prevention (CDC) has published strategies for the clinical management of skin infections caused by MRSA. The major points in the CDC strategies are:

- Incise and drain wounds
  - In the case of moderate furuncles, abscesses, and septic joints
  - Consider applying moist heat to small furuncles, which may promote their drainage
- Collect specimens from wound-drainage fluids for culture and sensitivity studies
- Select appropriate antibiotic regimens to target *S. aureus*, using:
  - Cephalexin or dicloxacillin
  - Other options, consisting of clindamycin, doxycycline, minocycline, trimethoprim–sulfamethoxazole, or linezolid
  - Check local susceptibility patterns when selecting an antibiotic
- Hospitalize patients with signs and symptoms of severe illness
- Teach patients good hygiene, including handwashing and disposal of contaminated bandages
- Teach patients about decolonization for their household members and close contacts, with:
  - Nasal mupirocin, which may also be used on fingernails and toenails daily

- Antiseptic body washes
- Avoidance of close contact with daycare centers or athletic practice facilities until wounds are healed
- Teach prevention to limit the spread of MRSA, by:
  - Handwashing with antimicrobial soap
  - Wearing gloves to manage wounds
  - Disposing of contaminated dressings and any articles contaminated with blood, nasal discharge, urine, or pus
  - Cleaning surfaces with diluted bleach solution consisting of 1 tablespoon of bleach in 1 quart of water
  - Laundering any contaminated linens in hot water and bleach

## Simple Laceration Repair

Trauma-induced lacerations are classified into four categories:

1. Clean
2. Clean-contaminated
3. Contaminated
4. Dirty or infected

Most fresh trauma injuries to soft tissue are considered contaminated wounds. Microorganisms multiply so rapidly that within 6 hours a contaminated wound may become an infected wound. Treatment guidelines related to the duration of a laceration are:

- Most lacerations may be closed if they are less than 6 hours old
- Lacerations of the face, scalp, and fingers may be closed within 24 hours if copious irrigation is completed before wound closure
- Any wound older than 24 hours should not be closed because of the increased risk of infection

Tetanus prophylaxis should be provided if the patient has not been vaccinated against tetanus in the past 5 years. If the patient was vaccinated but this was clearly done more than 5 years ago, administer Td toxoid (dose: 0.5 mL).

**COACH CONSULT**

Take extra caution to gently probe any trauma-induced laceration, particularly those with a poor history of how they occurred. Cases of wound infections have been reported when foreign objects such as bullet fragments, dirt, gravel, or other such items have not been removed from the wound bed before suturing.

**COACH CONSULT**

When selecting suture size and tensile strength, remember that size 5-0 (00000) is smaller in diameter than size 4-0. Knot tensile strength is the force in pounds that the suture can withstand before it breaks when knotted.

Steps in simple laceration repair include:

- Cleansing the wound and gently probing it for foreign objects
- Determining whether trauma has caused damage to nerves and tendons in the wound bed area
- Preparing equipment and supplies:
  - Sutures: Determine the size and type of sutures you will need according to the type of the wound. Table 4–3 provides specific information on suture selection
  - Needle holders, scissors, pick ups
  - Anesthetic solution

### Table 4–3 Selection of Suture Type and Size by Laceration Location

| LOCATION | SUTURE TYPE | SUTURE SIZE | DURATION (DAYS) |
|---|---|---|---|
| Scalp | Nylon | 3-0 to 5-0 | 7 |
| Eyelid | Prolene or silk | 6-0 to 7-0 | 3–5 |
| Conjunctiva | Plain gut | 7-0 to 8-0 | Absorbed |
| Face | Nylon | 5-0 to 7-0 | 3–5 |
| Mucus membranes | Plain or chromic gut | 3-0 to 5-0 | Absorbed |
| Near joints | Nylon | 4-0 to 6-0 | 10–14 |
| Chest | Nylon | 3-0 to 5-0 | 7–10 |
| Abdomen | Nylon | 3-0 to 5-0 | 7–10 |
| Arm | Nylon | 3-0 to 5-0 | 7–10 |
| Leg | Nylon | 3-0 to 5-0 | 7–10 |
| Fingertip | Nylon | 5-0 to 6-0 | 10–12 |
| Foot/toe | Nylon | 4-0 to 5-0 | 1–14 |
| Subcutaneous tissue | Dexon or Vicryl | 3-0 to 5-0 | Absorbed |
| Muscle | Dexon or Vicryl | 3-0 to 5-0 | Absorbed |
| Back | Nylon | 3-0 to 5-0 | 12–14 |

- Gloves
- Sterile field
- Dressings, tape

## Suture Technique

- Interrupted, individual stitches. Advantages:
  - More secure closure
  - May be used if wound is infected
- Continuous, running stitches. Advantages:
  - Allows rapid placement of sutures
  - Strong because tension is distributed evenly along the length of the suture strand
- Subcuticular stitches. Advantages:
  - In the dermis, beneath the epithelial layer
  - Short, lateral stitches for the full length of the wound
  - Helps to minimize scarring and hold skin edges in close approximation

Figure 4–3 provides an example of wound healing with and without sutures.

### ALERT

Avoid use of epinephrine on the fingers, toes, nose, and penis. Critical pointers for particular anesthetic solution include:
- Procaine: Do not exceed 1000 mg in an adult
- Lidocaine: Do not exceed 500 mg in an adult
- Bupivacaine: Do not exceed 200 mg in an adult
- Mepivacaine: Do not exceed 500 mg in an adult
- Tetracaine: Do not exceed 50 mg in an adult

### COACH CONSULT

If a patient presents with a laceration on the hand or forearm, carefully check all digits for range of motion and muscle strength before suturing. Lacerations that damage tendons in these areas require orthopedic consultation for effective wound closure and healing.

## (a) Primary intention

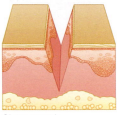
Clean wound

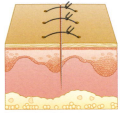
Sutured early

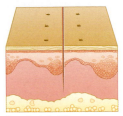
Results in hairline scar

## (b) Secondary intention

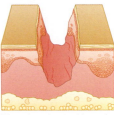
Wound gaping and irregular

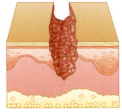
Granulation occurring

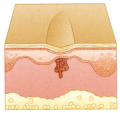
Epithelium fills in scar

## (c) Tertiary intention

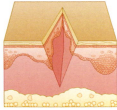
Wound not sutured

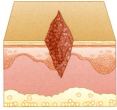
Granulation partially fills
in wound

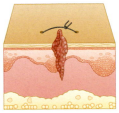
Granulating tissue
sutured together

**FIGURE 4-3:** Wound healing with and without sutures.

# 5 Pharmacology Helpful Aids

# CHAPTER 5

# Helpful Aids in Pharmacology

Pharmacotherapeutic agents offer health care providers a beneficial tool in disease management. It is possible to select from many pharmaceuticals when prescribing therapeutic medications. When selecting a pharmaceutical appropriate for a specific patient, the NP must be knowledgeable about specific indications for the use, dosages, precautions, and interactions of drugs and adverse reactions to different drugs. Consideration should always be given to the uniqueness of each individual patient and any special circumstances associated with that patient. This chapter presents helpful topics for the NP in prescribing pharmaceuticals, including:

- Cytochrome P450 interactions
- Antibiotic use by classes and pathogens
- Insulin preparations by type, onset of action, and peak effect
- Proper crushing or chewing of medications
- Common drug equivalents
- Approximate practical equivalents
- Schedule of controlled drugs
- Pregnancy categories

## Cytochrome P450 Interactions

Metabolism of drugs takes place mainly in the liver and small intestines, but also occurs in the kidneys, lungs, and brain. The body's enzyme system contains a group of isoenzymes called the cytochrome P450 (CYP) system, which is essential for drug metabolism. The nomenclature of the cytochrome P450 system classifies its member isoenzymes (CYP) according to their family, subfamily, and the individual gene that encodes each of these isoenzymes. For example, the isoenzymes CYP3A4 belong to family 3, subfamily A, and gene 4.

Drug interactions involving CYP are caused by inhibitors and inducers. Inhibitors compete with other drugs for a particular enzyme, thus affecting the optimal level of metabolism of the drugs that the enzyme metabolizes, which in many cases affects the individual's response to a particular drug, including the possibility of making the drug ineffective. A strong inhibitor is one that causes more than a fivefold increase in the area under the curve (AUC) for the time-versus-concentration of a drug, which is equivalent to more than an 80% decrease in clearance of the drug. A moderate inhibitor is one that causes between a two- to fivefold increase in the plasma AUC for a drug, or a 50% to 80% decrease in its clearance. A weak inhibitor is one that causes more than a 1.25-fold but less than a twofold increase in the plasma AUC values for a drug, or a 20% to 50% decrease in its clearance. Inhibitors and the strengths of their effects on plasma drug levels are shown in Table 5–1.

Inducers stimulate the production of an enzyme, thus increasing the rate of drug metabolism by the enzyme and causing the enzyme's substrate drug to be cleared out of the system faster. This will also affect an individual's response to a drug, such as by making the drug ineffective because it has not been in the system long enough to have an effect. Inducers of CYP450 enzymes are shown in Table 5–2.

## Antibiotics

Antibiotics have the ability to kill bacteria (bactericidal) or inhibit the growth of bacteria (bacteriostatic). When selecting an appropriate antimicrobial agent for treating an infection, the NP must:

- Question the patient about underlying medical conditions such as diabetes, immunosuppression, past medications, or intravenous (IV) drug use, which may predispose the patient to infection or help to identify the most likely pathogen causing the infection

# Table 5–1 Cytochrome P450 Inhibitors

| CYP3A4,5,7 (NEARLY 50% OF DRUG METABOLISM) | CYP2D6 (NEARLY 25% OF DRUG METABOLISM) | CYP2C8/9 (NEARLY 15% OF DRUG METABOLISM) |
|---|---|---|
| **Strong** <br> • Indinavir <br> • Nelfinavir <br> • Ritonavir <br> • Clarithromycin <br> • Itraconazole <br> • Ketoconazole <br> • Nefazodone <br> • Saquinavir <br> • Telithromycin | **Strong** <br> • Bupropion <br> • Fluoxetine <br> • Paroxetine <br> • Quinidine | **Strong** <br> • Gemfibrozil <br> • Fluconazole |
| **Moderate** <br> • Aprepitant <br> • Erythromycin <br> • Fluconazole <br> • Grapefruit juice <br> • Verapamil | **Moderate** <br> • Duloxetine <br> • Derbinafine | **Moderate** <br> • Trimethoprim <br> • Amiodarone |
| **Moderate-Weak** <br> • Diltiazem | | |
| **Weak** <br> • Cimetidine | **Weak** <br> • Amiodarone <br> • Cimetidine <br> • Sertraline | |
| **Others** <br> • Amiodarone <br> • NOT azithromycin <br> • chloramphenicol <br> • Delavirdine <br> • Diethyl-dithiocarbamate <br> • Fluvoxamine <br> • Gestodene <br> • Imatinib <br> • Mibefradil <br> • Mifepristone <br> • Norfloxacin <br> • Norfluoxetine | **Others** <br> • Celecoxib <br> • Chlorpheniramine <br> • chlorpromazine <br> • Cinacalcet <br> • Citalopram <br> • Clemastine <br> • Clomipramine <br> • Cocaine <br> • Diphenhydramine <br> • Doxepin <br> • Doxorubicin <br> • Escitalopram | **Others** <br> • Glitazones <br> • Montelukast <br> • Quercetin <br> • Fenofibrate <br> • Fluvastatin <br> • Fluvoxamine <br> • Isoniazid <br> • Lovastatin <br> • Phenylbutazone <br> • Probenicid <br> • Sertraline <br> • Sulfamethoxazole |

*Continued*

## Table 5–1  Cytochrome P450 Inhibitors—cont'd

| CYP3A4,5,7 (NEARLY 50% OF DRUG METABOLISM) | CYP2D6 (NEARLY 25% OF DRUG METABOLISM) | CYP2C8/9 (NEARLY 15% OF DRUG METABOLISM) |
|---|---|---|
| • Star fruit<br>• Voriconazole | • Goldenseal<br>• Halofantrine<br>• Histamine H1 receptor antagonists<br>• Hydroxyzine<br>• Levomepromazine<br>• Methadone<br>• Metoclopramide<br>• Mibefradil<br>• Midodrine<br>• Moclobemide<br>• Perphenazine<br>• Ranitidine<br>• Red-haloperidol<br>• Ritonavir<br>• Ticlopidine<br>• Tripelennamine | • Sulfaphenazole<br>• Teniposide<br>• Voriconazole<br>• Zafirlukast |

Adapted from Indiana University Department of Medicine Division of Clinical Pharmacology Web site: http://medicine.iupui.edu/clinpharm/ddis/ClinicalTable.asp

## Table 5–2  Inducers of Cytochrome P450 Enzymes

| CYP1A2 | CYP2B6 | CYP2C9 | CYP2E1 | CYP3A4, 5, 7 |
|---|---|---|---|---|
| Tobacco | Phenobarbital<br>Phenytoin<br>Rifampin | Rifampin<br>Secobarbital | Ethanol<br>Isoniazid | Carbamazepine<br>Phenobarbital<br>Phenytoin[2]<br>Pioglitazone<br>Rifabutin<br>Rifampin<br>St. John's wort<br>Troglitazone[1] |

Adapted from Indiana University Department of Medicine Division of Clinical Pharmacology Web site: http://medicine.iupui.edu/clinpharm/ddis/ClinicalTable.asp

- Determine where the infection was acquired, whether in the community or a hospital, since this may help narrow the list of possible pathogens causing the infection. Empirical therapy should be directed toward the most likely organisms infecting a specific body site

- Base the choice of available pharmacotherapeutic options on two criteria:
  1. Effectiveness in eradicating the causative organism of an infection
  2. Producing the least harmful or adverse effects

The following sections outline common pathogens and their body sites of invasion, along with recommendations for treating the infections they cause.

## Skin and Soft-Tissue Infections
- Cellulitis/erysipelas
- Diabetic foot infections
- Folliculitis
- Furuncle/carbuncle
- Impetigo
- Paronychia

### *Common Pathogens*
- *Staphylococcus aureus*
- *Streptococcus* spp.
- Enterobacteriaceae
- *Pseudomonas aeruginosa*
- *Enterococcus*
- Anaerobes

### *Recommendations for Treatment*
Superficial infections (cellulitis, cellulitis involving blisters and shallow ulcers) are typically caused by *S. aureus* or beta-hemolytic streptococci. Folliculitis associated with whirlpools, hot tubs, and heated swimming pools is typically caused by *P. aeruginosa.*

Infections of ulcers that are chronic or have been previously treated with antibiotics may be caused by aerobic gram-negative bacilli as well as by staphylococci or streptococci.

Deep soft-tissue infections, osteomyelitis, and gangrene are more often polymicrobial, including aerobic gram-negative bacilli and anaerobes (anaerobic streptococci, *Bacteroides fragilis* group, and *Clostridium* spp.), but *S. aureus* is also common as a single pathogen in such infections.

Antibiotics are indicated for cellulitis and deep infections after debridement. IV antibiotics are generally not needed except for severe infections, those with concomitant bacteremia, or infections causing systemic toxicity.

- **Methicillin-sensitive *S. aureus* (MSSA) (oral):** Cephalexin 500 mg PO qid, dicloxacillin 500 mg PO qid, clindamycin 300 to 450mg PO tid, amoxicillin/clavulanate 875 mg PO bid.
- **Methicillin-resistant *S. aureus* (MRSA) (oral [check susceptibilities]):** Clindamycin 300 to 450mg PO tid, trimethoprim–sulfamethoxazole (TMP–SMX) 1 or 2 DS tablets PO bid, minocycline 100 mg PO bid, or linezolid 600 mg PO bid
- **Consider decolonization for recurrent soft tissue infections:** 2% Mupirocin ointment applied to the nares twice daily for 5 days with or without Hibiclens washes
- **Rifampin:** May be added to oral agents for MRSA in patients with recurrent soft-tissue infections; rifampin should *never* be used as monotherapy
- **Streptococcal infections (without other infecting or ganisms, e.g., erysipelas):** Penicillin V 500 mg PO qid for 10 days, amoxicillin 500 mg PO tid for 10 days, penicillin G benzathine 1.2 million U IM as a single dose, or cephalexin 500 mg PO qid for 10 days
- **Penicillin allergy:** Azithromycin 500 mg PO for 1 day, followed by 250 mg PO qd for 4 days; clarithromycin 250 mg PO bid for 7 to10 day; or clindamycin 300 mg PO tid for 7 to 10 days

For acute paronychia, oral antibiotics alone are not sufficient if there is abscess; incision and drainage are required. Most authorities support the use of oral antibiotics in acute paronychia even with adequate incision and drainage.

Preferred antibiotics for acute paronychia are:

- **Amoxicillin–clavulanate:** 500 mg PO tid or 875 mg bid for 7 days or until infection resolves
- **If the patient has a penicillin allergy:** Clindamycin 300 mg PO q6h for 7 days or until infection resolves
- **Alternatives (ineffective if anaerobes are suspected as pathogens):** Dicloxacillin 250 to 500 mg PO qid or cephalexin (Keflex) 500 mg PO q6h for 7 days or until infection resolves

## Bite Wounds
- Bats, Cats, Dogs, Human

### *Common Pathogens*
- *Pasteurella multocida* (cats and dogs)
- *Capnocytophaga canimorsus* (dogs)
- *Eikenella corrodens* (humans)

- *Streptococcus* spp. (all bites), especially *S. anginosus*
- *Staphylococcus aureus* (all bites)
- *Staphylococcus intermedius* (dogs)
- Anaerobes (all bites), especially *Prevotella* spp.

## Recommendations for Treatment

Principles: (1) clean and débride the wound, (2) treat with antibiotics (for severe early or late and infected bites), usually amoxicillin/clavulanate (875 mg PO bid), (3) administer tetanus toxoid, (4) if bite is an animal bite, consider rabies (rare except with bat exposure in the United States).

To clean a bite wound, use copious soap and water, alcohol, and povidone-iodine; for a puncture wound use high-pressure irrigation with a 20-mL syringe and #18 needle. Débride necrotic tissue; immobilize and elevate a bitten extremity.

For wound closure, suturing is usually not needed except for early uninfected wounds and facial wounds; use adhesive strips to approximate wound edges.

If the patient's history includes tetanus vaccination, give three or fewer than three doses of tetanus-diphtheria (Td) toxoid, or if the cause of the wound is unknown and the wound is minor, give a Td series of 0.5 mL at presentation, 1 to 2 months, and 6 to 12 months for a total of three doses. For severe bite injuries give a Td series and tetanus immune globulin.

## Antibiotic Prophylaxis and Treatment

Indications for antibiotic prophylaxis in severe injuries < 8 hours old; crush injuries; injuries with bone or joint penetration; wounds of the face, hands, or genitals; or injuries to an immunosuppressed host:

- **Preferred prophylaxis:** Amoxicillin/clavulanate (Augmentin) 875/125 mg PO bid for 7 days
- **Alternative:** Moxifloxacin (Avelox) 400 mg PO qd for 7 days
- **Alternatives:** Amoxicillin, doxycycline, cefuroxime (active against most oral flora of humans and animals)
- **Outpatient treatment (preferred):** Amoxicillin/clavulanate (Augmentin) either 875/125 mg PO bid or 2000 (XR)/125 mg PO bid
- **Outpatient alternative:** Moxifloxacin 400 mg PO qd or azithromycin 500 mg PO followed by 250 mg PO qd

## Eye/Orbit

- Conjunctivitis
- Blepharitis

## Common Pathogens

- *Staphylococcus aureus*
- *Haemophilus influenzae*
- *Neisseria gonorrhoeae*
- *Chlamydophila trachomatis*

## Recommendations for Treatment

For bacterial conjunctivitis, give all doses of antibiotics while the patient is awake. Ointments may blur vision for 20 min after being administered. Use only systemic antibiotics for gonorrheal/chlamydial disease.

- **Trimethoprim–polymyxin B (Polytrim) solution**: 1 drop q3h for 7 to 10 days
- **Bacitracin–polymyxin B (Polysporin) ophthalmic solution:** 1 drop q3–4h for 7 to 10 days
- **Sulfacetamide (Bleph-10) 10% solution:** 1 or 2 drops q2–3h for 7 to 10 days; taper to twice daily with improvement. Some staphylococcus strains may be resistant
- **Erythromycin ophthalmic ointment:** 1/2-inch qid inside lower lid for 5 to 7 days. Some staphylococcus strains may be resistant.
- **Fluoroquinolones:** Use for more serious cases, especially if *Pseudomonas* is suspected (contact lens wearers) or corneal ulcers exist
- **Levofloxacin (Quixin) 0.5% solution:** 1 or 2 drops q2h for 2 days, then 1 or 2 drops qid for 5 days; or ofloxacin (Ocuflox) 0.3% solution: 1 or 2 drops q2–4h for 2 days, then 1 or 2 drops qid for 5 days; or ciprofloxacin (Ciloxan) 0.3% solution: 1 or 2 drops q2h for 2 days, then 1 or 2 drops q4h for 5 days
- **Bacitracin-neomycin-polymyxin B (Neosporin Ophthalmic) solution:** 1 to 2 drops q4h for 7 to 10 days. Up to 10% of patients are allergic to neomycin.
- **Tobramycin (Tobrex) 0.3% solution:** 1 or 2 drops q4h for 7 days or gentamicin (Garamycin, Genoptic) 0.3% solution 1 or 2 drops q4h for 7 days

## Ear

- Otitis externa

## Common Pathogens

- *Pseudomonas aeruginosa*
- *Staphylococcus aureus*

### Recommendations for Treatment

Typical indications for topical antibiotic therapy are otalgia, swelling, and otorrhea. Add oral antibiotics for recurrent infections, severe signs and symptoms, poorly controlled diabetes, and immunocompromised patients.

- **Neomycin/polymyxin/hydrocortisone (Cortisporin Otic):** 4 drops tid for 7 to 10 days (prescribe as suspension and not as solution, which burns)
- **Ofloxacin (Floxin):** 10 drops qd or bid for 7 to 10 days (used with tympanic membrane [TM] perforation or tympanostomy tube)
- **Ciprofloxacin 0.3%/dexamethasone 0.1% (Ciprodex):** 4 drops bid for 7 to 10 days (used with TM perforation or tympanostomy tube)
- **Tobramycin (Tobradex ophthalmic):** 3 or 4 drops tid for 7 days (use only if TM is intact)
- **Gentamicin (Garamycin ophthalmic):** 3 or 4 drops tid for 7 days (use only if TM is intact)
- **Acetic acid/propylene glycol/hydrocortisone 1% (VoSol HC):** 4 to 6 drops tid for 10 days

## Ear

- Otitis media
- *Common Pathogens*
- *Streptococcus pneumoniae*
- *Haemophilus influenzae*

### Recommendations for Treatment (Adults)

Address risk factors for eustachian tube dysfunction: Smoking, allergies, sinusitis, reflux.

- Amoxicillin: 500 mg PO tid for 7 to 10 days
- Cefuroxime (Ceftin): 500 mg PO bid for 7 to 14 days
- Ceftriaxone: 1 g IM (Rocephin) qd for 3 doses
- Cefpodoxime: 200 mg PO bid for 7 to 10 days
- Alternative therapy (if patient has beta-lactam allergy or initial therapy fails): Cefdinir 300 mg PO bid or 600 mg PO qd; clindamycin 300 mg PO tid or qid + levofloxacin (Levaquin) 500 mg PO qd or moxifloxacin (Avelox) 400 mg PO qd, all for 7 to 10 days
- Amoxicillin/clavulanate use as primary therapy for patients who are immunocompromised or have diabetes.

## Throat

- Pharyngitis

### Common Pathogens
- *Streptococcus pyogenes* (Group A streptococcus)
- *Neisseria gonorrhoeae* (rare)

### Recommendations for Treatment
- **Penicillin VK:** 250 mg PO qid or 500 to 1000 mg PO bid, each for 10 days, or penicillin benzathine 1.2 million units IM in a single dose
- **If patient has penicillin allergy:** Erythromycin estolate 500 mg PO bid or tid for 10 days, or azithromycin (Z-pack) PO or clarithromycin (Biaxin) XR, Biaxin XR 1 g once daily PO or 500 mg PO bid for 5 days
- **Cefpodoxime (Vantin):** 200 mg bid PO for 5 days
- **Cefadroxil (Duricef):** 500 mg bid PO for 5 days
- **Loracarbef (Lorabid):** 200 mg bid for 5 days

## Nose
- Sinusitis/Rhinosinusitis, Acute

### Common Pathogens
- *Streptococcus pneumoniae*
- *Haemophilus influenzae*

Less common pathogens in acute sinusitis and rhinosinusitis are *Moraxella catarrhalis, S. aureus*, and anaerobes.

### Recommendations for Treatment
Classification of sinusitis:
- **Acute:** < 4 weeks
- **Subacute:** 4 to 12 weeks
- **Chronic:** > 12 weeks

Most sinusitis is viral or allergic; the usual indication for antibiotic treatment is symptoms lasting > 7 days. Antibiotic treatment is indicated in the presence of nasal purulence and symptoms that are severe or persist for > 10 days or are worse at 7 days.

Nearly all antibiotic treatment for sinusitis is empiric. For severe, nonresponsive sinusitis or sinusitis in a patient with a history of recent antibiotic use, a fluoroquinolone (levo-, or moxifloxacin) or amoxicillin/clavulanate should be used.

- **Preferred treatment:** Amoxicillin 0.5 to 1.5 g PO tid for 10 to 14 days; amoxicillin/clavulanate 825/125 mg PO bid; or cefpodoxime 200 to 400 mg bid for 10 to 14 days
- **Alternate treatment:** Azithromycin 2 g as a single dose or 500 mg PO qd for 3 days; clarithromycin 500 mg PO bid for 14 days; or doxycycline 100 mg PO bid or TMP–SMX DS bid PO for 10 to 14 days

- **Fluoroquinolones:** Levofloxacin (Levaquin) 500 mg qd or moxifloxacin (Avelox) 400 mg qd, with either drug given for 5 to 10 days

## Nose
- Sinusitis/Rhinosinusitis, Subacute/Chronic

### Common Pathogens
The bacteriology of chronic sinusitis is less well defined than that of acute sinusitis (in which the most common pathogens are *S. pneumoniae, H. influenzae ,* and *M. catarrhalis*), although flare-ups of chronic sinusitis may be caused by the usual acute pathogens. In cases of polymicrobial infection, gram-negative organisms and possibly anaerobes are found more often. *Pseudomonas aeruginosa* and *S. aureus* are more common in nosocomial infections and those in patients who are immunocompromised.

### Recommendations for Treatment
- **Preferred:** Amoxicillin/clavulanate (Augmentin) 875 mg PO bid for 3 to 6 weeks
- **Alternatives:** Clindamycin (Cleocin) 300 mg PO tid for 3 to 6 weeks
- **Cefuroxime axetil (Ceftin):** 500 mg PO bid for 3 to 6 weeks
- **Cefprozil (Cefzil):** 500 mg PO bid for 3 to 6 weeks
- **Clarithromycin (Biaxin):** 500 mg PO bid for 3 to 6 weeks
- **Levofloxacin (Levaquin):** 500 mg PO qd for 3 to 6 weeks
- **Moxifloxacin (Avelox):** 400 mg PO qd for 3 to 6 weeks

## Respiratory System
- Pneumonia/Community Acquired

### Common Pathogens
- *Streptococcus pneumoniae*
- *Haemophilus influenzae*
- *Moraxella catarrhalis*
- *Chlamydophila pneumoniae*
- *Legionella* spp.
- *Mycoplasma pneumoniae*

### Recommendations for Treatment
Antibiotics for the empirical treatment of community-acquired pneumonia in adults are:
- **Outpatient and uncomplicated pneumonia**: Doxycycline or a macrolide
- **Doxycycline:** 100 mg bid PO for 7 to 10 days

- **Azithromycin:** 500 mg PO qd for 3 days (Tri-pak) or 2 g PO as a single dose (Zmax)
- **Clarithromycin:** 1 g (XR) PO qd or 500 mg bid PO for 7 days
- **Outpatients and patients with comorbidities (chronic obstructive pulmonary disease [COPD], diabetes, congestive heart failure [CHF], etc), and/or those who have had recent antibiotic therapy: The antibiotics named previously, or fluoroquinolone or a ketolide**
- **Fluoroquinolone:** Levofloxacin 750 mg/d PO for 5 days or moxifloxacin 400 mg qd PO for 7 days
- **Telithromycin:** 800 mg qd PO for 7 to 10 days

Pathogen-specific antibiotic treatment:

- *Streptococcus pneumoniae* **(penicillin sensitive):** Amoxicillin, ceftriaxone, cefotaxime, cefpodoxime, cefprozil, or a macrolide until the patient has been afebrile for 3 days
- *Streptococcus pneumoniae* **(penicillin resistant):** Levofloxacin, moxifloxacin, vancomycin, linezolid, or telithromycin
- **Mycoplasma or chlamydia:** A macrolide or doxycycline for 7 days
- **Legionella:** Azithromycin for 3 to 5 days or a fluoroquinolone for 7 days
- *Haemophilus influenzae***:** Doxycycline, a second or third generation cephalosporin, or a fluoroquinolone for 1 to 2 weeks
- **Influenza:** Rimantadine, zanamivir, or oseltamivir for 5 days
- **Anaerobes:** Clindamycin, amoxicillin/clavulanate (Augmentin), ampicillin/sulbactam (Unasyn), or piperacillin/tazobactam (Zosyn)

## Genitourinary System

- Acute Urinary Tract Infection/Cystitis (Uncomplicated)

### Common Pathogens

- *Escherichia coli* (80% to 90% of genitourinary [GU] infections)
- *Staphylococcus saprophyticus* (0 to 2% of GU infections, with much higher rates in young women)

More than 95% of uncomplicated urinary tract infections (UTIs) are due to a single organism. Organisms less common than *E. coli* or *S. saprophyticus* in causing UTI include other Enterobacteriaceae, *P. aeruginosa*, groups B and D streptococci, enterococci, *H. influenzae* (rarely), anaerobes, Salmonella, Shigella, adenovirus type 11, ureaplasma, and mycoplasma. In sexually active women, dysuria without pyuria suggests a sexually transmitted disease (STD) rather than UTI.

Risk factors for acute uncomplicated UTI in premenopausal women are (1) coitus, (2) a history of UTI, (3) spermicide exposure, and (4) recent antimicrobial use.

Risk factors for recurrent uncomplicated UTI in premenopausal women are the same as those given above, as well as (a) a maternal history of UTI or (b) a history of childhood UTI (both of which are factors consistent with a hereditary predisposition to UTI).

UTIs are common among women of all ages; the incidence of uncomplicated cystitis is 0.5 to 0.7 episodes per woman/year. The prevalence of asymptomatic bacteruria is 5% to 6% among healthy, sexually active, nonpregnant women, and it increases with age.

## Recommendations for Treatment

TMP–SMX and TMP alone are first-line antibiotics for treating uncomplicated UTIs because they are inexpensive and there is a critical need to reserve fluoroquinolones for use in complicated UTIs. Overuse of TMP–SMX or TMP in acute cystitis may lead to resistance.

Nitrofurantoin is encouraged for use (see Longer Duration Therapy) because of high rates of resistance to TMP–SMX among *E. coli* (>10% in all regions of the United States examined) and because it is a fluoroquinolone-sparing agent for women with mild to moderate symptoms who are allergic to TMP–SMX, have had an antibiotic prescription in the previous 3 months (except for nitrofurantoin), or live in a locality in which the prevalence of *E. coli* resistance to TMP–SMX is >20% among women with uncomplicated UTIs.

Older women with acute bacterial cystitis should be managed with a longer antibiotic regimen; TMP–SMX should never be used as empirical therapy in this age group.

If *S. saprophyticus* is the suspected or known cause of a UTI, more prolonged therapy (7 days) should be used because of its greater efficacy.

## Short-Course Therapy, Empirical

- **Trimethoprim–sulfamethoxazole DS (Bactrim/Septra):** 1 tablet PO bid for 3 days (preferred for empirical therapy if local prevalence of *E. coli* resistance to TMP–SMX is <10% to 20%; if it is >10% to 20%, use a fluoroquinolone). Check at least once every 6 months with a local laboratory for resistance rates.
- **Trimethoprim:** 300 mg PO qd for 3 days (do not use if resistance to TMP–SMX is >10% to 20%). Check every 6 months with a local laboratory for *E. coli* resistance rates
- **Norfloxacin:** 400 mg PO bid for 3 days for women with severe symptoms and allergy to TMP–SMX, or who have had an antibiotic prescription in the last 3 months (except for a fluoroquinolone), or who live in locality in which *E. coli* resistance to norfloxacin is >20% among women with acute uncomplicated UTIs

- **Ciprofloxacin:** 250 mg PO bid for 3 days for women with severe symptoms and allergy to TMP–SMX, or who have had an antibiotic prescription in the last 3 months (except a fluoroquinolone), or who live in locality in which *E. coli* resistance to ciprofloxacin is >20% among women with acute uncomplicated UTIs
- **Ofloxacin:** 200 mg PO bid for 3 days for women with severe symptoms and allergy to SMX, or who have had an antibiotic prescription in the last 3 months (except a fluoroquinolone), or who live in locality in which *E. coli* resistance to ofloxacin is >20% among women with acute uncomplicated UTIs
- **Amoxicillin/clavulanate**: 500/125 mg PO bid for 3 days (a higher percentage of organisms are resistant to amoxicillin alone). This regimen is inferior to ciprofloxacin, and if amoxicillin/clavulanate is used, longer duration therapy is indicated

### *Longer Duration Therapy*
- **Nitrofurantoin macrocrystals:** 50 or 100 mg qid PO for 7 days; nitrofurantoin monohydrate macrocrystals 100 mg bid PO for 7 days
- **Amoxicillin/clavulanate:** 500/125 mg PO bid for 7 days (a higher percentage of organisms are resistant to amoxicillin alone)
- **TMP– SMX (Bactrim DS):** 1 tablet PO bid for 5 to 7 days (preferred for empirical therapy if prevalence of *E. coli* resistance to TMP–SMX is <10% to 20%; if >20% use a fluoroquinolone)
- **Trimethoprim:** 100 mg PO bid for 7 days
- **Cephalexin:** 250 mg PO tid for 7 days
- **Norfloxacin:** 400 mg PO bid for 7 days
- **Ciprofloxacin:** 250 mg PO bid for 7 days
- **Amoxicillin:** 250 mg PO tid for 7 days

### *Treatment in Women With Diabetes Mellitus*
- Do *not* use short-course (3-day) therapy in patients with diabetes
- Treat for 7 to 10 days with any agent outlined in Longer Duration Therapy section

## Genitourinary System
- Acute Pyelonephritis, Uncomplicated

### *Common Pathogens*
- *Escherichia coli*
- *Staphylococcus saprophyticus*
- *Proteus* spp.

### Recommendations for Treatment

Initial empirical treatment for acute pyelonephritis should be modified according to the results of urine culture and sensitivity tests and blood culture. Completion of 14 days of fully effective treatment is the key to resolution of infection.

### Empiric Outpatient Treatment

- **Ciprofloxacin:** 500 mg PO bid for 14 days
- **Ofloxacin:** 200 mg PO bid for 14 days
- **Levofloxacin:** 500 mg PO qd for 14 days
- **Norfloxacin:** 400 mg PO bid for 14 days
- **Alternatives:** Ceftriaxone 1 g IM as a single dose, followed by an oral fluoroquinolone to complete 14 days of treatment
- **Gentamicin:** 2 mg/kg IM or IV as a single dose, followed by an oral fluoroquinolone to complete 14 days of treatment
- **Ciprofloxacin:** 400 mg IV as a single dose, followed by an oral fluoroquinolone to complete 14 days of treatment
- **Levofloxacin:** 500 mg IV as a single dose, followed by an oral fluoroquinolone to complete 14 days of treatment

Adapted from Johns Hopkins Point of Care IT Center ABX Guide Web site.

## Penicillins

Penicillins are used for treating respiratory, genitourinary (GU), skin, soft-tissue, bone, joint, and intra-abdominal infections. Other uses for penicillins include the treatment of tetanus, meningitis, pneumonia, Lyme disease, anthrax, botulism, gas gangrene, gonorrhea, syphilis, and bacterial septicemia. Penicillins are also used as prophylaxis in patients with bacterial endocarditis or valvular heart disease and who are undergoing dental procedures or minor upper respiratory tract surgery.

### Penicillinase-Sensitive Penicillins

Penicillinase-sensitive penicillins are natural, first generation penicillins. These drugs are considered bactericidal against the following organisms:

- **Gram-positive:** Streptococci, enterococci, non-penicillinase-producing staphylococci.
- **Gram-negative:** Non-penicillinase-producing strains of *N. gonorrhoeae* and *N. meningitidis*

> **COACH CONSULT**
>
> Penicillinase-sensitive penicillins include:
> - Penicillin G benzathine (Biclinnin LA)
> - Penicillin G potassium aqueous
> - Penicillin G procaine (Wycillin)
> - Penicillin VK (Veetids)

• **Certain anaerobic oral flora:** *Actinomyces israelii, Pasteurella multocida, Listeria monocytogenes, Treponema pallidum*

### Penicillinase-Resistant Penicillins

Penicillinase-resistant penicillins are narrow-spectrum antibiotics. These second generation drugs are effective against the following bacteria:

• **Gram-positive:** *S. aureus*; Streptococcus groups. A, B, G, C; *S. epidermidis*

### Aminopenicillins

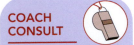
Aminopenicillins are broad-spectrum drugs and are considered third generation penicillins. These drugs are effective against the following organisms:

• **Gram-positive:** Streptococci, enterococci, non-penicillinase-producing staphylococci
• **Gram-negative:** Non-penicillinase-producing strains of *N. gonorrhoeae* and *N. meningitidis*
• **Anaerobic flora:** *A. israelii, P. multocida, L. monocytogenes, T. pallidum*

### Antipseudomonal Penicillins

Antipseudomonal penicillins are fourth generation antibiotics and are considered extended-spectrum penicillins. This class of drugs is effective against the following bacteria:

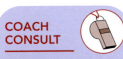
• **Gram-positive:** Streptococci, enterococci, non-penicillinase-producing staphylococci
• **Gram-negative:** P. aeruginosa, Klebsiella, Non-penicillinase-producing strains of *N. gonorrhoeae* and *N. meningitidis*, Enterobacter spp., *M. catarrhalis, H. influenzae, E. coli, P. mirabilis* and *P. vulgaris*, Providencia sp., Morganella sp., Citrobacter sp., Acinetobacter sp.
• **Anaerobes:** *Bacteroides fragilis*, Clostridium (not *C. difficile*)

## Cephalosporins

Cephalosporins are related to penicillins both pharmacologically and in their chemical structure. There are four generations of cephalosporins. Each successive generation of cephalosporin drugs has greater activity than the previous generation against gram-negative organisms and anaerobes, as well as greater stability against beta-lactamase enzymes and greater ability to enter the cerebrospinal fluid (CSF). Cephalosporins are indicated for treating infections caused by susceptible organisms that invade the respiratory, urinary, and biliary tracts and skin, soft tissue, or bone. They are also used to treat more serious infections such as septicemias, meningitis, endocarditis, peritonitis, acute pelvic inflammatory disease, and gonorrhea, and for patients undergoing surgical procedures associated with a high risk of infection, such as biliary, cardiovascular, obstetric and gynecologic, and orthopedic surgical procedures.

### First Generation Cephalosporins

First generation cephalosporins have good gram-positive coverage but have limited action against gram-negative bacteria. These drugs do not reach effective concentrations in the CSF. This class of cephalosporins is effective against the following bacteria:

- **Gram-positive:** Streptococcus groups A, B, C, G, *S. pneumoniae*, viridans Streptococcus, methicillin-sensitive *S. aureus*
- **Gram-negative:** *N. gonorrhoeae*, *H. influenzae*, *E. coli*, *Klebsiella* sp., *P. mirabilis*

### Second Generation Cephalosporins

The second generation cephalosporins have different spectra of activity, and in most cases susceptibility tests should be done for each of these drugs before they are used. None of these drugs is active against *P. aeruginosa*, and they do not reach effective concentrations in the CSF. The second generation cephalosporins are effective against the following organisms:

- **Gram-positive:** Streptococcus groups A, B, C, G, *S. pneumoniae*, viridans Streptococcus, *S. aureus* (not MRSA)
- **Gram-negative:** *M. catarrhalis*, *H. influenzae*, *E. coli*, *Klebsiella* sp., *P. mirabilis* and *P. vulgaris*, *Providencia* sp., *Morganella* sp.

### Third Generation Cephalosporins

The third generation cephalosporins are indicated for infections caused by organisms susceptible to the first and second generation cephalosporins. They also extend the spectrum of cephalosporin activity to include gram-negative organisms. The third generation cephalosporins reach clinically effective

**COACH CONSULT**

Drugs belonging to the first generation cephalosporins include:
- Cephalexin (Keflex)
- Cefazolin (Ancef)
- Cefadroxil (Duricef)
- Cephradine (Velosef)

**COACH CONSULT**

Drugs belonging to the second generation cephalosporins are:
- Cefaclor (Ceclor)
- Cefotetan disodium (Cefotan)
- Cefoxitin sodium (Mefoxin)
- Cefuroxime axetil (Ceftin)
- Cefuroxime sodium (Kefurox, Zinacef)
- Cefprozil (Cefzil)
- Loracarbef (Lorabid)

**COACH CONSULT**

Cefuroxime does penetrate into the CSF.

**COACH CONSULT**

Drugs belonging to the third generation cephalosporins are:
- Cefdinir (Omnicef)
- Ceftibuten (Cedax)
- Cefixime (Suprax)
- Cefoperazone (Cefobid)
- Cefotaxime (Claforan)
- Cefpodoxime sodium (Vantin)
- Ceftazidime (Fortaz)
- Cefditoren (Spectracef)
- Ceftizoxime (Cefizox)
- Ceftriaxone (Rocephin)

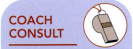

**COACH CONSULT**

The following are examples of sulfonamides:
- Sulfadiazine (Microsulfon)
- Sulfamethoxazole (Gantanol, Urobak)
- Sulfisoxazole
- Trimethoprim–sulfamethoxazole (TMP-SMX, Bactrim, co-trimoxazole, Septra)

concentration in the CSF. Some parenteral forms of these drugs are effective against *P. aeruginosa*. The following are organisms against which the third generation cephalosporins have activity:

- **Gram-positive:** Streptococcus groups A, B, C, G; *S. pneumoniae*; viridians streptococci
- **Gram-negative:** *N. gonorrhoeae*, *M. catarrhalis*, *H. influenzae*, *E. coli*, *Klebsiella* sp., *P. mirabilis* and *P. vulgaris*, *Providencia* sp., *Citrobacter*, *Enterobacter*, *Serratia*

### Fourth Generation Cephalosporins

Cefepime (Maxipime) is the only fourth generation cephalosporin drug now available. It is considered a broad-spectrum antibiotic because of its activity against both gram-positive and gram-negative organisms. It is administered parenterally and has a greater spectrum of activity and greater stability against beta-lactamase enzymes than do other cephalosporins.

## Sulfonamides

Sulfonamide drugs are bacteriostatic and are used in the treatment of UTIs, otitis media (OM), and bronchitis, as well as malaria, ulcerative colitis, dermatitis herpetiformis, chlamydial infections, nocardiosis, gonorrhea, and protozoal infections. These drugs are also used prophylactically in patients with a history of rheumatic fever, patients allergic to penicillin, adults and children infected with human immunodeficiency virus (HIV), granulocytopenic patients, and patients with traveler's diarrhea. The sulfonamide drugs provide active coverage against the following organisms:

- **Gram-positive:** Streptococcus groups A, B, C, G; *S. pneumoniae*; *Enterococcus faecalis*; *S. aureus* (MSSA and MRSA)
- **Gram-negative:** *E. coli*, *Klebsiella* sp., *Enterobacter* sp., *Salmonella* sp., *Shigella* sp., *Serratia marcescens*

## Tetracyclines

Tetracyclines are bacteriostatic but are considered the drugs of first choice for treating Rocky Mountain spotted fever, typhus fever, Q fever, trachoma, lymphogranuloma venereum urethritis, cervicitis, pneumonia, peptic ulcer disease, brucellosis, and cholera. Tetracyclines can also be used to treat acne, sinusitis, tularemia, anthrax, yaws and plague, tetanus, rat-bite fever, tropical sprue, and cystitis. Doxycycline is used prophylactically for persons traveling to areas of the world where malaria is prevalent. Tigecycline is a parenteral form of tetracycline. It belongs to a new class of antibiotics called glycycylines and is approved for treating complicated intra-abdominal infections and skin and skin-structure infections.

Tetracycline drugs provide active coverage against the following bacteria:

- **Gram-positive:** Streptococcus groups A, B, C, G; *S. pneumoniae*; *S. aureus* (MSSA, MRSA)
- **Gram-negative:** *N. gonorrhoeae, N. meningitidis, M. catarrhalis, H. influenzae, Aeromonas, Klebsiella* sp., *Salmonella* sp., *Shigella* sp., *Brucella* sp., *Legionella* sp.
- **Miscellaneous:** *Chlamydophila* sp., *Mycoplasma pneumoniae, Rickettsia* sp.
- **Anaerobes:** Actinomyces, *Bacteroides fragilis, Prevotella melaninogenicus, Clostridium* (not *C. difficile*), *Peptostreptococcus* sp.

**COACH CONSULT**

Tetracycline drugs administered orally can be better absorbed by taking them on an empty stomach.

**COACH CONSULT**

The following are examples of tetracycline drugs:
- Doxycycline (Doryx, Doxy, Monodox, Vibramycin, Vibra-Tabs)
- Minocycline (Minocin)
- Tetracycline (Achromycin V, Panmycin, Sumycin, Tetracyn)
- Tigecycline (Tygacil)

## Quinolones

The quinolones constitute a very potent broad-spectrum class of antibiotics. This class of drugs is indicated in treating bacterial infections of the respiratory, GU, and gastrointestinal (GI) tracts. Quinolones are also used to treat:

- Infections of bones and joints
- Skin and soft tissues
- Multi-drug-resistant tuberculosis caused by atypical mycobacteria
- Acquired immune deficiency syndrome (AIDS)
- Fever in patients with neutropenia and cancer

Quinolones are active against the following bacterial organisms:

- **Gram-positive:** Streptococcus groups A, B, C, G; *S. pneumoniae*; viridians Streptococcus; *E. faecalis*; *S. aureus* (MSSA); *S. epidermidis*
- **Gram-negative:** *N. gonorrhoeae, N. meningitidis, M. catarrhalis, H. influenzae, E. coli, Klebsiella* sp., *Enterobacter* sp., *Serratia* sp., *Salmonella* sp., *Shigella* sp., *P. mirabilis, P. vulgaris, Providencia* sp., *Morganella* sp., *Aeromonas* sp., *Acinetobacter* sp., *P. aeruginosa, Legionella* sp.
- **Miscellaneous:** *Chlamydia* sp., *M. pneumoniae*
- **Anaerobes:** Gemifloxacin provides coverage of most *Peptostreptococcus, Porphyromonas,* and *Fusobacterium* species, although its activity against other gram-negative anaerobes appears to be variable

**COACH CONSULT**

The following are examples of quinolone antibiotics:
- Ciprofloxacin (Cipro)
- Gemifloxacin (Factive)
- Levofloxacin (Levaquin)
- Lomefloxacin (Maxaquin)
- Moxifloxacin (Avelox, Vigamox)
- Norfloxacin (Chibroxin, Noroxin)
- Ofloxacin (Floxin)
- Sparfloxacin (Zagam)

**COACH CONSULT**

The following are examples of macrolide antibiotics:
- Azithromycin (Zithromax)
- Clarithromycin (Biaxin, Biaxin XL)
- Dirithromycin (Dynabec)
- Erythromycin base (E-Base, E-Mycin, EryC, Ery-Tab)
- Erythromycin ethylsuccinate (E.E.S., Ery-Ped)
- Erythromycin lactobinate (Erythrocin)
- Erythromycin stearate (Erythrocin Stearate)

## Macrolides

The macrolide antibiotics are bacteriostatic; at higher concentrations they may be bactericidal to some bacteria. The macrolides are indicated for infections of the upper and lower respiratory tract, skin, and soft tissue caused by susceptible organisms and for pertussis, diphtheria, intestinal amebiasis, pelvic inflammatory disease (PID), nongonococcal urethritis, syphilis, Legionnaires' disease, and rheumatic fever. Macrolides are often used for patients who are allergic to beta-lactam antibiotics. This class of antibiotic is also used for prophylaxis in dental procedures. Macrolides are effective against the following bacteria:

- **Gram-positive:** Streptococcus groups A, B, C, G; *S. pneumoniae*; *S. aureus* (MSSA); *L. monocytogenes*
- **Gram-negative:** *M. catarrhalis, N. gonorrhoeae, N. meningitidis, H. influenzae, Legionella* sp.
- **Anaerobes:** *Actinomyces, Clostridium* (not *C. difficile*), *Peptostreptococcus*
- **Miscellaneous:** *Chlamydophila* sp., *M. pneumoniae, M. avium*

Erythromycin stimulates smooth muscle and increases GI motility; it is therefore beneficial in conditions such as diabetic gastroparesis.

## Aminoglycosides

Aminoglycosides are narrow-spectrum antibiotics that are used to treat serious gram-negative infections, especially those caused by *P. aeruginosa*, *E. coli*, *Klebsiella*, *Serratia*, and *P. mirabilis*. This class of drugs is used to treat systemic infections of the:

- Blood stream
- Respiratory tract
- Bones and joints
- Skin and soft tissue
- Intra-abdominal area

## Carbapenems

Carbapenems are a class of antibiotics used to treat moderate to severe infections ranging from intra-abdominal infections to community-acquired pneumonia, complicated UTIs, acute pelvic infections, and complicated skin and soft-tissue infections in patients with diabetes. This class of drugs is effective against most gram-positive organisms (except MRSA) and highly effective against most gram-negative organisms and anaerobes.

## Miscellaneous Antibiotics

Aztreonam (Azactam) is a monobactam. It is the only drug in its class and has activity against most gram-negative organisms, but provides no coverage against gram-positive organisms or anaerobes.

Clindamycin (Cleocin) is indicated only for gram-positive anaerobic infections such as serious respiratory infections, bacterial endocarditis, toxoplasmosis, acne, serious skin and soft-tissue infections, septicemia, intra-abdominal infections, and infections of the female pelvis and genital tract. Clindamycin is also used as prophylaxis against bacterial endocarditis and in patients allergic to penicillin or those who do not tolerate erythromycin. This drug is also used in patients who are having minor respiratory tract surgery or dental procedures.

Chloramphenicol (Chloromycetin) is a broad-spectrum antibiotic that provides good coverage against gram-positive and gram-negative organisms. It is used to treat meningitis; bacteremia; and skin, intra-abdominal,

CNS, and soft-tissue infections when it is not feasible to use less toxic drugs.

Linezolid (Zyvox) is the first of a new class of drugs called oxazolidinones. It is used to treat infections caused by MRSA and vancomycin-resistant *Enterococcus faecium* (VREF).

Telithromycin (Ketek) is the first drug of its class, known as ketolides. Telithromycin is used to treat mild to moderate community-acquired pneumonia. It has activity against the following organisms: Streptococcus groups A, C, G; *S. pneumoniae*; MSSA; *N. meningitidis*; *M. catarrhalis*; *H. influenzae*; *Legionella* sp; *Chlamydophila* sp.; *M. pneumoniae*; *Rickettsia* sp.; *Peptostreptococcus* sp.

**ALERT**

Vancomycin has serious adverse effects such as ototoxicity, nephrotoxicity, and superinfection.

Vancomycin is a narrow-spectrum drug that is bactericidal. It is indicated in the treatment of infections caused by the following organisms, all of which are gram-positive: Streptococcus groups A, B, C, G; *S. pneumoniae*; *E. faecalis* and *E. faecium*; MSSA and MRSA; *S. epidermidis*; *Corynebacterium jeikeium*; and *L. monocytogenes*. It is effective against the following anaerobes: Actinomyces, *C. difficile* and other *Clostridium* spp., and *Peptostreptococcus* sp.

## Insulin Therapies

The American Diabetes Association/European Association for the Study of Diabetes (ADA/EASD) and American College of Endocrinology/American Association of Clinical Endocrinologists (ACE/AACE) have produced guidelines for achieving and maintaining glucose levels as close as possible to the normal range. When a patient's levels of glycosylated hemoglobin (HbA$_{1c}$) reach >8.5%, the ADA recommends that analog insulin therapy be initiated. The ADA recommends target HbA$_{1c}$ levels of <7%. In individuals not experiencing hypoglycemia, the ADA recommends an HbA$_{1c}$ <6%. The AACE further recommends that HbA$_{1c}$ levels be maintained at ≥6.5%. Patients must be well informed and confident enough in the management of their diabetes to self-adjust their food intake, exercise, or insulin dose in response to glucose levels and to understand the consequences of not doing so. The insulin preparations are shown in Table 5–3.

National guidelines published by the ADA and other international authorities on diabetes recommend a specific approach to managing hyperglycemia in individuals with type 2 diabetes. The overall objective in

## Table 5–3 Insulin Preparations

| PREPARATION | BRAND | ROUTE | ONSET (HOURS) | PEAK (HOURS) | DURATION (HOURS) |
|---|---|---|---|---|---|
| **RAPID ACTING** | | | | | |
| Insulin Aspart | NovoLog | SC, IV, CSII | <0.25 | 1–3 | 3–5 |
| Insulin Glulisine | Apidra | SC, IV | <0.25 | 1 | 2–4 |
| Insulin Lispro | Humalog | SC | <0.25 | 1 | 3.5–4.5 |
| **SHORT ACTING** | | | | | |
| Insulin injection regular (R) (OTC) | Humulin R U-100 | SC, IM, IV | 0.5 | 2–4 | 6–8 |
| | Novolin R | SC, IM, IV | 0.5 | 2.5–5 | 8 |
| **INTERMEDIATE ACTING** | | | | | |
| Insulin Isophane Suspension (NPH) (OTC) | Humulin N | SC | 1–2 | 6–12 | 18–24 |
| | Novolin N | SC | 1.5 | 4–12 | 24 |
| **SHORT AND INTERMEDIATE ACTING MIXTURES** | | | | | |
| Insulin Aspart Protamine/Insulin Aspart | Novo Log Mix 70/30 | SC | <0.25 | 1–4 | 24 |
| Insulin isophane suspension (NPH)/ regular insulin (R) | Humulin 50/50 | SC | 0.5 | 3–5 | 24 |
| Insulin isophane suspension (NPH)/ regular insulin (R) | Novolin 70/30 | SC | 0.5 | 2–12 | 24 |
| | Humulin 70/30 | SC | 0.5 | 2–12 | 24 |
| Insulin lispro protamine/ insulin lispro | Humalog Mix 50/50 | SC | <0.25 | 1 | 16 |
| | Humalog Mix 75/25 | SC | <0.25 | 0.5–1.5 | 24 |

*Continued*

## Table 5–3 Insulin Preparations—cont'd

| PREPARATION | BRAND | ROUTE | ONSET (HOURS) | PEAK (HOURS) | DURATION (HOURS) |
|---|---|---|---|---|---|
| **LONG ACTING** | | | | | |
| Insulin detemir | Levemir | SC | 1 | None | 24 |
| Insulin glargine | Lantus | SC | 1.1 | None | >24 |

Insulin isophane (OTC); regular insulin (R) (OTC).

CSII: continuous subcutaneous insulin infusion; IM: intramuscular injection; Inh: inhalation; IV: intravenous infusion; OTC: over the counter; SC: subcutaneous injection.

Injectable insulins listed in the table are available in a concentration of 100 U/mL; Humulin R, in a concentration of 500 U/mL for SC injection only, is available by prescription from Eli Lilly, Inc., for insulin-resistant patients who are hospitalized or under close medical supervision.

Adapted from Monthly Prescribing Reference. Haymarket Publishing Inc. Web site: http://www.empr.com

managing type 2 diabetes is to achieve and maintain glycemic levels as close to the nondiabetic range as possible. Interventions should be changed and medications rapidly titrated upward to allow for the safety of the individual patient. The following is a summary of recommendations from the ADA and EASD:

- Intervention at the time of diagnosis with metformin, in combination with lifestyle changes, diet therapy, and exercise
- Continuing timely augmentation of therapy with additional agents (including early initiation of insulin therapy) as a means of achieving and maintaining recommended levels of glycemic control (i.e., $HbA_{1c} < 7\%$ for most patients)

Oral medications approved for treating type 2 diabetes are shown in Table 5–4. It is not unusual to use multiple medications to achieve recommendations for glycemic control.

## Crushing or Chewing Medications

Dosage forms currently used for some drugs may change these drugs' release or efficacy if the dosage form is crushed or chewed. Drugs in these dosage forms may contain a controlled-release, extended-release, long-acting, or sustained-release mechanism that delivers these drugs at a slower rate than with conventional tablet or capsule dosage forms. The modified delivery systems may change the frequency with which

## Table 5-4  Oral Antidiabetic Agents

| DRUG CLASS | GENERIC NAME | BRAND | STRENGTH AND FORM |
|---|---|---|---|
| Alpha-glucosidase inhibitors | Acarbose | Precose | 25 mg tablets |
| | Miglitol | Glyset | 25 mg tablets |
| | | | 50 mg tablets<br>100 mg tablets |
| Amino acid derivatives | Nateglinide | Starlix | 60 mg tablets<br>120 mg tablets |
| Biguanides | Metformin | Fortamet | 500 mg extended-release tablets<br>1000 mg extended-release tablets |
| | | Glucophage | 500 mg tablets<br>850 mg tablets<br>1000 mg tablets |
| | | Glucophage XR | 500 mg extended-release tablets<br>750 mg extended-release tablets |
| | | Glumetza | 500 mg extended-release tablets |
| | | Riomet | 500 mg/5mL oral solution |
| Bile acid sequestrant | Colesevelam | Welchol | 625 mg tablets |
| Dipeptidyl peptidase | Sitagliptin | Januvia | 25 mg tablets<br>50 mg tablets<br>100 mg tabs |
| Combination dipeptidyl peptidase-4 inhibitor + biguanide | Sitagliptin + metformin | Janumet | 50 mg/500 mg tablets<br>50 mg/1000 mg tablets |

| Table 5–4 Oral Antidiabetic Agents—cont'd | | | |
|---|---|---|---|
| **DRUG CLASS** | **GENERIC NAME** | **BRAND** | **STRENGTH AND FORM** |
| Meglitinides | Repaglinide | Prandin | 0.5 mg tablets<br>1 mg tablets<br>2 mg tablets |
| Sulfonylureas<br>First generation | Chlorpropamide | Diabinese | 100 mg scored tablets<br>250 mg scored tablets |
| Sulfonylureas<br>Second<br>generation | Glimepiride | Amaryl | 1 mg scored tablets<br>2 mg scored tablets<br>4 mg scored tablets |
| | Glipizide | Glucotrol | 5 mg scored tablets<br>10 mg scored tablets |
| | | Glucotrol XL | 2.5 mg ext-rel tablets<br>5 mg ext-rel tablets<br>10 mg ext-rel tablets |
| | Glyburide | Diaßeta | 1.25 mg scored tablets<br>2.5 mg scored tablets<br>5 mg scored tablets |
| | | Micronase | 1.25 mg scored tablets<br>2.5 mg scored tablets<br>5 mg scored tablets |
| | Glyburide,<br>micronized | Glynase<br>Pres Tab | 1.5 mg scored tablets<br>3 mg scored tablets<br>6 mg scored tablets |
| Combination<br>sulfonylurea +<br>biguanide | Glipizide +<br>metformin<br>(mg glipizide/<br>mg metformin) | Metaglip | 2.5 mg/250 mg tablets<br>2.5 mg/500 mg tablets<br>5 mg/500 mg tablets |
| | Glyburide +<br>metformin<br>(mg glyburide/<br>mg metformin) | Glucovance | 1.25 mg/250 mg tablets<br>2.5 mg/500 mg tablets<br>5 mg/500 mg tablets |

## Table 5–4 Oral Antidiabetic Agents cont'd

| DRUG CLASS | GENERIC NAME | BRAND | STRENGTH AND FORM |
|---|---|---|---|
| Thiazolidinediones | Pioglitazone | Actos | 15 mg tablets<br>30 mg tablets<br>45 mg tablets |
| | Rosiglitazone | Avandia | 2 mg tablets<br>4 mg tablets<br>8 mg tablets |
| Combination thiazolidinedione + biguanide | Pioglitazone + metformin | Actoplus Met | 15 mg/500 mg tablets<br>15 mg/850 mg tablets |
| | Rosiglitazone + metformin (mg rosiglitazone/ mg metformin) | Avandamet | 2 mg/500 mg tablets<br>4 mg/500 mg tablets<br>2 mg/1000 mg tablets<br>4 mg/1000 mg tablets |
| Combination thiazolidinedione + sulfonylurea | Pioglitazone + glimepiride (mg pioglitazone/ mg glimepiride) | Duetact | 30 mg/2 mg tablets<br>30 mg/4 mg tablets |
| | Rosiglitazone + glimepiride (mg rosiglitazone/ mg glimepiride) | Avandaryl | 4 mg/1 mg tablets<br>4 mg/2 mg tablets<br>4 mg/4 mg tablets |

Adapted from Monthly Prescribing Reference Haymarket Publishing Inc., 2009; http://www.empr.com/Diabetes-Treatment/article/123836/

a drug has to be prescribed and the duration of its availability for utilization by the body. Many drug dosage forms should not be crushed, chewed, or dissolved, since this may interfere with the absorption of these drugs. The names of drugs and drug dosage form to which these various considerations apply may contain abbreviations that indicate the unique mechanism for drug delivery, such as CD, CR, ER, LA, SR, and XL. Medications that have an outer coating, such as enteric-coated medications, should not be chewed, crushed, or divided. Table 5–5 contains some frequently used medications that should not be chewed, crushed, or divided.

## Table 5–5 Medications That Should Not Be Crushed or Chewed

**ALLERGIC DISORDERS**

**Sustained release:**
Chlor-Trimeton 8HR/12HR
**Orally disintegrating tablets:**
Alavert ODT, Clarinex Reditabs, Claritin Reditabs

**CARDIOVASCULAR SYSTEM**

**Sustained release:**
Adalat CC, Advicor, Afeditab CR, Aggrenox, Altoprev, Calan SR, Cardene, SR, Cardizem CD, Cardizem LA, Cardizem, Cardura XL, Cartia XL, Coreg CR, Covera HS, Dilacor XR, Dilatrate SR, DynaCirc CR, Imdu, Inderal LA, Innopran XL, Isoptin SR, Lescol XL, Lexxel, Niaspan, Nifediac CC9, Norpace CR, Plendil, Procanbid, Procardia XL, Quinidine Gluconate ER, Quinidine Sulfate ER, Ranexa, Rythmol SR, Sular, Tarka, Tiazac, Toprol XL, Trental, Verelan, Verelan PM
**Sublingual:**
Isordil SL, Nitroquick, Nitrostat
**Miscellaneous:**
Lanoxicap

**CENTRAL NERVOUS SYSTEM**

**Sustained release:**
Adderall XR, Ambien CR, Budeprion SR, Carbatrol, Compazine Spansules, Concerta, Cymbalta, Depakene, Depakote, Depakote ER, Depakote Sprinkles, Dexedrine Spansule, Dilantin, Effexor XR, Eskalith CR, Equetro, Focalin XR, Invega, Lithobid, Metadate CD, Metadate ER, Methylin ER, Paxil CR, Phenytek, Prozac Weekly, Razadyne ER, Ritalin LA, Ritalin SR, Seroquel XR, Sinemet CR, Somnote, Tegretol XR, Tranxene SD, Topamax, Wellbutrin SR/XL, Xanax XR
**Orally disintegrating tablets:**
Abilify DiscMelt, Aricept ODT, FazaClo, Klonopin Wafers, Niravam, Parcopa, Remeron Solutab, Risperdal M-Tabs, Zelapar, Zyprexa Zydis
**Miscellaneous:**
Keppra, Strattera, Zonegran

**DERMATOLOGICAL/EAR/EYE DISORDERS**

**Sustained release:**
Diamox, Doryx, Oracea, Solodyn
**Miscellaneous:**
Accutane, Minocin, Propecia

**ENDOCRINE SYSTEM**

**Sustained release:**
Fortamet, Glipizide ER, Glucophage XR, Glucotrol XL, Glumetza, Zemplar
**Buccal:**
Striant

Table 5–5 **Medications That Should Not Be Crushed or Chewed—cont'd**

## ENDOCRINE SYSTEM

**Miscellaneous:**
Sensipar

## GASTROINTESTINAL TRACT

**Sustained release:**
Colestid, Donnatal Extentabs, Levbid, Lialda, Pentasa
**Enteric coated:**
Aciphex, Asacol, Azulfidine EN-tabs, Correctol, Creon, Dulcolax, Entocort EC, Fleet, Nexium, Pancrease MT1, Pancrecarb MS, Prevacid1, Prilose, Protonix
**Orally disintegrating tablets:**
Prevacid Solutab, Zofran ODT
**Sublingual:**
Levsin SL
**Miscellaneous:**
Amitiza, Marinol, Pepto-Bismol Caplet

## IMMUNE SYSTEM/NEOPLASM

**Sustained release:**
Myfortic
**Miscellaneous:**
Cellcept, Temodar, Zolinza

## INFECTIONS AND INFESTATIONS

**Sustained release:**
Augmentin XR, Biaxin XL, Ceclor CD, Cipro XR, Doryx, Ery-Tab, Flagyl ER, Proquin XR
**Enteric coated:**
Eryc, Videx EC
**Miscellaneous:**
Aptivus, Ceftin, Ketek, Lamprene, Minocin, Mycelex Troche, Valcyte

## MUSCULOSKELETAL DISORDERS

**Sustained release:**
Indocin SR, Lodine XL, Mestinon Timespan, Naprelan, Norflex, Oruvail XR, Tylenol Arthritis, Voltaren XR
**Enteric coated:**
Arthrotec, Azulfidine EN-tabs, Bayer Arthritis, EC-Naprosyn, Ecotrin, Sulfazine EC, Voltaren
**Miscellaneous:**
Actonel, Actonel+ Ca, Boniva, Dolobid, Evista, Feldene, Fosamax, Fosamax+ D

*Continued*

## Table 5–5  Medications That Should Not Be Crushed or Chewed—cont'd

### NUTRITION

**Sustained release:**
Bontril Slow Release, Diethylpropion SR, Fero-Folic, Ferro-Sequels, Ionamin, K-Dur, Klor-Con, Klor-Con M6, Klotrix, K-Tab, Mag-Tab SR, Micro-K1, Prelu-2, Slo-Niacin, Slow-Fe, Slow Fe+ Folic Acid, Slow K
**Miscellaneous:**
K-Lyte

### PAIN AND PYREXIA

**Sustained release:**
Actiq (lozenge), Avinza, Kadian, MS Contin, Opana ER, Oramorph Sr, Oxycontin, Topamax, Ultram ER
**Orally disintegrating tablets:**
Maxalt-MLT, Zomig ZMT
**Buccal:**
Fentora

### POISONING AND DRUG DEPENDENCE

**Sustained release:**
Zyban
**Enteric coated:**
Campral
**Sublingual:**
Suboxone, Subutex
**Miscellaneous:**
Commit (lozenge), Exjade

### RESPIRATORY TRACT

**Sustained release:**
Alavert D-12, Allegra-D, Clarinex-D, Claritin-D, Accuhist LA, Bromfed PD/SR, Bromfenex, Bromfenex PD, Deconamine SR, Duratuss A/GP/PE, Entex LA/PSE, Extendryl SR/JR, Humibid, Mucinex, Prolex-D/PD, Sudafed12/24HR, Theo-24, Uniphyl, Zyrtec-D
**Miscellaneous:**
Tessalon

### UROGENITAL SYSTEM

**Sustained release:**
Detrol LA, Ditropan XL, Enablex, Flomax, Sanctura-XR, Uroxatral
**Enteric coated:**
Urocit-K
**Miscellaneous:**
Avodart, Proscar, Renagel, Vesicare

Adapted from Monthly Prescribing Reference Haymarket Marketing Inc., Publishing, 2009; http://media.haymarketmedia.com/Documents/2/DNCC_1065.pdf

# Approximate Practical Equivalents

Weight and measure equivalents are handy references when the need arises to convert drug dosages. Table 5–6 provides the NP with easy access to common approximate practical equivalents.

## Table 5–6  Approximate Practical Equivalents

| WEIGHT EQUIVALENTS | |
|---|---|
| 1 grain | 65 mg |
| 1 mg | 0.015 grains |
| 1 g | 15.432 grains |
| 1 g | 0.035 ounces |
| 1 ounce avoirdupois (oz) | 28.35 g |
| 1 ounce apothecary | 31.1 g |
| 1 pound avoirdupois (lb) | 454 g |
| 1 pound avoirdupois (lb) | 0.45 kg |
| 1 kg | 2.2 pounds avoirdupois (lb) |
| VOLUME EQUIVALENTS | |
| 1 mL | 16.23 minims |
| 1 cc* | 1.0 mL |
| 1 fluidram† | 3.7 mL |
| 1 teaspoonful† | 5 mL |
| 1 tablespoonful | 15 mL |
| 1 fluid ounce | 29.57 mL |
| 1 wineglassful (2 fl oz) | 60 mL |
| 1 teacupful (4 fl oz) | 120 mL |

*Continued*

## Table 5–6 **Approximate Practical Equivalents—cont'd**

| VOLUME EQUIVALENTS | |
|---|---|
| 1 tumblerful (8 fl Z) | 240 mL |
| 1 pint (pt or O or Oct) | 473 mL |
| 1 quart | 946 mL |
| 1 L | 33.8 fluid ounces |
| 1 gallon (gal or C or cong) | 3785 mL |

* cc and mL are equivalent.
† On prescription, a fluidram is assumed to contain a teaspoonful, which is 5 mL.

| WEIGHT-TO-VOLUME EQUIVALENTS | |
|---|---|
| 1 mg/dL | 10 mcg/mL<br>1 mg percent (mg %) |
| 1% solution | 10 mg/mL |
| 1 part per million (ppm) | 1 mg/L |

| LINEAR EQUIVALENTS | |
|---|---|
| 1 millimeter | 0.04 inches |
| 1 inch | 25.4 millimeters |
| 1 inch | 2.54 centimeters |
| 1 meter | 39.37 inches |
| 1 inch | 0.025 meters |

Adapted from Monthly Prescribing Reference Haymarket Marketing Inc. Publishing, 2009; http://www.empr.com/Approximate-Practical-Equivalents/article/123355

## Schedules of Controlled Drugs

A controlled drug is one whose use and distribution are tightly controlled because of its abuse potential or risk. Controlled drugs are also known as scheduled drugs. Controlled drugs are ranked in the order of their risk for abuse and are placed in specific schedules by the U.S. Drug Enforcement

Administration (DEA). Drugs with the greatest potential for abuse are assigned to Schedule I and those with the least potential for abuse are assigned to Schedule V. These schedules are commonly abbreviated as C-I, C-II, C-III, C-IV, and C-V. Some examples of drugs in these schedules are shown in Box 5–1.

---

### Box 5–1  Schedule of Controlled Drugs

- **Schedule I:** Drugs with a high risk for abuse. These drugs have no safe, accepted medical use in the United States. Some examples are heroin, marijuana, lysergic acid diethylamide (LSD), phencyclidine (PCP), and crack cocaine.
- **Schedule II:** Drugs with a high risk for abuse but which also have safe and accepted medical uses in the United States. Products marked CII have a high potential for abuse that may lead to severe psychological or physical dependence. Prescriptions for these drugs must be written in ink or typewritten and signed by the prescribing practitioner. Verbal prescriptions cannot be made except in a genuine emergency, and a written prescription must be provided to the dispensing pharmacist within 72 hours after such verbal prescription. No prescriptions for these drugs can be renewed. Drugs in Schedule II include certain narcotic, stimulant, and depressant drugs. Some examples are morphine, cocaine, oxycodone (Percodan), methylphenidate (Ritalin), and dextroamphetamine (Dexedrine).
- **Schedule III:** These drugs have less of an abuse risk than those in Schedule II. Drugs in Schedule III also have safe and accepted medical uses in the United States. Use of these drugs may lead to moderate or low physical dependence or high psychological dependence. Prescriptions for drugs in Schedule III can be oral or written, and may be renewed up to five times within 6 months. Some examples of drugs in Schedule III are anabolic steroids, butalbital (Fiorinal), and hydrocodone combination products <15 milligrams per dosage unit (mg/du) (Lorcet, Lortab, Vicodin, Vicoprofen, Tussionex, Norco).
- **Schedule IV:** These drugs have a low abuse potential, but their use may lead to limited physical or psychological dependence. Prescriptions for these drugs may be oral or written, and may be renewed up to five times within 6 months. Some examples of drugs in Schedule IV are alprazolam (Xanax), zolpidem (Ambien), and zopiclone (Lunesta).
- **Schedule V:** These drugs have a low abuse potential, may or may not require a prescription, and are subject to state and local regulation. Some examples are 2.5 mg/25 mcg preparations of diphenoxylate (Lomotil) (tablets: 2.5 mg diphenoxylate and 0.025 mg atropine: liquid:2.5 mg diphenoxylate and 0.025 mg atropine per teaspoonful), and codeine preparations of 200 mg/100 mL or 100 g (Robitussin A-C, Pediacof)

# Pregnancy Categories

When pregnancy appears as a contraindication or precaution to the use of a drug, the safety of the drug is usually qualified by its inclusion in a specific category. These categories are shown and described in Table 5–7.

| Table 5–7 **Categories for Drug Use in Pregnancy** | |
| --- | --- |
| **CATEGORY** | **DESCRIPTION** |
| A | Adequate, well-controlled studies in pregnant women have not shown an increased risk of fetal abnormalities. |
| B | Animal studies have revealed no evidence of harm to the fetus, but there are no adequate and well-controlled studies in pregnant women. or Animal studies have shown an adverse effect, but adequate and well-controlled studies in pregnant women have failed to demonstrate a risk to the fetus. |
| C | Animal studies have shown an adverse effect and there are no adequate and well-controlled studies in pregnant women. or No animal studies have been conducted and there are no adequate and well-controlled studies in pregnant women. |
| D | Adequate and well-controlled or observational studies in pregnant women have demonstrated a risk to the fetus. However, the benefits of treatment with the drug may outweigh the potential risk. |
| X | Adequate and well-controlled or observational studies in animals or pregnant women have demonstrated positive evidence of fetal abnormalities. The use of the product is contraindicated in women who are or may become pregnant. |

# 6 Medical References

# CHAPTER 6

# Medical References

This chapter contains an assortment of medical references for use in the clinical assessment of patients. It describes the Glasgow Coma Scale (GCS) for adults and children, scoring guidelines for the Apgar test, reporting scales for adult patients with attention deficit-hyperactivity disorder (ADHD), the scale for calculating the International Prostate Symptoms Score (IPSS), a pelvic pain and urgency scale, and a fibromyalgia self-report scale. It also provides an outline for recording a patient history and conducting a physical examination. Additional information is provided on laboratory values in anemia and hepatitis, depression scales, and general information on fractures and sprains. The chapter concludes with an overview of commonly used herbal products.

## Glasgow Coma Scale

The GCS provides a score in the range of 3 to 15 to allow the clinician to assess mental status. Scores ranging from 3 to 8 are seen in patients in comatose states. A score of 9 to 11 is indicative of moderately severe head injury; and a score of 12 or more may indicate a minor injury. Scores on the GCS are recorded for three areas of response: eye opening, verbal response, and motor response. The three response scores are added together to yield the coma score. Table 6–1 provides the GCS scoring for an adult head-injury patient; Table 6–2 provides GCS scoring adjusted for children and infants.

## Table 6–1 Glasgow Coma Scale

| SCALE | BEHAVIOR | SCORE |
|---|---|---|
| Eye opening response | Spontaneous, opens eyes with blinking at baseline | 4 points |
| | Opens eyes to verbal command, speech, or shout | 3 points |
| | Opens eyes to pain, not applied to face, but to other body areas | 2 points |
| | None | 1 point |
| Verbal response | Oriented | 5 points |
| | Confused conversation, able to answer questions, coherent speech | 4 points |
| | Inappropriate responses, jumbled phrases | 3 points |
| | Incomprehensible speech/sounds | 2 points |
| | None | 1 point |
| Motor response | Obeys commands for movement | 6 points |
| | Purposeful movements in response to painful stimulus | 5 points |
| | Withdraws from painful stimulus | 4 points |
| | Abnormal spastic flexion, decorticate posturing | 3 points |
| | Extensor response, decerebrate posturing | 2 points |
| | None | 1 point |

## Apgar Scores

The Apgar score is used to evaluate infants for activity, pulse, grimace, appearance, and respiration status at 1 min and 5 min after birth. Apgar scores based on these variables range from 0 to 10. A score of 7 at 1 min after birth is considered good health. The 5-min score should be at least 7, reflecting appropriate fetal adjustment after birth. Table 6–3 presents a simple algorithm for applying an Apgar score to a newborn.

## Table 6–2 Glasgow Coma Scale for Children and Infants (Verbal Response)

| SCORE | 2–5 YEARS | 0–23 MONTHS |
|---|---|---|
| 5 | Appropriate words or phrases | Smiles or coos appropriately |
| 4 | Inappropriate words | Cries but is consolable |
| 3 | Persistent cries and screams | Persistent inappropriate crying and screaming |
| 2 | Grunts | Grunts or is agitated or restless |
| 1 | No response | No response |

Adapted from Northeast Center for Special Care: http://www.northeastcenter.com/modified-glasgow-coma-scale-for-infants-and-children.htm

## Table 6–3 Apgar Scores for Newborn Assessment

| APGAR CRITERION | 0 | 1 | 2 |
|---|---|---|---|
| Color (appearance) | Blue/pale | Normal color, but hands and feet are bluish | Normal color all over, hands and feet pink |
| Pulse | Absent | <100 | >100 |
| Reflex (grimace) | None | Grimace, facial movement only with stimulation | Cough/sneeze, pulls away |
| Tone (activity) | Limp, no movement | Some flexion, arms and legs flexed with little movement | Active, spontaneous movement |
| Respirations | Absent | Slow/irregular, weak cry | Crying/good rate |

## Prostate Symptoms Test for Men

The American Urological Association has developed a questionnaire to assess the symptoms of urological problems in male patients. The questionnaire is known as the IPSS. Each of the seven questions in the questionnaire is scored from 0 to 5; total scores are tallied to determine the severity of symptoms. A score of 0 to 7 represents mild symptoms; a score of 8 to 19 represents moderate symptoms; and a score of 20 to 35 represents severe symptoms. Table 6–4 contains the IPSS questions for bothersome bladder symptoms in men. The first seven questions deal with the bothersome symptoms of prostate enlargement. The final question on the tool inquires about quality of life related to bladder symptoms.

## Table 6–4 International Prostate Symptom Score

| QUESTIONS | RESPONSES | SCORE |
|---|---|---|
| **UROLOGY QUESTIONS** | | |
| 1. How often have you had a sensation of not emptying your bladder completely after you have finished urinating? | Not at all<br>Less than 1 time in 5<br>Less than half the time<br>About half the time<br>More than half the time<br>Almost always | 0<br>1<br>2<br>3<br>4<br>5 |
| 2. How often have you had to urinate again within 2 hours after you finished urinating? | Not at all<br>Less than 1 time in 5<br>Less than half the time<br>About half the time<br>More than half the time<br>Almost always | 0<br>1<br>2<br>3<br>4<br>5 |
| 3. How often have you stopped and started urinating several times while urinating? | Not at all<br>Less than 1 time in 5<br>Less than half the time<br>About half the time<br>More than half the time<br>Almost always | 0<br>1<br>2<br>3<br>4<br>5 |
| 4. How often have you found it difficult to postpone urination? | Not at all<br>Less than 1 time in 5<br>Less than half the time<br>About half the time<br>More than half the time<br>Almost always | 0<br>1<br>2<br>3<br>4<br>5 |
| 5. How often have you had a weak urinary stream? | Not at all<br>Less than 1 time in 5<br>Less than half the time<br>About half the time<br>More than half the time<br>Almost always | 0<br>1<br>2<br>3<br>4<br>5 |

| QUESTIONS | RESPONSES | SCORE |
|-----------|-----------|-------|
| **Table 6–4 International Prostate Symptom Score—cont'd** | | |
| 6. How often have you had to push or strain to begin urination? | Not at all<br>Less than 1 time in 5<br>Less than half the time<br>About half the time<br>More than half the time<br>Almost always | 0<br>1<br>2<br>3<br>4<br>5 |
| 7. How often have you had to get up at least once in the night to urinate? | Not at all<br>Less than 1 time in 5<br>Less than half the time<br>About half the time<br>More than half the time<br>Almost always | 0<br>1<br>2<br>3<br>4<br>5 |
| **QUALITY OF LIFE QUESTION** | | |
| If you had to spend the rest of your life with your urinary condition just the way it is right now, how would you feel? | Delighted<br>Pleased<br>Mostly satisfied<br>Mixed<br>Mostly dissatisfied<br>Unhappy<br>Terrible | |

Source: http://www.usrf.org/questionnaires/AUA_SymptomScore.html

## Pelvic Pain and Urgency/Frequency Scale

The pelvic pain and urgency/frequency scale provides a mechanism for the self-reporting and assessment of male and female genitourinary symptoms on both a symptom scale and a bothersome symptom scale. Questions on the scale assess urinary frequency as well as issues relating to pelvic pain in seven questions. Table 6–5 presents the Pelvic Pain and Urgency/Frequency Patient Symptom Scale. Symptom scores and bothersome-symptom scores are combined for a total patient score. Scores range from 1 to 35. A score of <10 is considered normal; a score of 10 to 14 indicates a 74% likelihood of pelvic disease; a score of 15 to 19 indicates a 76% likelihood of disease; and a score of 20 or more indicates a 91% likelihood of pelvic disease.

## Table 6–5 Pelvic Pain and Urgency/Frequency Patient Symptom Scale

|  |  | 0 | 1 | 2 | 3 | 4 | SYMPTOM SCORE | BOTHER SCORE |
|---|---|---|---|---|---|---|---|---|
| 1 | How many times do you go to the bathroom during the day? | 3–6 | 7–10 | 11–14 | 15–19 | 20+ |  |  |
| 2a | How many times do you go to the bathroom at night? | 0 | 1 | 2 | 3 | 4+ |  |  |
| 2b | If you get up at night to go to the bathroom, does it bother you? | Never | Occasionally | Usually | Always |  |  |  |
| 3a | Do you now or have you ever had pain or symptoms during or after sexual intercourse? | Never | Occasionally | Usually | Always |  |  |  |
| 3b | Has pain or urgency ever made you avoid sexual intercourse? | Never | Occasionally | Usually | Always |  |  |  |
| 4 | Do you have pain associated with your bladder or in your pelvis (vagina, labia, lower abdomen, urethra, perineum, testes, or scrotum)? | Never | Occasionally | Usually | Always |  |  |  |

|  |  | | | | |
|---|---|---|---|---|---|
| 5a | If you have pain, is it usually | Mild | Moderate | Severe | |
| 5b | Does your pain bother you? | Never | Occasionally | Usually | Always |
| 6 | Do you still have urgency after going to the bathroom? | Never | Occasionally | Usually | Always |
| 7a | If you have urgency, is it usually | Mild | Moderate | Severe | |
| 7b | Does your urgency bother you? | Never | Occasionally | Usually | Always |
| 8 | Are you sexually active? Yes _____ No _____ | | | | |
| | Symptom score = 1, 2a, 3a, 4, 5a, 6, 7a | | | | |
| | Bother score = 2b, 3b, 5b, 7b | | | | |
| | Total score = Symptom score + Bother score | | | | |

© C. Lowell Parsons

## Fibromyalgia Symptom Intensity Scale

The Fibromyalgia Symptom Intensity Scale (FSIS) is an excellent tool to use with patients with fibromyalgia in the clinic setting. Patients can complete the self report of their symptom intensity while waiting for the health care clinician, and then be ready to discuss their symptom management with the clinician. This tool would also provide excellent documentation of progress or lack of progress in patient symptom management if data were collected at each office visit. Table 6–6 presents the FSIS.

Table 6–6 **Fibromyalgia Symptom Intensity Scale**

HOW MUCH OF A PROBLEM HAS FATIGUE OR TIREDNESS BEEN FOR YOU IN THE PAST WEEK? PLEASE WRITE IN THE BOX BELOW THE NUMBER THAT BEST DESCRIBES THE SEVERITY OF YOUR FATIGUE ON A SCALE OF 0-100 WITH 0 REPRESENTING FATIGUE IS NOT A PROBLEM AND 100 REPRESENTING FATIGUE IS A MAJOR PROBLEM

Fatigue is no problem                                    Fatigue is a major problem

PLEASE INDICATE BELOW THE AMOUNT OF PAIN AND/OR TENDERNESS YOU HAVE HAD OVER <u>THE PAST 7 DAYS</u> IN EACH OF THE JOINT AND BODY AREAS LISTED BELOW. PLEASE MARK AN X IN THE BOX THAT BEST DESCRIBES YOUR PAIN OR TENDERNESS. BE SURE TO MARK BOTH THE RIGHT SIDE AND THE LEFT SIDE SEPARATELY. IF YOU HAVE HAD NO PAIN OR TENDERNESS IN A PARTICULAR JOINT OR BODY PART, MARK "NONE." THERE SHOULD BE AN ANSWER FOR EVERY JOINT OR BODY PART LISTED.

| JOINTS | NONE | MILD | MODERATE | SEVERE |
|---|---|---|---|---|
| Shoulder, left | ☐ | ☐ | ☐ | ☐ |
| Shoulder, right | ☐ | ☐ | ☐ | ☐ |
| Hip, left | ☐ | ☐ | ☐ | ☐ |
| Hip, right | ☐ | ☐ | ☐ | ☐ |
| Jaw, left | ☐ | ☐ | ☐ | ☐ |
| Jaw, right | ☐ | ☐ | ☐ | ☐ |
| Lower back | ☐ | ☐ | ☐ | ☐ |
| Upper back | ☐ | ☐ | ☐ | ☐ |
| Neck | ☐ | ☐ | ☐ | ☐ |
| Head | ☐ | ☐ | ☐ | ☐ |

| JOINTS | NONE | MILD | MODERATE | SEVERE |
|---|---|---|---|---|
| **Table 6–6  Fibromyalgia Symptom Intensity Scale—cont'd** | | | | |
| **OTHER BODY AREAS** | | | | |
| Upper arms, left | ☐ | ☐ | ☐ | ☐ |
| Upper arms, right | ☐ | ☐ | ☐ | ☐ |
| Lower arms, left | ☐ | ☐ | ☐ | ☐ |
| Lower arms, right | ☐ | ☐ | ☐ | ☐ |
| Upper leg, left | ☐ | ☐ | ☐ | ☐ |
| Upper leg, right | ☐ | ☐ | ☐ | ☐ |
| Lower leg, left | ☐ | ☐ | ☐ | ☐ |
| Lower leg, right | ☐ | ☐ | ☐ | ☐ |
| Chest | ☐ | ☐ | ☐ | ☐ |
| Abdomen | ☐ | ☐ | ☐ | ☐ |

Source: National Data Bank for Rheumatic Diseases, www.arthritis-research.org

## Adult Attention Deficit-Hyperactivity Disorder Self-Report Scale

The Adult ADHD Self-Report Scale (ASRS) provides patients with a quick scale with which to report symptoms, impairments, and history to aid the clinician in identifying and managing adult ADHD. Components of the scale are based on the 18 criteria for ADHD given in the *Diagnostic and Statistical Manual of Mental Disorders, 4th Edition* (DSM IV) published by the American Psychiatric Association. The six questions in Part A of the scale are most predictive of symptoms consistent with ADHD; part B contains the remaining 12 questions. If a patient has four or more marks in the darker-shaded boxes in Part A, the score is highly consistent with adult ADHD. The frequency cues in Part B provide additional information to aid the clinician in the analysis of patient symptoms, but these responses are not scored in the tool. Table 6–7 shows the questions in the Adult ADHD Self Report Scale.

## Table 6–7 Adult Attention Deficit-Hyperactivity Disorder Self-Report Scale

Please answer the questions below, rating yourself on each of the criteria shown using the scale on the right side of the page. As you answer each question, place an X in the box that describes how you have felt and conducted yourself over the past 6 months. Please give this completed checklist to your health care provider to discuss during today's appointment.

| PART A | NEVER | RARELY | SOMETIMES | VERY OFTEN | OFTEN |
|---|---|---|---|---|---|
| 1. How often do you have trouble wrapping up the final details of a project, once the challenging parts have been done? | ☐ | ☐ | ☐ | ☐ | ☐ |
| 2. How often do you have difficulty getting things in order when you have to do a task that requires organization? | ☐ | ☐ | ☐ | ☐ | ☐ |
| 3. How often do you have problems remembering appointments or obligations? | ☐ | ☐ | ☐ | ☐ | ☐ |
| 4. When you have a task that requires a lot of thought, how often do you avoid or delay getting started? | ☐ | ☐ | ☐ | ☐ | ☐ |
| 5. How often do you fidget or squirm with your hands or feet when you have to sit down for a long time? | ☐ | ☐ | ☐ | ☐ | ☐ |
| 6. How often do you feel overly active and compelled to do things, as if you were driven by a motor? | ☐ | ☐ | ☐ | ☐ | ☐ |

## Table 6–7  Adult Attention Deficit-Hyperactivity Disorder Self-Report Scale—cont'd

| PART B | NEVER | RARELY | SOMETIMES | OFTEN | VERY OFTEN |
|---|---|---|---|---|---|
| 7. How often do you make careless mistakes when you have to work on a boring or difficult project? | ☐ | ☐ | ☐ | ☐ | ☐ |
| 8. How often do you have difficulty keeping your attention when you are doing boring or repetitive work? | ☐ | ☐ | ☐ | ☐ | ☐ |
| 9. How often do you have difficulty concentrating on what people say to you even when they are speaking to you directly? | ☐ | ☐ | ☐ | ☐ | ☐ |
| 10. How often do you misplace or have difficulty finding things at work or at home? | ☐ | ☐ | ☐ | ☐ | ☐ |
| 11. How often are you distracted by activity or noise around you? | ☐ | ☐ | ☐ | ☐ | ☐ |
| 12. How often do you leave your seat in meetings or other situations in which you are expected to remain seated? | ☐ | ☐ | ☐ | ☐ | ☐ |
| 13. How often do you feel restless or fidgety? | ☐ | ☐ | ☐ | ☐ | ☐ |

*Continued*

## Table 6–7 Adult Attention Deficit-Hyperactivity Disorder Self-Report Scale

| PART B | NEVER | RARELY | SOMETIMES | OFTEN | VERY OFTEN |
|---|---|---|---|---|---|
| 14. How often do you have difficulty unwinding and relaxing when you have time to yourself? | ☐ | ☐ | ☐ | ☐ | ☐ |
| 15. How often do you find ourself talking too much when you are in social situations? | ☐ | ☐ | ☐ | ☐ | ☐ |
| 16. When you are in a conversation, how often do you find yourself finishing the sentences of people you are talking to? | ☐ | ☐ | ☐ | ☐ | ☐ |
| 17. How often do you have difficulty waiting your turn in situations when turn taking is required? | ☐ | ☐ | ☐ | ☐ | ☐ |
| 18. How often do you interrupt others when they are busy? | ☐ | ☐ | ☐ | ☐ | ☐ |

From the World Health Organization (WHO).

## History and Physical Examination Template

The outline shown here for a history and physical examination provides structure and organization designed to permit the clinician to organize medical documentation.

- Name, age, race, sex, and occupation
- Referral source
- Chief complaint

- History of presenting complaint
- Past medical history
  - General
  - Childhood illnesses
  - Adult illnesses
  - Injuries
  - Hospitalizations
  - Surgeries
- Medicines
- Allergies
- Immunization status
- Social status
  - Marital
  - Children
  - Education
  - Sexual history
  - Psychological
  - Occupational exposure
  - Tobacco/alcohol use
- Review of systems
  - General
  - Skin
  - Head/ear, nose, and throat (ENT)
  - Respiratory
  - Cardiac/circulatory
  - Gastrointestinal
  - Genital/gynecological
  - Musculoskeletal
  - Neurological
  - Endocrine
  - Hematological
  - Psychiatric
- Physical examination
  - Vital signs
  - General survey
  - Skin
  - ENT/head
  - Lungs and thorax
  - Breast
  - Cardiac

- Abdomen
- Genitourinary/rectal
- Musculoskeletal
- Neurological

## Hamilton D Scale

The Hamilton D scale is a 21-item scale that patients can answer in the office before seeing the NP. The items address mood, somatic issues, activity, and general feelings inventory. Items on the Hamilton D scale are ranked on a scale of 0 to 4 and include:

- Depressed mood (sadness, hopeless, helpless, worthless)
- Feelings of guilt
- Suicide
- Insomnia
- Work and activities
- Psychomotor (slowness of thought and speech, concentration ability, motor activity)
- Agitation
- Anxiety
- Somatic complaints (gastrointestinal [GI] and general)
- Changes in weight
- Insight
- Hypochondriasis
- General symptoms (loss of libido, sexual performance issues)
- Diurnal variation
- Depersonalization and derealization
- Paranoid symptoms
- Obsessive compulsive symptoms

## Anemia Chart

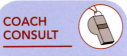

**COACH CONSULT**

Adults need about 180 mg of elemental iron daily during anemic states. Children need about 3 mg/kg/day.

Anemias are classified as microcytic, normocytic, or macrocytic on the basis of the mean corpuscular volume (MCV) in the patient's complete blood count (CBC) report. The initial work-up for anemia should include a thorough patient history of all related symptoms, a complete physical examination, and laboratory values (CBC, hemoglobin [Hgb] and hematocrit [Hct], and MCV). Table 6–8 provides diagnostic help with differentiating anemias on the basis of their classification.

# Table 6–8 Classification of Anemias

| ANEMIA | SERUM Fe³⁺ | TIBC | FERRITIN | Hct | MCV | RBC MORPHOLOGY | COMMENTS |
|---|---|---|---|---|---|---|---|
| Iron deficiency | ↓ | ↑ | ↓↓ <30 ng/mL Is suggestive | ↓ | Normal but later ↓ | Hypochromic Microcytic | Responds to iron replacement |
| Chronic disease | ↓ | ↑ | Normal or high | ↓ But >25% | Normal Slight ↓ | Nondiagnostic | Causes: Cancer, chronic infection, liver disease |
| Vitamin B₁₂ deficiency | X | X | High | ↓ May be low (10%–15%) | ↑↑ >110 fL Can be normal | Anisocytosis Poikilocytosis Howell–Jolly bodies | Glossitis, peripheral neuropathy 12 Nl B 100–250 pg/mL |
| Folic acid deficiency | X | X | High | ↓ May be low (10%–15%) | ↑↑ >110 fL May be normal | Anisocytosis Poikilocytosis Howell–Jolly bodies | Get B12 level to differeniate from B12 def. Always supplement both, just in case |
| Hemolytic anemia | X | X | X | ↓↓ | ↑ | Anisocytosis Poikilocytosis | Hct will fall by about 3%/week until cause is resolved |

*Continued*

## Table 6–8 Classification of Anemias—cont'd

| ANEMIA | SERUM Fe³⁺ | TIBC | FERRITIN | Hct | MCV | RBC MORPHOLOGY | COMMENTS |
|---|---|---|---|---|---|---|---|
| Sideroblastic | ↑↑ May be ≥180 mcg/dL | Normal to low | Normal to high | X | Normal or slightly high | Sideroblasts Basophilic stippling | Alcoholism, lead poisoning, benzene poisoning, irradiation, chemotherapy, rifampin, pyrazinamide |
| Spherocytosis | X | X | X | Normal or low | | Spherocytes | ↑↑ MCHC/spleen fx Fragile spherocytes = hemolysis |
| Sickle cell | X | X | X | X | Normal to low | Sickled RBCs | Sickledex = quick screen Hbg electrophoresis is definitive |
| Beta-thalassemia | Normal or high | Normal to low | Normal or high | ↓↓May be <10% | Normal to low | Target cells Basophilic stippling | Look for family hx Recessive trait |
| G6PD deficiency | X | X | X | During acute phase may be markedly ↓↓ | Episode ↑ | Bite cells Heinz bodies | Common in African American men G6PD enzyme deficiency = Dx |

Hct: hematocrit; G6PD: glucose-6-phosphate dehydrogenase; Hbg: hemoglobin; hx: history; MCV: mean corpuscular volume; RBC: red blood cell; TIBC: total iron-binding capacity; X = values not generally used in the diagnosis of this type of anemia.

# Hepatitis Chart

Diagnoses of the different types of hepatitis are determined by the presence of the various antigens and antibodies shown in the following list:

- IgM antibodies are seen in cases of recent infection
- IgG antibodies, which indicate a previous infection
- Hepatitis B surface antigen (HBsAg), which indicates an acute or chronic infection with hepatitis B
- Hepatitis B core antigen (HBeAg), which is present in the high-infectivity stage of hepatitis B
- IgM anti-Hbc, which is the earliest indicator of acute hepatitis B infection. HBsAg and hepatitis B e-antigen (HBeAg) will appear earlier than IgM anti-Hbc but are more difficult to detect and more expensive to identify
- Anti-HBe, which indicates a resolution of acute hepatitis B infection
- Anti-HBsAg, interpreted as demonstrating immunity to hepatitis B virus (after infection or immunization)

Table 6–9 provides further diagnostic information related to testing for the various other types of hepatitis.

**COACH CONSULT**

In all types of hepatitis, alanine aminotransferase (ALT) levels are higher than aspartate aminotransferase (AST) levels.

**COACH CONSULT**

Hepatitis D virus is transmitted only after infection with hepatitis B virus (HBV). Consider testing for hepatitis D virus (HDV) in sexually active, gay men who have HBV infection.

# Fracture Types

The primary types of bone fracture visible on x-ray films include greenstick, transverse, complete, spiral, hairline, oblique, and comminuted fractures. These are defined as follows:

- **Closed fracture:** No broken skin
- **Comminuted fracture:** More than two fragments of bone, highly unstable
- **Complete fracture:** Complete fracture through the width of a bone
- **Complex fracture:** Severe damage to soft tissue surrounding the fractured bone
- **Compound fracture:** Bone breaks and fragments of bone penetrating soft tissues and breaking through skin

## Table 6–9 Hepatitis Tests

| HEPATITIS TYPE | ACUTE DISEASE MARKERS | CHRONIC DISEASE MARKERS | MARKERS OF RECOVERY |
|---|---|---|---|
| A | IgM anti-HAV antibody | None | IgG anti-HAV antibody |
| B | IgM anti-HBc (core) antibody HBsAg | HBsAg HBcAg (high infectivity) | Anti-HBsAg antibody |
| C | PCR shows HCV RNA Anti-HCV antibody (may be negative early in disease) | Anti-HCV antibody | Undetectable HCV RNA |
| D | Anti-HDV antibody | Total anti- HDV antibody | None |
| E | IgM anti-HEV antibody | None | None |

HAV: hepatitis A virus; HBsAg: hepatitis B surface antigen; HBc: hepatitis B virus core antigen; HCV: hepatitis C virus; HDV: hepatitis D virus; HEV: hepatitis E virus.

Information from Hollier, A. (2006). Adult and Family NP Certification Review Book. Lafayette, LA: APEA Publishers

- **Compression fracture:** Impact fracture
- **Greenstick fracture:** Incomplete fracture in which only one side of a bone is broken; the bone may be bent. More common in children
- **Hairline fracture:** Incomplete fracture with minimal trauma to bone and no significant bone displacement; appears as a crack in the bone
- **Oblique fracture:** A fracture that runs at an angle
- **Spiral fracture:** A break caused by a twisting type of motion; highly unstable
- **Transverse fracture:** A bone break that gives rise to a transverse break or fissure within the bone at a right angle to the lengthwise aspect of the bone

Fractures can be displaced or nondisplaced. Displacement refers to pieces of a fractured bone that have moved from their original location in the intact bone. Displacement falls into three subcategories:

- **Translation displacement:** Sideways movement of the fracture
- **Angulation displacement:** The extent of bending of a bone at a fracture site, described in degrees of angulation

- **Shortening displacement:** The extent to which a fracture is collapsed, measured in centimeters. Also called bayonette apposition

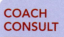

**COACH CONSULT**

A hip fracture may be present in the absence of hip pain or the pain may be referred to the knee. Compare leg lengths in a patient who has had a fall to identify potential hip fractures, one leg will often be longer than the other, or will rotate outward on the affected side.

## Closed Fractures

Closed fractures leave the skin intact and without a wound related to the fracture. There are three AO classifications for fractures:

- **Type A AO classification:**
  - Extra-articular
  - Avulsion fracture, complete fracture, comminuted fracture
- **Type B AO classification:**
  - Intra-articular single-condyle fractures
  - Simple fracture, crush/depression fracture, comminuted fracture
- **Type C AO classification:**
  - Intra-articular with both condyles fractured
  - Simple fracture, crush/depression fracture, comminuted-split depression fracture

## Open Fractures

Open fractures present with an open wound resulting from the underlying fracture. Open fractures are classified into one of three grades according to the Gustilo classification system, with the third grade having three subsets:

- **Grade 1 open fracture:**
  - Wound size <1 cm with minimal soft-tissue damage
  - Wound bed is clean
  - Simple bone injury
  - Average time for bone healing 21 to 28 weeks
- **Grade 2 open fracture:**
  - Wound size >1 cm with moderate soft-tissue damage
  - Moderate contamination of wound bed
  - Fracture displays moderate comminution
  - Average healing time 26 to 28 weeks
- **Grade 3A open fracture:**
  - Wound size is >10 cm with crushed tissue and contamination
  - The fractured bone can be covered with soft tissue
  - Average healing time is 30 to 35 weeks

- **Grade 3B open fracture:**
  - Wound size is >10 cm with crushed tissue and contamination
  - Soft tissue is inadequate and coverage of the fracture requires a regional tissue flap
  - Average healing time 30 to 35 weeks
- **Grade 3C open fracture:**
  - Fracture with major vascular injury requiring repair
  - In some cases it will be necessary to consider amputation

## Salter-Harris Classification

The Salter-Harris fracture classifications represent fractures across the growth plates or physes of bones. This classification system is used for pediatric fractures that involve the growth plate, which are graded from type I through type V. The characteristics of the different grades are as follows:

- **Type I Salter-Harris Fracture:** A fracture that occurs across the physis, without metaphysical or epiphysial injury
- **Type II Salter-Harris Fracture:** A fracture that occurs across the physis and extends into the metaphysis
- **Type III Salter-Harris Fracture:** A fracture that occurs across the physis and extends into the epiphysis
- **Type IV Salter-Harris Fracture:** A fracture that occurs through the metaphysis, physis, and epiphysis
- **Type V Salter-Harris Fracture:** A fracture that results from a crush injury to the physis

## Specific Fracture Types

Following are some specific types of fractures related to the mechanisms by which they occur or their locations.

- **Articular fractures:** These fractures involve joint surfaces. When treating these fractures, be sure to look for ligament injuries as well
- **Colles' fracture:** Colles' fracture is a fracture of the radius from 2 to 3 cm proximal to the wrist joint and with dorsal displacement. It is also known as a silver-fork fracture. The most

common cause of such fractures is falling onto an outstretched hand, with the force of the fall translated upward to the glenohumeral articulation of the shoulder. Classically, there is a "dinner fork" deformity of the wrist

- **Smith's fracture:** Smith's fracture is a fracture of the radius from 2 to 3 cm proximal to the wrist joint and with volar displacement, or a Colles' fracture but with displacement in the reverse direction
- **Boxer's fracture:** A boxer's fracture involves the fifth metacarpal area following impact against a clenched fist. It can also involve the fourth metacarpal bone. The fracture is in the metacarpal neck, metacarpal neck, with the metacarpal head tilting in the volar direction, causing the joint to lie in hyperextension and the collateral ligaments to become slack
- **Dancer's fracture:** The dancer's fracture, or Jones fracture, involves the fifth metatarsal bone of the foot, or the base of the small toe. The fracture is spiral through the base of the fifth metatarsal and occurs about 1 to 2 cm from the tip and is commonly caused by a tendon pulling away a small portion of the bone. It generally results from an inversion injury caused by missteps off the demi-pointe position in ballet. X-rays of the foot should be made with the foot in full flexion for best visibility of this fracture

**COACH CONSULT**

Differentiating among fractures, dislocations, sprains, and strains can be difficult in the clinical setting. If in doubt, always get an x-ray of the injured limb. In assessing a specific joint complaint, always remember to evaluate the joints above and below the affected joint for related injuries. Table 6–10 provides a comparison of types and symptoms of musculoskeletal injuries.

## Sprain Classifications

Sprains are graded as I, II, or III, depending on the nature of the impact that causes them and the resulting damage to the affected joint. A sprain is an injury to a muscle or tendon usually associated with its improper use or overuse.

- **Grade I/minor incomplete tear:** Ligament pain, but the joint is stable and without excessive edema
- **Grade II/significant incomplete tear:** Ligament pain with noted joint

**COACH CONSULT**

Nonsteroidal anti-inflammatory drugs (NSAIDs) provide pharmacological relief of pain and reduce inflammation in sprains and should be recommended unless contraindicated.

**COACH CONSULT**

A good exercise therapy for ankle sprains involves having the patient "write" the letters of the alphabet with the sprained ankle, repeating this exercise several times a day after the initial injury or insult has passed. Patients may generally begin this exercise within 2 or 3 days after a sprain.

instability upon examination, but an endpoint of movement of the affected joint is felt

- **Grade III/complete tear:** Ligament and muscle pain without stability or an endpoint of movement of the joint served by the ruptured ligament. Severe pain and inability to bear weight

  All sprains respond well to RICE:
- **R**est with limited or no weight-bearing for several days
- **I**ce applied at 20-min intervals
- **C**ompression dressing to minimize edema and provide support to the ankle
- **E**levation for several days after the injury

## Common Herbal and Folk Remedies

Patients are increasingly turning to herbal therapies to supplement their medical regimens. It is essential to maintain a complete listing of all prescription and herbal medications that a patient is taking. Many drug–drug

| Table 6–10 Symptoms of Musculoskeletal Injury | | | | |
|---|---|---|---|---|
| **SYMPTOM** | **FRACTURE** | **DISLOCATION** | **SPRAIN** | **STRAIN** |
| Pain | Severe | Moderate to severe | Mild to moderate | Mild to moderate |
| Swelling | Moderate to severe | Mild | Mild to severe | Mild to moderate |
| Bruising | Mild to severe | Mild to severe | Mild to severe | Mild to severe |
| Deformity | Variable | Marked | None | None |
| Function | Loss of function | Loss of function | Limited | Limited |
| Tenderness | Severe | Moderate to severe | Moderate | Moderate |
| Crepitus | Present | Absent | Absent | Absent |

Adapted from Hancock, J. The Practitioner's Pocket Pal Ultra Rapid Medical Reference. Miami, FL: MedMasters Inc., 2002

interactions are possible with inappropriate combinations of drugs. Home remedies are common in many cultures across the United States. These are commonly passed down from one generation to the next to aid in symptom management at home. Table 6–11 is a listing of home remedies commonly encountered in practice.

Herbal preparations are available on an over-the-counter (OTC) basis in stores across the United States. These preparations are not controlled by the U.S. Food and Drug Administration (FDA) and may therefore have considerable differences in preparation and content from one provider to another. Examples of commonly used herbal preparations include:

- Black cohosh, which has estrogenic effects. Adverse reactions include nausea, vomiting, dizziness, and weakness
- Types of buckthorn, which can produce severe watery diarrhea and may contribute to spinal demyelination and paralysis
- Bush tea contains pyrrolizidine and is a known hepatotoxic agent
- *Cassia* spp. contain botanical laxatives and diuretics; they can produce significant electrolyte disturbances from excessive diarrhea

### Table 6–11 Commonly Used Home Remedies

| HERBAL REMEDY | USES | EFFICACY | SAFETY PROFILE + YES - NO |
|---|---|---|---|
| Garlic | HTN, antibiotic, cough syrup, tripida | + | +++ |
| Lead/mercury oxides | Empacho, teething | – | – |
| Damiana | Aphrodisiac, chickenpox | 0 | + |
| Wormwood | Worms, colic, diarrhea, cramps | + Purgative | – |
| Eucalyptus (Vicks Vapor Rub) | Coryza, asthma, bronchitis, TB | + Respiratory 0 TB | + |
| Chaparral | Arthritis (poultice), tea for cancer, venereal disease, TB, cramps, analgesic | + Poultice 0 as tea | – Internal |

*Continued*

## Table 6–11 Commonly Used Home Remedies—cont'd

| HERBAL REMEDY | USES | EFFICACY | SAFETY PROFILE + YES - NO |
|---|---|---|---|
| Mullein | Cough suppression, asthma, coryza, TB | + cough 0 asthma, TB, coryza | ++ If right species is used |
| Chamomile | Nausea, flatus, colic, anxiety, eyewash | + Except eyewash = 0 | ++ If patient has no allergy |
| Oregano | Coryza, expectorant, worms, menstrual difficulties | 0/+ Except worms = 0 | + |
| Passion flower | Anxiety, HTN | +++ Sedative | ++ If right species is used |
| Bricklebush | Adult-onset diabetes, gallbladder disease | ??? | ??? |
| Rue | Antispasmodic, abortifacient, insect repellant | ??? | – (internal, external) |
| Sage | Prevention of hair loss, coryza, diabetes | ??? | – |
| Linden flower | Sedative, HTN, diaphoresis | + Sedative, other ??? | – |
| Trumpet flower | Adult-onset diabetes, gastric symptoms, chickenpox | ??? | ??? |
| Spearmint | Dyspepsia, flatus, colic | ++ | + |
| Aloe vera | External: cuts, burns Internal: purgative, immune stimulant | External +++ Internal +/? | External +++ Internal --- |
| Sapodilla | Insomnia, HTN, malaria | ??? | ??? |

HTN: hypertension; TB: tuberculosis
   + Safety documented; – indicates low safety profile; ? no safety data available

- Chamomile teas can produce allergies similar to those seen with ragweed, asters, and chrysanthemums. One cup of tea may cause hives, respiratory distress, or an anaphylactic reaction
- Chromium II chelated is an isomer of niacin and is typically used to reduce blood lipid levels by aiding in glucose and fat metabolism
- Comfrey is a Russian tea used as a digestive aid. It has been linked to liver damage
- Cranberry will produce acidic urine
- Eucalyptus oil can cause seizures, apnea, aspiration, and bronchospasm if ingested. Very low doses can be fatal to children
- American mistletoe has potential vasopressor effects
- Garlic is believed to be effective as an antibiotic against gram-negative and gram-positive bacteria and to reduce lipid levels
- *Gingko biloba* is an herb used in Oriental medicine to treat asthma, bronchitis, peripheral vascular disease, and problems of the central nervous system (CNS). Toxicity from this herb may present as headache and GI upset
- Kava-kava contains methysticum, which produces ataxia, blurred vision, CNS intoxication, deafness, jaundice, and dermatosis
- Juniper is a hallucinogen that can produce renal toxicity and GI irritation
- Licorice produces mineral corticoid effects, sodium retention, edema, hypertension, and hypokalemia
- Ma huang is a Chinese product consisting of ephedra and can have dangerous cardiac effects
- Mandrake contains scopolamine and hyoscyamine, which have anticholinergic effects
- Melaleuca oil is used for dermatological conditions but can produce CNS depression
- Mormon tea contains ephedrine
- Morning glory seeds are hallucinogenic
- Nutmeg is a weak monoamine oxidase (MAO) inhibitor
- Oleander tea contains cardiac glycosides that can produce arrhythmias and cardiac arrest
- Pennyroyal has oxytocic properties; it can be used as an abortifacient and in the regulation of menstruation
- Periwinkle contains vinca alkaloids used in treating cancer

- Pokeweed contains saponins, triterpenes, and glycoproteins, all of which may induce changes in vision, respiratory depression, and seizures
- Sassafras, which is derived from root bark, was originally used as an antiseptic, an aromatic, a diuretic, a stimulant, and a vasodilator. The FDA has banned sassafras for internal use due to identified carcinogenic properties
- Saw palmetto is used for benign prostatic hyperplasia
- Senna is used as a natural laxative
- St. John's wort has both MAO inhibitory and serotonin-specific reuptake inhibitory properties
- Yohimbe is used as an aphrodisiac and a hallucinogen. Overdoses may cause hypertension, weakness, and paralysis

# 7 Documentation

# CHAPTER 7

# Documentation

A concise, accurate medical record is essential to recording pertinent facts, findings, and observations about a patient's health. Accuracy and completeness of documentation are required to attain timely reimbursement for services rendered. The medical record serves as a tool for both continuity of care and communication between health care providers when multiple practitioners are providing care for an individual.

The following principles should be followed with regard to the medical record:

- All entries should be complete and legible
- Patient encounters should include
    - Chief complaint
    - Relevant history, physical examination findings, and prior diagnostic tests
    - Assessment, clinical impression, and diagnosis
    - Medical plan of care
    - Identity of the health care provider, date of encounter
- Rationales for orders should be easily inferred if not documented
- Past and present diagnoses should be accessible to the health care provider
- Identification of health risk factors should be included
- Evaluation of patient progress and outcomes of treatments should be evident
- Current Procedural Terminology (CPT) codes and International Classification of Diseases–9th Clinical Modification (ICD-9-CM) codes should be supported by the documentation in the medical record

**COACH CONSULT**

The medical record is a compilation of data including a patient history, review of systems, past and present illnesses, examinations, tests, treatments, and outcomes, in chronological order.

**259**

# Evaluation and Management Services

The descriptors for the levels of evaluation and management (E &M) services recognize seven components used in defining the levels of care: History, examination, medical decision making, counseling, coordination of care, nature of the presenting problem, and practitioner time. The first three components are the key components for selecting a level of E &M service.

One of five CPT codes may be selected to bill for outpatient visits by a new patient:

- **99201:** This is generally a self-limiting or minor problem that requires 10 minutes of face-to-face provider time with the patient. Documentation must include:
  - A problem-focused history
  - A problem-focused examination
  - Straightforward medical decision making
- **99202:** For conditions of minor to moderate severity, requiring 20 minutes of face-to-face provider time. Documentation must include:
  - An expanded problem-focused history
  - An expanded problem-focused examination
  - Straightforward medical decision making
- **99203:** For a presenting problem of moderate severity, requiring 30 minutes of face-to-face provider time. Documentation must include:
  - A detailed history
  - A detailed examination
  - Medical decision making of low complexity
- **99204:** For presenting problems of moderate to high severity, requiring 45 minutes of face-to-face provider time. Documentation must include:
  - A comprehensive history
  - A comprehensive examination
  - Medical decision making of moderate complexity
- **99205:** For problems of moderate to major severity, requiring 60 minutes of face-to-face provider time. Documentation must include:
  - A comprehensive history
  - A comprehensive examination
  - Medical decision making of high complexity

# Documentation of History

The levels of E &M services for a patient history are based on the patient's chief complaint (CC); a history of the patient's present illness (HPI); a review of the patient's body systems (ROS); and the patient's past, family, and social history (PFSH).

## Chief Complaint
The chief complaint is a concise statement that describes the symptoms, problem, or condition for which the patient has presented to the clinic on the date of presentation. It is usually recorded in the patient's own words.

## History of Present Illness
The history of the patient's present illness is a chronological description of the illness and generally includes the following features of the illness:

- Body location
- Quality
- Severity
- Duration
- Timing
- Context
- Modifying factors
- Associated signs and symptoms

**COACH CONSULT**

A brief HPI consists of from one to three elements of the HPI. An extended HPI should have at least four elements of the HPI, or the status of at least three chronic or inactive conditions.

## Review of Systems
The ROS is an inventory of body systems obtained by a series of questions attempting to identify signs and symptoms that the patient may be experiencing. The ROS questions include specific signs and symptoms for each of the following body systems:

- Constitutional
- Eyes
- Ears, nose, mouth, throat
- Cardiovascular
- Respiratory
- Gastrointestinal
- Musculoskeletal
- Genitourinary

- Integumentary
- Neurological
- Psychiatric
- Endocrine
- Hematological/lymphatic
- Allergic/immunological

## Past, Family, and/or Social History

The past history includes the patient's past experiences with illness, operations, injuries, and treatments. The family history is a review of medical events in the patient's family, including hereditary diseases. The social history includes an age-appropriate review of past and current activities.

The past, family, and/or social history (PFSH) is not required for some categories of E & M services. They are relevant for patient visits following hospitalization, follow-up inpatient consultations, and subsequent nursing facility care.

A summary of the documentation requirements for each component of the patient history is provided in Table 7–1.

### Table 7–1 Requirements for Documentation of Patient History by Level of Care

| LEVEL OF CARE | HISTORY OF PRESENT ILLNESS | REVIEW OF SYSTEMS | PAST, FAMILY, AND/OR SOCIAL HISTORY | TYPE OF HISTORY |
|---|---|---|---|---|
| 99201 | Brief | N/A | N/A | Problem-focused |
| 99202 | Brief | Problem-pertinent | N/A | Expanded problem-focused |
| 99203 | Extended | Extended | Pertinent | Detailed |
| 99204 and 99205 | Extended | Complete | Complete | Comprehensive |

# Documentation of Physical Examination

There are four levels of physical examination for E &M service coding:

1. **Problem focused:** A limited examination of the body area or organ system affected by illness
2. **Expanded problem focused:** A limited examination of the affected body area or organ system and any symptomatic or related body areas or organ systems
3. **Detailed:** An extended examination of the affected body area or organ system and any other symptomatic or related body areas or organ systems.
4. **Comprehensive:** A general multisystem examination or complete examination of a single organ system and other symptomatic or related body areas or organ systems.

Requirements for a general multisystem examination are outlined in Table 7–2. An example of levels of physical examination would be seen in an expanded problem-focused examination for a patient complaining of symptoms of rhinitis. The requirements for an expanded problem-focused examination are that at least one body system or area be assessed and that at least six bullet points be included. Bullet points are key indicators identified on the documentation requirement chart with a bullet mark. For the patient with rhinitis, the health care provider may elect to include the following six bullet points: (1) recording of at least three vital signs (sitting blood pressure [BP], pulse rate, and weight); (2) otoscopic examination; (3) examination of the nasal mucosa; (4) examination of the oropharynx; (5) external inspection of the ears and nose; and (6) auscultation of the heart. Documentation of these six bullet points would yield sufficient information for an expanded problem-focused examination.

When documenting multisystem and single-organ-system examinations, make sure to remember the following tips:

- Specific abnormal and relevant negative findings of the examination of the affected or symptomatic body area or organ system should be documented in detail
- Abnormal or unexpected findings of the examination of any asymptomatic body area or organ system should be described
- A brief statement or notation, indicating "negative" or "normal" is sufficient to document normal findings related to unaffected areas or asymptomatic body areas or organ systems. However, an entire organ system should not be documented with a statement such as "negative"

## Table 7–2 General Multisystem Examination

| TYPE OF EXAMINATION | DESCRIPTION |
|---|---|
| Problem-focused | Include performance and documentation of from one to five elements identified by a bullet point in one or more organ systems or body areas |
| Expanded problem-focused | Include performance and documentation of at least six elements identified by a bullet point in one or more organ systems or body areas |
| Detailed | Include at least six organ systems or body areas. For each system or area selected, identify performance and documentation of at least two elements by a bullet point. May include performance and documentation of at least 12 elements identified by a bullet point in two or more organ systems or body areas |
| Comprehensive | Include at least nine organ systems or body areas. For each system or area selected, all elements of the examination identified by a bullet point should be performed unless specific directions limit the content of the examination. For each area/system, document at least two elements identified by a bullet point |

The elements for a general multisystem examination are listed in Table 7–3.

The documentation guidelines for the patient history identify 10 single-organ-system examinations, focused on the following systems or organs:

1. Cardiovascular
2. Ear, nose, and throat
3. Eye
4. Genitourinary
5. Hematological/lymphatic/immunological
6. Musculoskeletal
7. Neurological
8. Psychiatric
9. Respiratory
10. Skin

Included in each body system or area are bulleted points or elements of examination that may be included in an assessment of that body system or area. A problem-focused single-organ-system examination should include from one to five bulleted points. Expanded problem-focused examinations should have documentation of at least six bulleted examination points. Detailed examinations include at least 12 elements identified by a

## Table 7–3 General Multisystem Examination Bullet Points

| SYSTEM/BODY AREA | ELEMENTS OF EXAMINATION |
|---|---|
| Constitutional | • Measurement of any three of the following seven vital signs: (1) sitting or standing BP, (2) supine BP, (3) pulse rate and regularity, (4) respiration, (5) temperature, (6) height,(7) weight<br>• General appearance of patient: Development, nutrition, body habitus, deformities, attention to grooming |
| Eyes | • Inspection of conjunctiva and eyelids<br>• Examination of pupils and irises: Reaction to light, accommodation, size, and symmetry<br>• Ophthalmoscopic examination of optic discs, including: size, C/D ratio, appearance; and posterior segments including vessel changes, exudates, and hemorrhages |
| Ears, nose, mouth, and throat | • External inspection of ears and nose: Overall appearance, scars, lesions<br>• Otoscopic examination of external auditory canal and tympanic membrane<br>• Assessment of hearing: Whispered voice, finger rub, tuning forks<br>• Inspection of nasal mucosa, septum, and turbinates<br>• Inspection of lips, teeth, and gums<br>• Examination of oropharynx, oral mucosa, salivary glands, hard and soft palates, tongue, tonsils, and posterior pharynx |
| Neck | • Examination of neck: Masses, overall appearance, symmetry, tracheal position<br>• Examination of thyroid: Enlargement, tenderness, masses |
| Respiratory | • Assessment of respiratory effort: Intercostal muscle retractions, use of accessory muscles, diaphragmatic movement<br>• Percussion of chest: Dullness, flatness, hyperresonance<br>• Palpation of chest: Tactile fremitus<br>• Auscultation of lungs: Breath sounds, adventitious sounds |
| Cardiovascular | • Palpation of heart: Location, size, thrills<br>• Auscultation of heart with notation of abnormal sounds/murmurs<br>• Examination of:<br>  • Carotid arteries: Pulse amplitude, bruits<br>  • Abdominal aorta: Size, bruits<br>  • Femoral arteries: Pulse amplitude, bruits<br>  • Pedal pulses: Pulse amplitude<br>  • Extremities: Edema and/or varicosities |

*Continued*

## Table 7–3 General Multisystem Examination Bullet Points—cont'd

| SYSTEM/BODY AREA | ELEMENTS OF EXAMINATION |
|---|---|
| Chest (breasts) | • Inspection of breasts: Symmetry, nipple discharge<br>• Palpation of breasts and axillae: Masses, lumps, tenderness |
| Gastrointestinal | • Examination of abdomen with notation of masses or tenderness<br>• Examination of liver and spleen<br>• Examination for presence or absence of bowel sounds<br>• Examination (when indicated) of anus, perineum and rectum, including sphincter tone, presence of hemorrhoids, rectal masses<br>• Stool sample for occult blood when indicated |
| Genitourinary | Male:<br>• Examination of scrotal contents: Hydrocele, spermatocele, tenderness of cord, testicular mass<br>• Examination of penis<br>• Digital rectal examination of prostate gland: Size, symmetry, nodularity, tenderness<br>Female:<br>• Examination of external genitalia, including appearance, hair distribution, and lesions; and vagina, including appearance, estrogen effect, discharge, lesions, pelvic support, cystocele, rectocele<br>• Examination of urethra: Masses, tenderness, scarring<br>• Examination of bladder: Fullness, masses, tenderness<br>• Cervix: General appearance, lesions, discharge<br>• Uterus: size, contour, position, mobility, tenderness, consistency, descent or support<br>• Adnexa/parametria: Masses, tenderness, organomegaly, nodularity |
| Lymphatic | Palpation of lymph nodes in two or more areas<br>• Neck<br>• Axillae<br>• Groin<br>• Other |
| Musculoskeletal | • Examination of gait and station<br>• Inspection and/or palpation of digits and nails: Clubbing, cyanosis, inflammatory conditions, petechiae, ischemia, infections, nodes |

Table 7–3 **General Multisystem Examination Bullet Points—cont'd**

| SYSTEM/BODY AREA | ELEMENTS OF EXAMINATION |
|---|---|
| Musculoskeletal (cont'd) | • Examination of joints, bones, and muscles of one or more of the following six areas: (1) head and neck; (2) spine, ribs, and pelvis; (3) right upper extremity; (4) left upper extremity; (5) right lower extremity; and (6) left lower extremity. Examination includes:<br>• Inspection and/or palpation with notation of any misalignment, asymmetry, crepitation, defects, tenderness, masses, effusions<br>• Assessment of range of motion with notation of any pain, crepitation, or contracture<br>• Assessment of stability with notation of any dislocation, subluxation, or laxity<br>• Assessment of muscle strength and tone (flaccid, cogwheel, spastic) with notation of any atrophy of abnormal movements |
| Skin | • Inspection of skin and subcutaneous tissues: Rash, lesions, ulcers<br>• Palpation of skin and subcutaneous tissue: Induration, subcutaneous nodules, tightening |
| Neurological | • Cranial nerve test with notation of any deficits<br>• Examination of deep tendon reflexes with notation of pathological reflexes (Babinski sign)<br>• Examination of sensation: Touch, pain, vibration, proprioception |
| Psychiatric | • Description of patient's judgment and insight<br>• Brief assessment of mental status including:<br>• Orientation to time, place, person<br>• Recent and remote memory<br>• Mood and affect: Depression, worry, agitation |

C/D ratio: cup-to-disc ratio.

bullet, and comprehensive examinations include all of the bulleted items in the examination.

# Complexity of Medical Decision Making

Medical decision making refers to the establishment of a diagnosis and management plan for a patient's condition. The complexity of this process is determined by the following factors:

- The number of possible diagnoses and/or the number of management options that must be considered, including:
  - Number and types of problems addressed by the provider

- Complexity of establishing a diagnosis
- Management decisions that are made by the provider
- The number and/or complexity of medical records, diagnostic tests, and other information that must be obtained, reviewed, and analyzed, including:
  - Decisions to obtain and review old records and/or obtain histories from sources other than the patient
  - Discussion of contradictory or unexpected test results with the provider who performed or interpreted the test
  - Personal reviews of images, tracings, or specimens by the provider who ordered a test or other procedure to supplement the information provided by the physician who prepared or interpreted the report of the test or procedure
- The risk of significant complications, morbidity, and/or mortality from diagnostic procedures or possible management options, as well as from comorbidities associated with the patient's presenting problem(s).

## ICD-9-CM Coding

Guidelines for coding and reporting with the International Classification of Diseases 9th Revision-Clinical Modification (ICD-9-CM) are available from the Centers for Medicare and Medicaid Services (CMS) and the National Center for Health Statistics (NCHS). ICD-9 codes are either three, four, or five digits long, with the first three digits representing the heading of a category of codes that may be further subdivided according to the fourth or fifth digit.

V codes are available to deal with encounters for circumstances other than a disease or injury. Examples might include:
- A person who is not sick encounters a health care service for some specific purpose, such as to receive prophylactic care, health screenings, or counseling on a health-related topic
- A person with a resolving disease or injury or with a chronic long-term condition encounters a health care service for specific aftercare of that disease or injury
- Circumstances or problems that influence a person's health status but do not in themselves constitute a current illness or injury
- Indication of birth for newborns

Categories of V codes include:
- Contact/exposure to a communicable disease, without symptoms
- Inoculations and vaccinations

- Patient status, including that of being a carrier of a disease or having the sequelae or residua of a past disease or condition

## Current Procedural Terminology Modifiers

Current procedural terminology (CPT) modifiers are two-digit numbers identified by the addition of a hyphen and the modifier number to the basic CPT code. Modifiers indicate that a service or procedure that was performed has been altered in some manner, such as by the performance of multiple procedures or an increase or decrease in the level of service provided at a patient visit. Table 7–4 gives examples of some commonly used CPT modifiers.

> Although a release of ICD-10-CM is now available for public viewing, the codes in ICD-10-CM are not currently valid for any purpose or use. There is now an anticipated implementation date for the ICD-10-CM of October 1, 2013.

Examples of use of a CPT modifier might include:

- Use of a -25 CPT modifier for a patient who presents with a nosebleed that requires packing to stop the bleeding and who during the same visit is evaluated for hypertension and whose medical regimen is adjusted
- Selection of a -22 CPT modifier for a child who presents for removal of a foreign object in the ear and who also has a large amount of cerumen removed from its ear during removal of the foreign object. This would represent an expanded service and would therefore justify the use of the modifier
- Possible use of a -32 modifier for a patient whose insurance provider requires a confirmatory consultative visit before a surgical procedure

### Table 7–4 Current Procedural Terminology Modifiers

| CPT MODIFIER | EXPLANATION OF USE OF THIS MODIFIER |
| --- | --- |
| -21 | Designates a prolonged E & M service, time is more than generally spent for a given category |
| -22 | Unusual service or procedure, the procedure becomes greater than normally expected |
| -25 | Separate E & M service on the same date by the same provider |

*Continued*

## Table 7-4 Current Procedural Terminology Modifiers—cont'd

| CPT MODIFIER | EXPLANATION OF USE OF THIS MODIFIER |
|---|---|
| -26 | Performance of a professional component of a procedure without the full scope of E & M; for example, a radiologist can use this modifier for reading an x-ray film |
| -32 | A mandated service |
| -50 | Bilateral code, performance of a procedure on two sides in the same visit |
| -51 | Multiple procedures at the same visit by the same provider |
| -52 | Reduced services; used when a full procedure cannot be completed because of complications with the patient (pain level, mental competence, etc) |
| -76 | A repeat procedure by the same provider |

E & M: evaluation and management.

## Electronic Medical Records

Often, providers will undercode a patient visit to avoid scrutiny by third-party payers. Improper coding and billing has led to sanctions and financial penalties, which are most undesirable. Electronic health care records can assist providers in the task of determining the level of service provided at a patient visit. Electronic medical record (EMR) software improves coding accuracy through automatic calculation of the level of service based on the documentation entered for each patient visit. The general outcome is more effective billing and coding, which in turn leads to higher reimbursement rates with fewer sanctions and penalties.

Some issues to consider in purchasing EMR software include:

- Training of staff and providers in keeping electronic records
- Ability to personalize documentation to the practice site
- Protection of privacy of patient records from electronic pirates
- Computer technology failures, including disconnects and battery and online support failures
- Portability of computer access from one room to another

# 8 Pediatric Management Pearls

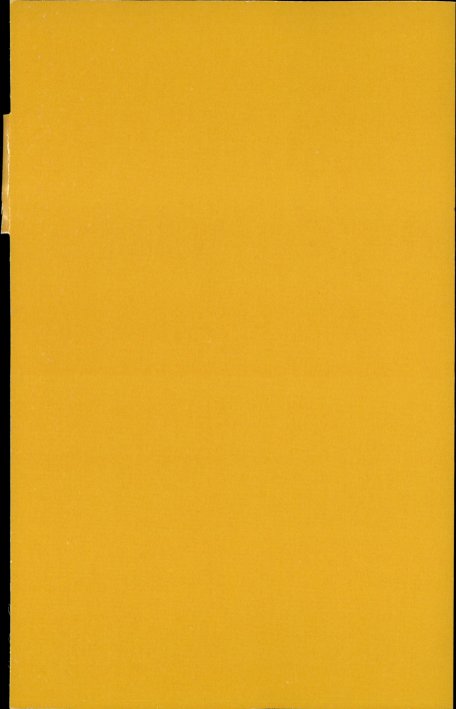

# CHAPTER 8

# Pediatric Management Pearls

The management of pediatric health care issues holds unique problems and issues distinct from those encountered in adult populations. Pediatric patients are not "little adults" and should not be treated as such in terms of their health care needs. This chapter addresses some common issues in pediatrics, including antibiotic usage and dosing, cough and cold management, well-child visits and developmental milestones, and an overview of commonly seen health care issues in pediatric populations.

## Pediatric Antibiotic Use and Dosing Guidelines

Clinicians everywhere are acutely aware of the need to limit antibiotic usage to clearly appropriate clinical cases in which bacterial or fungal infections are identified. Continued overuse or abuse of antibiotics will lead to increased antibiotic resistance. This section provides specific information about antibiotics that are appropriate for use in pediatrics. It includes a brief discussion of antibiotic usage, followed by a dosing chart for each antibiotic based on children's weights.

### Amoxicillin
Amoxicillin (Amoxil) is a broad-spectrum penicillin effective in the management of acute otitis media (OM) at a dosage of 80 to 90 mg/kg/day; as well as mild to moderate ear, nose, and throat (ENT) infections and skin or genitourinary infections, at 25 mg/kg/day in divided doses; and lower respiratory infections or severe ENT, skin, or genitourinary infections at

45 mg/kg/day in divided doses. Amoxicillin provides coverage of gram-positive organisms, including Streptococcus groups A, B, C, and G; *Staphylococcus aureus*, including methicillin-resistant *S. aureus* (MRSA); and *Enterococcus faecalis*.

Amoxicillin is available in several forms, including 200 mg and 400 mg chewable tablets; pediatric drops at a concentration of 50 mg/mL; and oral suspensions in varying strengths from 200 mg/5 mL to 400 mg/5 mL. Adult-strength amoxicillin is available as 500 mg and 875 mg tablets. Table 8–1 provides an amoxicillin dosing chart for children based on body weight.

## Azithromycin

Azithromycin (Zithromax) is a later generation macrolide antibiotic that may be used to treat infections caused by susceptible organisms, including acute bacterial exacerbations of chronic obstructive pulmonary disease (COPD), acute bacterial sinusitis, acute OM, community-acquired

| Table 8–1  **Pediatric Dosing Chart for Amoxicillin*** | | |
|---|---|---|
| **WEIGHT (LB)** | **DOSAGE 200 mg/5 mL tsp q12h** | **DISPENSE (mL)** |
| **MILD 25 mg/kg/day** | | |
| 20 | ½ | 50 |
| 30 | ¾ | 75 |
| 40 | 1 | 100 |
| **SEVERE 45 mg/kg/day** | | |
| 20 | 1 | 100 |
| 30 | 1½ | 150 |
| 40 | 2 | 200 |
| 50 | 2½ | 250 |
| Age <3 months: Maximum dose 30 mg/kg/day | | |

*Suspensions: 200 mg/5 mL; 250 mg/5 mL; 400 mg/5 mL
   Chewable tablets: 200 mg, 400 mg
   Pediatric drops: 50 mg/mL

pneumonia, pharyngitis, tonsillitis, uncomplicated skin and skin-structure infections, urethritis, cervicitis, chancroid in men, and *Mycobacterium avium*-complex disease. Azithromycin provides antibiotic coverage of gram-negative and gram-positive organisms as well as atypical organisms. As an oral suspension, it is available in two strengths: 100 mg/5 mL and 200 mg/5 mL. Table 8–2 provides a dosing chart for azithromycin based on patient weight.

## Cefadroxil

Cefadroxil (Duricef) has indications as a first generation cephalosporin antibiotic in the treatment of urinary tract infections (UTIs), skin and skin-structure infections, pharyngitis, tonsillitis, and impetigo. Cefadroxil is an effective antibiotic against most common gram positive organisms. It is available as a suspension in strengths of 250 mg/5 mL and 500 mg/5 mL. Table 8–3 is a pediatric dosing chart for cefadroxil based on patient weight.

## Cefdinir

Cefdinir (Omnicef) is a fourth generation cephalosporin antibiotic that can be used in treating community-acquired pneumonia, acute exacerbations of chronic bronchitis, acute sinusitis, pharyngitis, tonsillitis, uncomplicated skin and skin-structure infections, and acute OM. Fourth generation cephalosporins typically provide excellent coverage for both gram-positive and gram-negative organisms as well as those beta-lactamase producing organisms. As a suspension, cefdinir is available in strengths of 125 mg/5 mL and 250 mg/5 mL. It is not recommended for patients younger than 6 months of age. Table 8–4 includes dosing charts for cefdinir.

| Table 8–2 **Pediatric Dosing Chart for Azithromycin Oral Suspension** | | | |
|---|---|---|---|
| **WEIGHT** | **SUSPENSION STRENGTH** | **FIRST-DAY DOSING** | **DAY 2–5 DOSING** |
| Up to 22 lb | 100 mg/5 mL | 1 tsp | ½ tsp daily |
| 23–44 lb | 200 mg/5 mL | 1 tsp | ½ tsp daily |
| 45–66 lb | 200 mg/5 mL | 1½ tsp | ¾ tsp daily |
| 67–88 lb | 200 mg/5 mL | 2 tsp | 1 tsp daily |

## Table 8–3 Pediatric Dosing Chart for Cefadroxil*

| WEIGHT (LB) | DOSAGE | DISPENSE (mL) |
|---|---|---|
| **250 mg/5 mL SUSPENSION tsp q12h** | | |
| 20 | ½ | 50 |
| 30 | ¾ | 75 |
| 40 | 1 | 100 |
| **500 mg/5 mL SUSPENSION** | | |
| 40 | ½ | 50 |
| 50 | ⅔ | 75 |
| 60 | ¾ | 75 |
| 70 | ¾ | 75 |
| 80 | 1 | 100 |
| 90 | 1 | 100 |

*30 mg/kg/day in divided doses q12h.

## Table 8–4 Pediatric Dosing Chart for Cefdinir*

| WEIGHT (LB) | DOSAGE 250 mg/5 mL tsp q12h | DISPENSE | DOSAGE 125 mg/5 mL tsp q12h | DISPENSE |
|---|---|---|---|---|
| 20–25 | ½ | 60 | | |
| 26–33 | ¾ | 60 | | |
| 34–45 | 1 | 60 | ½ | 60 |
| 46–53 | 1¼ | 100 | ¾ | 60 |
| 54–65 | 1½ | 100 | 1¼ | 100 |
| 66–73 | 1¾ | 100 | 1½ | 100 |
| 74–85- | 2 | 120 | 1½ | 100 |
| 86–90 | 2¼ | 120 | 1¾ | 120 |

*14 mg/kg/day divided q12h.

## Cefixime

Cefixime (Suprax) is a third generation cephalosporin that provides antibiotic coverage for OM, pharyngitis, tonsillitis, acute bronchitis, uncomplicated UTIS, and cervical or urethral gonorrhea. Third generation cephalosporins provide weak coverage for gram-positive organisms but better coverage for gram-negative and beta-lactamase-producing organisms. Cefixime is available in suspension at 100 mg/5 mL and 200 mg/5 mL. It is not recommended for use in children younger than 6 months of age.

## Cefprozil

Cefprozil (Cefzil) is a second generation cephalosporin that is effective in the management of mild to moderate pharyngitis, tonsillitis, acute bronchitis, acute sinusitis, skin and skin-structure infections, and OM. Cefprozil is effective against most common gram-positive and gram-negative organisms. For pediatric patients it is provided in oral suspensions of 125 mg/5 mL and 250 mg/5 mL. It is not recommended for patients younger than 6 months of age. Table 8–5 provides a pediatric dosing chart for cefprozil.

| Table 8–5 **Pediatric Dosing Chart for Cefprozil\*** | | |
|---|---|---|
| WEIGHT (LB) | DOSAGE | DISPENSE (mL) |
| 125 mg/5 mL tsp q12h | | |
| 10 | ½ | 50 |
| 15 | ¾ | 75 |
| 20 | 1 | 100 |
| 250 mg/5 mL | | |
| 30 | ¾ | 75 |
| 40 | 1 | 100 |
| 60 | 1½ | 150 |
| 70 | 1¾ | 175 |

\*30 mg/kg/day bid.

## Ceftriaxone

Ceftriaxone (Rocephin) is an injectable fourth generation cephalosporin that provides coverage for susceptible pathogens in bacteremia, acute bacterial OM, lower respiratory tract infections, UTIs, skin and skin structure infections, pelvic inflammatory disease (PID), intra-abdominal infections, meningitis, and uncomplicated gonorrhea. It is not recommended for use in children younger than age 2 months. The recommended dosage formula for ceftriaxone in children is 50 to 75 mg/kg/day, with a maximum dosage of 2 g/day. Table 8–6 provides a dosing chart for ceftriaxone based on patient weight.

| Table 8–6 **Pediatric Dosing Chart for Ceftriaxone** | | |
|---|---|---|
| **WEIGHT (Kg)** | **WEIGHT (Lb)** | **RECOMMENDED DOSE (in mg)** |
| 1 | 2.2 | 50 |
| 2 | 4.4 | 100 |
| 3 | 6.6 | 150 |
| 4 | 8.8 | 200 |
| 5 | 11 | 250 |
| 6 | 13.2 | 300 |
| 7 | 15.4 | 350 |
| 8 | 17.6 | 400 |
| 9 | 19.8 | 450 |
| 10 | 22 | 500 |
| 11 | 24.2 | 550 |
| 12 | 26.4 | 600 |
| 13 | 28.8 | 650 |
| 14 | 30.8 | 700 |
| 15 | 33 | 750 |

## Table 8–6 Pediatric Dosing Chart for Ceftriaxone—cont'd

| WEIGHT (Kg) | WEIGHT (Lb) | RECOMMENDED DOSE (in mg) |
|:---:|:---:|:---:|
| 16 | 35.2 | 800 |
| 17 | 37.4 | 850 |
| 18 | 39.6 | 900 |
| 19 | 41.8 | 950 |
| 20 | 44 | 1000 |

## Cefuroxime

Cefuroxime (Ceftin) is a second generation cephalosporin indicated in the management of mild to moderate infections, including pharyngitis, tonsillitis, acute maxillary sinusitis, acute OM, bronchitis, uncomplicated skin and skin-structure infections, UTIs, gonorrhea, and early Lyme disease. Cefuroxime will provide coverage against most common gram-positive and gram-negative organisms. In suspension form it is available at 125 mg/5 mL and 250 mg/5 mL. Instruct parents to give cefuroxime with food. It is not recommended for infants younger than 3 months of age. Table 8–7 provides a pediatric dosing chart for cefuroxime.

## Clarithromycin

Clarithromycin (Biaxin) is a macrolide antibiotic recommended for the treatment of mild to moderate pharyngitis or tonsillitis, bronchitis, community acquired pneumonia, acute maxillary sinusitis, acute OM, and uncomplicated skin and skin-structure infections. Clarithromycin is effective against many gram-positive and gram-negative organisms, as well as some atypical organisms such as *Mycoplasma pneumoniae*, *Legionella pneumophila*, and *Chlamydia pneumoniae*. It is not recommended for children younger than 6 months of age. Clarithromycin is available in suspensions of 125 mg/5 mL and 250 mg/5 mL. Dosing guidelines are based on a formula that prescribes 15 mg/kg/day in two divided doses. Table 8–8 provides a pediatric dosing chart for clarithromycin based on body weight for twice-daily dosing regimens.

## Erythromycin

Erythromycin (Eryped) is an early generation macrolide antibiotic that has indications for upper and lower respiratory tract infections, skin and soft

## Table 8–7  Pediatric Dosing Chart for Cefuroxime

| WEIGHT (LB) | DOSAGE tsp/day | DISPENSE (mL) |
|---|---|---|
| MILD ILLNESS 20 mg/kg/day; 125 mg/5 mL | | |
| 15 | ½ | 50 |
| 22 | ¾ | 75 |
| 28 | 1 | 100 |
| 40 | 1¼ | 125 |
| 50 | 1¾ | 175 |
| SEVERE ILLNESS 20 mg/kg/day (250mg/5 mL) | | |
| 20 | ½ | 50 |
| 30 | ¾ | 75 |
| 40 | 1 | 100 |
| 50 | 1¼ | 125 |
| Age <3 months: Not recommended. | | |

## Table 8–8  Pediatric Dosing Chart for Clarithromycin*

| CHILD'S WEIGHT | | DOSAGE IN 5-mL TEASPOON GIVEN TWICE DAILY | | |
|---|---|---|---|---|
| Kg | LB | DOSE | STRENGTH | BOTTLE SIZE |
| 9 | 20 | ½ tsp | 125 mg/5 mL | 50 mL |
| 17 | 37 | 1 tsp<br>½ tsp | 125 mg/5 mL<br>250 mg/5 mL | 100 mL<br>50 mL |
| 25 | 55 | ½ tsp | 250 mg/5 mL | 50 mL |
| 33 | 73 | ¾ tsp | 250 mg/5 mL | 100 mL |

| Table 8–8 **Pediatric Dosing Chart for Clarithromycin*—cont'd** | | | |
|---|---|---|---|
| **PEDIATRIC DOSING AS TABLETS** | | | |
| **Kg** | **LB** | **STRENGTH** | **NUMBER OF TABLETS†** |
| >33 | 73 | 250 mg | 20 tablets total, taking one twice daily x 10 days |
| Age <6 months: Not recommended | | | |

*For 10 days at 15 mg./kg/day in two divided doses daily.
†For 10 days in two divided doses per day.

tissue infections, GU tract infections, Legionnaire's disease, pertussis, and listeriosis. Erythromycin is effective against most gram-positive and atypical organisms. It is available as a chewable 200 mg tablet, as a pediatric drops (100 mg/2.5 mL dropper), or as a suspension of either 200 mg/5 mL or 400 mg/5 mL. Dosing is divided into two, three, or four evenly distributed doses per day. Table 8–9 provides a dosing chart by weight for erythromycin.

## Tetracycline

Tetracycline (Sumycin) can be given to children older than 8 years of age for the treatment of infections caused by tetracycline-sensitive organisms, including rickettsiae and *M. pneumoniae, Vibrio cholerae, Chlamydia psittaci*

| Table 8–9 **Pediatric Dosing Chart for Erythromycin*** | | | | |
|---|---|---|---|---|
| **WEIGHT (LB)** | **WEIGHT (Kg)** | **30 mg/kg/day** | **40 mg/kg/day** | **50 mg/kg/day** |
| **ERYPED 200 mg/5 mL SUSPENSION** | | | | |
| 10 | 4.5 | 1.5 mL bid | 2.5 mL bid | 3.5 mL bid |
| 20 | 9.1 | ¾ tsp bid | 1 tsp bid | 1¼ tsp bid |
| 30 | 13.6 | 1 tsp bid | 1¼ tsp bid | 1½ tsp bid |
| 40 | 18.2 | 1¼ tsp bid | 1½ tsp bid | 2tsp bid |
| **ERYPED 400 mg/5 mL SUSPENSION** | | | | |
| 50 | 22.7 | ¾ tsp bid | 1 tsp bid | 1¼ tsp bid |
| 60 | 27.3 | 1 tsp bid | 1¼ tsp bid | 1¾ tsp bid |

*From 30 to 50 mg/kg/day in divided doses.

(psittacosis), *Yersinia pestis* (plague), and *Shigella*. Tetracycline provides effective coverage for gram-negative organisms, MRSA, and atypical organisms. It is available as a suspension with 125 mg/5 mL. Caution parents of the potential damage that tetracycline can cause to tooth enamel, and about photosensitivity with this drug, whose use requires sunscreen for outdoor activities.

## Combination Drugs

### *Augmentin*

Augmentin, a combination of amoxicillin and clavulanic acid, is a broad-spectrum penicillin combined with a beta-lactamase inhibitor and is effective against some beta-lactamase-producing bacteria resistant to various other antibiotics. Augmentin will provide coverage of most gram-positive and gram-negative organisms in addition to beta-lactamase-producing organisms. It is recommended in the management of sinusitis, OM, lower respiratory tract and skin and skin-structure infections, and UTIs. It is available as a suspension (125 mg/tsp, 200 mg/tsp, 400 mg/tsp, and 600 mg/tsp), chewable tablets (200 mg, 250 mg, and 400 mg), and adult-strength tablets (250 mg, 500 mg, and 875 mg). Dosing is based on the amoxicillin component of the drug rather than the clavulanic acid component. Augmentin is not recommended for children younger than age 3 months. Advise parents to give Augmentin with food to minimize gastrointestinal (GI) complaints associated with this medication. Table 8–10 provides a pediatric dosing chart for Augmentin based on body weight.

### *Bactrim*

Bactrim (or Septra) is a combination of sulfamethoxazole and trimethoprim that is effective in the management of UTIs, traveler's diarrhea, acute OM in children, and acute exacerbations of chronic bronchitis. Bactrim and Septra are effective against common gram-negative organisms such as *Escherichia coli*, *Klebsiella*, *Salmonella*, *Proteus*, and MRSA. Neither product should be given to children younger than 2 months of age. Both Bactrim and Septra are available in suspension at a strength of 200 mg of sulfamethoxazole per 5 mL. Table 8–11 provides dosing information for Bactrim suspension based on weight; the same chart can be used when prescribing Septra suspension.

### *Pediazole*

Pediazole is a combination of erythromycin and sulfisoxazole. It is indicated for the treatment of acute OM in children older than 2 months of age. The dose is calculated based on the basis of the erythromycin component of the drug, at 50 mg/kg/day in three or four divided doses. Table 8–12 provides a

## Table 8–10 Pediatric Dosing Chart for Augmentin ES-600

| WEIGHT (LB) | DOSAGE 600 mg/5 mL tsp q12h | DISPENSE (mL) |
|---|---|---|
| 12–19 | ½ | 75 |
| 20–25 | ¾ | 100 |
| 26–33 | 1 | 100 |
| 34–39 | 1¼ | 150 |
| 40–47 | 1½ | 150 |
| 48–53 | 1¾ | 150 and 50 |
| 54–61 | 2 | 150 and 75 |
| 62–69 | 2¼ | 150 and 100 |
| 70–77 | 2½ | 150 and 150 |
| 78–85 | 2¾ | 150 and 150 |
| 86 | 3 | 150 and 150 |

Age <12 weeks: 30 mg/kg/day in two divided doses.
Age >12 weeks: 45 mg/kg/day in two divided doses.
Chewable tablets: 125 mg, 200 mg, 250 mg, 400 mg
Suspension: 200 mg/5 mL; 250 mg/5 mL; 400 mg/5 mL
Tablets XR: 250 mg, 500 mg, 875 mg, 1000 mg

## Table 8–11 Pediatric Dosing Chart for Bactrim*

| WEIGHT (LB) | DOSAGE 200 mg/5 mL tsp q12h | DISPENSE (mL) |
|---|---|---|
| 12–18 | ½ | 50 |
| 20 | ¾ | 75 |
| 25 | 1 | 100 |
| 35 | 1½ | 150 |
| 40 | 1¾ | 175 |
| 50 | 2 | 200 |

*40 mg/kg/day given q12h.

## Table 8–12 Pediatric Dosing Chart for Pediazole

| WEIGHT (Kg) | DOSE |
| --- | --- |
| <6 | 50 mg/kg in three or four doses |
| 6–8 | 2.5 mL q8h |
| 8–15 | 2.5 mL q6h |
| 16–23 | 5 mL q6h |
| 24–44 | 7.5 mL q6h |
| >45 | 10 mL q6h |

dosing chart for Pediazole based on body weight. Pediazole is contraindicated for children with allergies to sulfa drugs.

## Choosing an Antibiotic

Choosing an antibiotic for treating a particular infection depends on multiple factors, all of which must be considered:

- Cost of the antibiotic: Can the patient afford the drug of first choice? Is it covered by the patient's medicine card or insurance?
- Recent antibiotic use: Has the patient been treated with an antibiotic in the past 90 days? If this is the case, it is generally best to select an alternative antibiotic so as to minimize the potential for development of antibiotic resistance
- Convenience of dosing: Compliance with a medication regimen is much greater if the medication is dosed daily or twice daily as compared to three or four times a day. Furthermore, for a child who is in school, dosing more than two times a day may require special considerations to allow the child to take the mid-day dose of a medication
- Taste of the liquid medication: Compliance can be hampered by medications that have an unpleasant taste. Local pharmacists can now add multiple flavors to medications to enhance patient compliance with their use

Table 8–13 provides a comparison of pediatric antibiotics that includes pathogen coverage, indications, and cost factors for each medication.

# Pediatric Cough and Cold Preparations

A wide variety of prescription and over-the-counter cough, cold, and nasal medications are available. Selecting appropriate medications for pediatric populations requires knowledge of the properties and indications for each one, as well as of proper dosing of each medication. This section discusses nasal decongestants and intranasal steroids, as well as antitussives, expectorants, and antihistamines for use in pediatric patients.

## Nasal Decongestants

Most nasal decongestants act rapidly and provide relief of nasal and nasopharyngeal mucosal congestion caused by the common cold, hay fever, sinusitis, and allergies. A consistently safe approach to the management of nasal congestion in children under 2 years of age is to instill nasal saline dropwise into the nares and to follow this with gentle suction applied with an ear/nose syringe. Table 8–14 provides dosing information for common nasal decongestants in children.

## Intranasal Steroids

Intranasal steroids are available for use in children older than 4 to 6 years of age, depending on the manufacturer's safety guidelines. They are sold as nasal sprays and provide relief of seasonal or perennial rhinitis, prevent recurrence of nasal polyps, and are useful in treating nonallergenic rhinitis.

The NP is advised to use the lowest possible dose of an intranasal steroid to control symptoms and to use these sprays for only a short period. Typical side effects of intranasal steroid sprays include nasal irritation, burning, stinging, and headache. Table 8–15 provides dosing information for several intranasal steroids.

## Antitussives

Antitussives provide symptomatic relief of coughing through cough suppression. Most antitussives provide rapid relief of coughing and have a short half-life. Table 8–16 provides information about the use of common antitussives in children.

> **ALERT**
>
> Making clinical decisions about the pediatric use of cough and cold medications depends not only on the type of medication but also on the age of the child. Many antihistamines and decongestants are contraindicated in younger children.

> **ALERT**
>
> Nasal decongestant sprays should not be used for more than 5 days.

> **COACH CONSULT**
>
> The best antitussive for loosening and thinning mucus in children is water taken orally and in a quantity appropriate for a child's age.

## Table 8-13 Comparison of Pediatric Antibiotics by Efficacy and Cost Factors

| DRUG | ORGANISM COVERAGE | | FOOD WITH DRUG | COST | DRUG INDICATIONS | | | | | | | COMMENTS |
|---|---|---|---|---|---|---|---|---|---|---|---|---|
| | Gram + | Gram - | | | PHARYNGITIS | BRONCHITIS | CAP | SINUSITIS | OTITIS MEDIA | SKIN INFECTIONS | UTI | |
| Amoxil (amoxicillin) | + | | EF | $ | + | | | + | + | + | + | + with MRSA |
| Augmentin (amoxicillin/+ clavulanate) | Most | + | WF | $$$ | | | + | + | + | + | + | Beta-lactamase-producing bacteria |
| Bactrim (trimethoprim–sulfamethoxazole) + | | + | EF | $ | | + | | | + | | + | Traveler's diarrhea, shigellosis, P. carinii |
| Biaxin (clarithromycin) | + | + | EF | $$$$ | + | + | + | + | + | + | + | Mycoplasma, Legionella, Chlamydia |
| Ceftin (cefuroxime) | + | + | EF | $$$ | + | + | | + | + | + | + | |
| Cefzil (cefprozil) | + | + | EF | $$$$ | + | + | + | | + | + | | Early Lyme disease |
| Duricef (cefadroxil) | + | | EF | $$$ | + | + | | | | + | + | Impetigo |

| Drug | | | Food | Cost | | | | | | | Indications |
|---|---|---|---|---|---|---|---|---|---|---|---|
| Eryped (erythromycin as ethylsuccinate) | + | + | WF | $ | + | + | + | + | + | + | Legionnaire's disease; pertussis, listeriosis |
| Omnicef (cefdinir) | + | + | EF | $$$$ | | + | + | + | | | Beta-lactamase-producing organisms |
| Pediazole (erythromycin/sulfisoxazole) | | + | WF | $$ | | + | + | + | | | |
| Rocephin (ceftriaxone) | + | + | EF | $$$$ | + | + | + | + | + | + | PID, intra-abdominal infections, meningitis, uncomplicated gonorrhea |
| Sumycin (tetracycline) | Weak | + | WF | $ | + | | | | | + | Rickettsiae, M. pneumoniae, cholera, psittacosis, shigellosis, MRSA, atypicals, acne |
| Suprax (cefixime) | Weak | + | | $ | + | + | | | | + | Beta-lactamase-producing organisms, gonorrhea |
| Zithromax (azithromycin) | + | + | EF | $$ | + | + | + | + | + | + | Urethritis, canchroid, cervicitis, M. avium complex |

CAP: community-acquired pneumonia; EF = with or without food; MRSA: methicillin-resistant *S. aureus*; PID: pelvic inflammatory disease; WF = with food.

## Table 8–14 Nasal Decongestant Use in Pediatric Populations

| DRUG NAME | FORMULATIONS | DOSING GUIDANCE | ALERTS |
|---|---|---|---|
| Oxymetazoline | Afrin nasal spray | Age >6 years: Two sprays in each naris twice daily | Do not use for longer than 5 days Can cause rebound congestion |
| Phenylephrine | | Age 6–12 years: (0.125% solution) Two or three drops in each naris four times daily Spray: One or two sprays in each naris four times daily | Do not use for longer than 5 days Sprays preferred over drops |
| Pseudoephedrine | Afrin Sudafed Tablets, softgel capsules, liquid, drops | No safety data for children <12 years of age | Monitor BP Side effects: Anxiety, restlessness, GI upset |

BP: blood pressure; GI: gastrointestinal.

## Table 8–15 Pediatric Dosing Guidelines for Intranasal Steroids

| DRUG NAME | FORMULATIONS | DOSING GUIDANCE | ALERTS | SIDE EFFECTS |
|---|---|---|---|---|
| Beclomethasone | Beconase Vancerase | Age 6–12 years: One inhalation three times daily | No safety data for children <6 years of age Discontinue use if no improvement in 3 days | Nasal irritation, burning, stinging, dryness, headache, delayed wound healing |
| Budesonide | Rhinocort Rhinocort Aqua | Age >6 years: Two sprays in each naris twice daily | Discontinue use if no improvement in 3 weeks | Nasal irritation, burning, stinging, dryness, headache, delayed wound healing |

## Table 8–15 Pediatric Dosing Guidelines for Intranasal Steroids—cont'd

| DRUG NAME | FORMULATIONS | DOSING GUIDANCE | ALERTS | SIDE EFFECTS |
|---|---|---|---|---|
| Flunisolide | Nasalide Nasarel | Age 6–14 years: One or two sprays daily; age >14 years: Two sprays daily | Discontinue use if no improvement in 3 weeks | Nasal irritation, burning, stinging, dryness, headache, delayed wound healing |
| Fluticasone | Flonase | Age >4 years: One or two sprays daily | Not recommended for allergic rhinitis | Nasal irritation, burning, stinging, dryness, headache, delayed wound healing |
| Triamcinolone | Nasacort Nasacort AQ | Age >12 years: Two sprays daily | Use smallest dose possible Discontinue use if no improvement in 3 weeks | Nasal irritation, burning, stinging, dryness, headache, delayed wound healing |

## Table 8–16 Pediatric Dosing Guidelines for Antitussives

| DRUG NAME | FORMULATIONS | DOSING GUIDELINES | ALERTS |
|---|---|---|---|
| Benzonatate | Tessalon Perles Capsules: 100 mg, 200 mg | Age >10 years of age: 100–200 mg tid; maximum: 600 mg/24 hours | Sedation, headaches |
| Codeine | Codeine Tablets, solution | Age 6–12 years: 5–10 mg q6h ; maximum: 60 mg/day; age 2–6 years: 2.5–5 mg q6h; maximum: 30 mg/day | Sedation |
| Dextromethorphan | Robitussin Benylin Hold Vicks 44 Delsym Gelcaps, liquid, sustained action | Age 6–12 years: Maximum 60 mg/day; age 2–6 years: Maximum 30 mg/day | Do not use with persistent cough associated with smoking, asthma, or emphysema |

## Expectorants

Expectorants containing guaifenesin provide symptomatic relief of dry, nonproductive coughs. They are available in immediate-release and sustained-release preparations. Expectorants should not be used for persistent coughs related to asthma, smoking, or emphysema or for a cough with excessive secretion. The maximum daily dosing of guaifenesin for children is:

- **Immediate-release guaifenesin:**
  - Children 6 to 12 years of age: 100 to 200 mg q4h4, with a maximum dose of 1200 mg/24 hours
  - Children 2 to 6 years of age: 50 to 100 mg q4h with a maximum dose of 600 mg/24 hours
- **Sustained-release guaifenesin:**
  - Children 6 to 12 years of age: 500 to 600 mg q12h
  - Children 2 to 6 year of age: 275 to 300 mg q12h

**ALERT**

The U.S. Food and Drug Administration (FDA) has issued a recommendation to avoid the use of decongestants for children younger than age 2 years, and to avoid using antihistamines in children younger than 6 years of age.

### Antihistamines

Caution is advised in the use of antihistamines for any patient younger than 2 years of age. Recent studies describe sedation as the only consistent effect of antihistamine use in young children. Other reported side effects of antihistamines in children include paradoxical excitability, dizziness, respiratory depression, and hallucinations.

Older antihistamines, such as diphenhydramine (Benadryl), have more anticholinergic activity than newer ones and can work effectively when allergies are not the cause of an upper airway cough. Second generation antihistamines such as cetirizine (Zyrtec) and loratadine (Claritin) do not have much anticholinergic activity and will therefore be effective only for coughs caused by allergies. Newer antihistamines are helpful in managing allergic rhinitis. Table 8–17 presents dosing information for first and second generation antihistamines in children.

## Acetaminophen and Ibuprofen Dosing Charts

Acetaminophen (Tylenol) and ibuprofen (Motrin) are indicated as analgesic and antipyretic agents. Both are available in multiple formulations. Ibuprofen is additionally classified as a nonsteroidal anti-inflammatory

## Table 8–17 First and Second Generation Antihistamines: Dosing

| DRUG NAME | FORMULATIONS | DOSING GUIDELINES | ALERTS |
|---|---|---|---|
| **FIRST GENERATION ANTIHISTAMINES** | | | |
| Azatadine | Optimine Trinalin Repetab | Age >12 years: One or two tablets twice daily Repetab: One tablet bid | No safety data for children <12 years of age Drowsiness |
| Azelastine HCl | Astelin Nasal Spray | Age 5–12 years: One spray bid | Not recommended for children <5 years of age |
| Brompheniramine | Brovex Brovex CT | Age <6 years: 0.125 mg/kg PO q6h; age 6–12 years: 2 mg q4–6h, maximum 12 mg/day; age >12 years: 4 mg q4–6h, maximum 24 mg/day | Drowsiness Urinary retention Thickened bronchial secretions |
| Chlorpheniramine | Chlor-Trimeton | Age 6–12 years: Maximum 12 mg/day; age >12 years: Maximum 24 mg/day | Drowsiness Dry mouth |
| Clemastine | Tavist | Age >12 years: Maximum 8 mg/day | Drowsiness |
| Cyproheptadine | Periactin Tablets: 4 mg Syrup: 2 mg/5 mL | Age 2–6 years: 2 mg bid, maximum 12 mg/day; age 7–14 years: 4 mg bid | Drowsiness |
| Diphenhydramine | Benadryl Elixir, tablets, capsules, chewable tablets | Children >10kg: 12.5–25 mg/day in divided doses | Drowsiness |
| Hydroxyzine | Atarax Vistaril | Age <6 years: 50 mg daily in divided doses; age >6 years: 50–100 mg/day in divided doses | Drowsiness |

*Continued*

## Table 8–17 First and Second Generation Antihistamines: Dosing—cont'd

| DRUG NAME | FORMULATIONS | DOSING GUIDELINES | ALERTS |
|-----------|--------------|-------------------|--------|
| **SECOND GENERATION ANTIHISTAMINES** | | | |
| Cetirizine | Zyrtec Tablets and syrup | Age 2–5 years: 2.5 mg daily<br>Age >6 years: 5–10 mg/day | No safety data for children <2 years of age<br>Some sedative effect |
| Desloratadine | Clarinex tablets | Age >12 years: 5 mg daily | No safety data for children <12 years of age |
| Fexofenadine | Allegra | Age >12 years: 60 mg bid<br>Age 6–11 years: 30 mg bid | No safety data for children <6 years of age<br>Renal impairment: Cut dose in half |
| Loratadine | Claritin Tablets Reditabs | Age 2–5 years: 5 mg daily<br>Age 6–11 years: 10 mg daily | Take on empty stomach<br>No safety data for children <6 years of age |

drug (NSAID). For antipyretic indications of ibuprofen, the patient's temperature determines the dosage required. If, for example, the temperature is < 102.5°F, the dosage is 5 mg/kg/dose, if the temperature is > 102.5°F the dosage is 10 mg/kg/dose. Table 8–18 presents an acetaminophen dosing chart for children based on body weight. Table 8–19 is an ibuprofen dosing chart based on body weight.

## Vitamins and Minerals

Children require more nutrients than any other human age group to ensure that the immune system will have the strength to defend them against multiple viruses, bacteria, fungi, parasites, and other microorganisms, which children come into contact on a daily basis. Table 8–20 provides recommended daily allowances (RDAs) of vitamins for children by age group. Table 8–21 provides RDAs of calcium, iron, protein, and zinc for children by age group.

| AGE | WEIGHT | DROPS 80 mg/0.8 mL | ELIXIR 160 mg/5 mL | CHILDREN'S CHEWABLE TABLETS AND MELTAWAYS 80 mg | JUNIOR STRENGTH CHEWABLE TABLETS AND MELTAWAYS 160 mg |
|---|---|---|---|---|---|
| 0–3 Months | 6–11 lb (2.7–5 kg) | 40 mg ½ dropper | NA | NA | NA |
| 4–11 Months | 12–17 lb (5.5–7.7 kg) | 80 mg 1 dropper | ½ tsp children's liquid | NA | NA |
| 1–2 Years | 18–23 lb (8.2–10.4 kg) | 120 mg 1½ dropper | ¾ tsp children's liquid | 1½ children's meltaways | NA |
| 2–3 years | 24–35 lb (10.9–15.9 kg) | 160 mg 2 droppers | 1 tsp children's liquid | 2 children's chewable tablets or meltaways | 1 junior strength tablet or meltaway |
| 4–5 Years | 36–47 lb (16.3–21.3 kg) | 240 mg 3 droppers | 1 ½ tsp children's liquid | 3 children's chewable tablets or meltaways | 1½ junior strength tablets or meltaways |
| 6–8 Years | 48–59 lb (21.8–26.8 kg) | NA | 2 tsp children's liquid | 4 children's chewable tablets or meltaways | 2 junior strength tablets or meltaways |
| 9–10 Years | 60–71 lb (27.2–32.2 kg) | NA | 2 ½ tsp children's liquid | 5 children's chewable tablets or meltaways | 2½ junior strength tablets or meltaways |
| 11 Years | 72–95 lb (32.7–43.1 kg) | NA | 3 tsp children's liquid | 6 children's chewable tablets or meltaways | 3 Junior strength tablets or meltaways; or 1–1½ adult tab |
| 12 Years | 95 + lb (43.5 kg+) | NA | 4 tsp children's liquid | 8 children's chewable tablets or meltaways | 4 junior strength tablets or meltaways; or 2 adult tablets |

Table 8–18  **Acetaminophen Dosing Chart by Age**

Source: www.tylenol.com

## Table 8-19 Motrin (Ibuprofen) Dosing Chart by Age

| AGE | WEIGHT | DROPS 50 mg/ 1.25 mL | SUSPENSION 100 mg/5 mL | CHEWABLES 50 mg tablet | ADULT 200 mg tablet |
|-----|--------|----------------------|------------------------|------------------------|---------------------|
| 6-11 Months | 13-17 lb | 1 dropper | ½ tsp | 1 tablet | NA |
| 12–23 Months | 18–23 lb | 2 droppers | 1 tsp | 2 tablets | NA |
| 2–3 Years | 24–35 lb | 3 droppers | 1 ½ tsp | 3 tablets | NA |
| 4–5 Years | 36–47 lb | NA | 2 tsp | 4 tablets | NA |
| 6–8 Years | 48–59 lb | NA | 2 ½ tsp | 5 tablets | NA |
| 9–10 Years | 60–71 lb | NA | 3 tsp | 6 tablets | NA |
| 11–12 Years | 72–95 lb | NA | 4 tsp | 8 tablets | 1–2 tablets |

Source: www.motrin.com

## Nutritional Issues

The following sections provide guidance for the management of normal and abnormal growth and development in pediatric populations. They address issues such as failure to thrive, underweight, and obesity as nutritionally based disorders encountered in a pediatric practice and provide helpful hints for identifying these and other developmental problems throughout infancy, childhood, and adolescence.

### Developmental Milestones

The U.S. Health Resources and Services Administration's Bright Futures initiative has developed guidelines for supervising the health of infants, children, and adolescents, with a focus on developmental observations, age-appropriate interview questions for parents and children, physical examination and appropriate screening procedures, and anticipatory guidance for parents of children in each age category. Developmental milestones for the different pediatric age categories are presented in Box 8–1.

### Check Lists for Well Child Visits

Children should be scheduled for routine checkups from birth through adolescence. In many clinics these are managed through Early Periodic Screening, Diagnosis, and Treatment (EPSDT) programs sponsored by the

## Table 8-20 Recommended Daily Allowances of Vitamins in Children

| VITAMIN | 6 MONTHS | 6 MONTHS–1 YEAR | 1–3 YEARS | 4–6 YEARS | 7–10 YEARS | 11–14 YEARS | 15–18 YEARS |
|---|---|---|---|---|---|---|---|
| Vitamin A | 125 IU | 125 IU | 133 IU | 166 IU | 233 IU | F 266 IU<br>M 333 IU | F 266 IU<br>M 333 IU |
| Vitamin D | 300 IU | 1400 IU | 1400 IU | 1400 IU | 1400 IU | 1400 IU | 1400 IU |
| Vitamin K | 5–10 mcg | 5–10 mcg | 15 mcg | 20 mcg | 30 mcg | 45 mcg | F 55 mcg<br>M 65 mcg |
| Vitamin $B_1$ Thiamin | 0.3–0.4 mg | 0.3–0.4 mg | 0.3–0.4 mg | 0.9 mg | 1 mg | F 1.1 mg<br>M 1.5 mg | F 1.1 mg<br>M 1.5 mg |
| Vitamin $B_2$ Riboflavin | 0.4–0.5 mg | 0.4–0.5 mg | 0.8 mg | 1.1 mg | 1.2 mg | F 1.3 mg<br>M 1.5 mg | F 1.3 mg<br>M 1.8 mg |
| Vitamin $B_3$ Niacin | 5–6 mg | 5–6 mg | 9 mg | 12 mg | 13 mg | F 15 mg<br>M 17 mg | F 15 mg<br>M 20 mg |
| Vitamin $B_5$ Pantothenic acid | 2–3 mg | 2–3 mg | 3 mg | 3–4 mg | 4–5 mg | 4–7 mg | 4–7 mg |
| Vitamin $B_6$ Pyridoxine | 0.3–0.6 mg | 0.3–0.6 mg | 1 mg | 1.1 mg | 1.4 mg | F 1.4 mg<br>M 1.7 mg | F 1.5 mg<br>M 2 mg |

*Continued*

Table 8-20 Recommended Daily Allowances of Vitamins in Children—cont'd

| VITAMIN | 6 MONTHS | 6 MONTHS–1 YEAR | 1–3 YEARS | 4–6 YEARS | 7–10 YEARS | 11–14 YEARS | 15–18 YEARS |
|---|---|---|---|---|---|---|---|
| Vitamin $B_{12}$ Cyanocobalamin | 0.3–0.5 mcg | 0.3-0.5 mcg | 0.7 mcg | 1.0 mcg | 1.4 mcg | 2 mcg | 2 mcg |
| Biotin | 10–15 mcg | 10–15 mcg | 20 mcg | 25 mcg | 30 mcg | 30–100 mcg | 30–100 mcg |
| Folic acid | 25–35 mcg | 25–35mcg | 50 mcg | 75 mcg | 100 mcg | 150 mcg | F 180 mcg M 200 mcg |
| Vitamin C | 30–35 mg | 30–35 mg | 40 mg | 45 mg | 50 mg | 50 mg | 60 mg |
| Vitamin E | 3–4 IU | 3–4 IU | 6 IU | 7 IU | F 8 IU M 10 iU | F 8 IU M 10 IU | F 8 IU M 10 IU |

Source: www.fda.org

## Table 8-21 Recommended Daily Mineral Intakes for Children

| MINERALS AND PROTEIN | 0-3 MONTHS | 4-6 MONTHS | 7-9 MONTHS | 10-12 MONTHS | 1-3 YEARS | 4-6 YEARS | 7-10 YEARS | 11-14 YEARS | 15-18 YEARS |
|---|---|---|---|---|---|---|---|---|---|
| Calcium | 525 mg | 525 mg | 525 mg | 525 mg | 350 mg | 450 mg | 550 mg | F 800 mg<br>M 1000 mg | F 800 mg<br>M 1000 mg |
| Iron | 1.7 mg | 4.3 mg | 7.8 mg | 7.8 mg | 6.9 mg | 6.1 mg | 8.7 mg | F 14.8 mg<br>M 11.3 mg | F 14.8 mg<br>M 11.3 mg |
| Protein | 12.5 g | 12.7 g | 13.7 g | 14.9 g | 14.5 g | 19.7 g | 28.3 g | F 41.2 g<br>M 42.1 g | F 45.0 g<br>M 55.2 g |
| Zinc | 4.0 mg | 4.0 mg | 5.5 mg | 5.0 mg | 5.0 mg | 6.5 mg | 7.0 mg | F 9.0 mg<br>M 9.0 mg | F 7.0 mg<br>M 9.5 mg |

Source: www.fda.org

Box 8–1 **Developmental Milestones in Pediatrics**

Developmental milestones about which the NP will want to inquire in children of different age categories include:

- **1 Week:** Does the child respond to sound, look at faces, follow with his or her eyes, and respond to parents' voices?
- **1 Month:** The child should lift his or her head momentarily, move arms, legs, and head; and sleep 3 to 4 hours at a time. When crying, the child should be consoled by being spoken to or held
- **2 Months:** The child should coo and vocalize reciprocally, and pay attention to voices and sounds. He or she should smile, show pleasure with parents, lift head, neck, and upper chest while on stomach, and maintain some head control when in the upright position
- **4 Months:** The child should babble, coo, smile, and laugh. When lying on stomach he or she should hold head erect and raise body with hands, roll over, open hands, hold own hands, grasp a rattle, control head well, and reach for objects
- **6 Months:** The child should say "dada" and "baba," roll over, have no head lag when pulled to sit up, sit with support, grasp and mouth objects, recognize parents, and rake in small objects. The child should smile, laugh, squeal, and turn in response to sounds.The child may have first tooth
- **9 Months:** The child should respond to his or her name; understand a few words; babble, crawl, and creep; pokes with finger; shake, bang, throw, and drop objects; play peek-a-boo and pat-a-cake; and feed himself or herself with fingers. Anxiety in the presence of strangers is prevalent in this age group
- **12 Months:** The child should be able to pull up to stand, should cruise (walk holding onto furniture), may take a few steps alone, should bang blocks together, say two to four words, imitate vocalizations, drink from cup, look for dropped objects, wave "bye-bye," and self-feed
- **15 Months:** The child should be able to say three to six words, point to body parts, understand simple commands, walk well, stoop, climb stairs, stack two blocks, self-feed with fingers, drink from a cup, listen to a story, and express by pointing, pulling, or grunting
- **18 Months:** The child should be able to walk backward, throw a ball, say 15 to 20 words, use two-word phrases, pull a toy, stack three blocks, and use a spoon and cup. He or she should also be able to listen to a story and name objects in a picture, show affection, follow simple directions, and scribble
- **24 Months:** The child should be able to go up and down stairs, kick a ball, stack five blocks, use at least 20 words, follow two-step commands, and imitate adults

Center for Medicare and Medicaid Services (CMS). These programs are required in each state by CMS and may have multiple names such as in Louisiana the program is called KidMed; in Arkansas the title is ARKids First; Tennessee named their EPSDT program TENNder Care; the Kansas program is named KAN be Healthy; and the Texas program is Texas Healthy Steps. The EPSDT programs provide a venue in which developmental milestones are evaluated, monitoring is done of growth and development, appropriate immunizations are provided, and a physical examination is done. The timetable for these procedures established by Kid Med programs is appropriate for all healthy children, at 1 month, 2 months, 4 months, 6 months, 9 months, 1 year, and yearly after that. Table 8–22 provides a schedule for well-child visits from birth to 12 months, covering all required examinations and screenings recommended by Bright Futures. Table 8–23 provides scheduling for well-child visits and procedures for children from 2 through 21 years of age.

## Specific Pediatric Health-Care Issues

Pediatric health care includes a variety of health-care issues specific to pediatric populations. This section highlights some common pediatric health-care issues typically addressed in primary care settings.

### Anaphylaxis

Every clinic must be acutely aware of the propensity for anaphylactic reactions to medications given as injections. A prudent policy is to require that all patients who receive an injection of any medication be required to

## Table 8–22 Well-Child Physical Examination Schedule: Birth to 12 Months

| EXAMINATION | 1 MONTH | 2 MONTHS | 4 MONTHS | 6 MONTHS | 9 MONTHS | 12 MONTHS | 15 MONTHS | 18 MONTHS |
|---|---|---|---|---|---|---|---|---|
| Head circumference | X | X | X | X | X | | | |
| Length | X | X | X | X | X | X | X | X |
| Skin | X | X | X | X | X | X | X | X |
| Gait | | | | | | X | X | X |
| Heart murmurs | X | X | X | X | X | X | | |
| Red reflex | X | X | | | | | | |
| Hip dysplasia | X | X | X | X | X | X | | |
| Testes descent | X | X | | | | | | |
| Neurological reflexes | X | X | X | | X | | | |
| Muscle tone | X | X | | | X | | | |
| Use of extremities | X | X | | | | | | |
| Abuse/neglect | X | X | X | X | X | X | X | X |
| Other | Thrush Cradle cap Diaper dermatitis | Abdominal Masses Torticollis Metatarsus adductus | Tendon reflexes Muscle tone | Parachute reflex for hemiparesis Tooth eruption | Parachute reflex for hemiparesis | Tooth eruption Dental caries Bruising | Tooth eruption Dental caries Bruising | Dental caries |

| Table 8–23 Well-Child Physical Examination Schedule: 2 Years to 21 Years | | | | | | | | | | | | |
|---|---|---|---|---|---|---|---|---|---|---|---|---|
| EXAMINATION | 2 YEARS | 3 YEARS | 4 YEARS | 5 YEARS | 6 YEARS | 8 YEARS | 10 YEARS | 11–14 YEARS | 15–17 YEARS | 18–21 YEARS |
| Height | X | X | X | X | X | X | X | X | X | X |
| Weight | X | X | X | X | X | X | X | X | X | X |
| BMI | X | X | X | X | X | X | X | X | X | X |
| Teeth | X | X | X | X | X | X | X | X | | |
| Signs of abuse | X | X | X | X | X | X | X | X | X | X |
| Vision | | X | X | X | X | X | X | | | |
| Hearing | | X | X | X | X | X | X | | | |
| BP | | | X | X | X | X | X | X | X | X |
| PPD | | X* | X* | X* | X* | X* | X* | | | |
| Urinalysis | | | | X | | | | | | |
| Lead intoxication | | X | X | X | X | | | | | |
| Hyperlipidemia | | X | X | X | X | X | X | | | |
| Scoliosis | | | | | | | X | X | X | X |

Continued

| Table 8–23 Well-Child Physical Examination Schedule: 2 Years to 21 Years—cont'd | | | | | | | | | | | |
|---|---|---|---|---|---|---|---|---|---|---|---|
| EXAMINATION | 2 YEARS | 3 YEARS | 4 YEARS | 5 YEARS | 6 YEARS | 8 YEARS | 10 YEARS | 11–14 YEARS | 15–17 YEARS | 18–21 YEARS |
| Early puberty | | | | | | X | X | X | X | X |
| Tanner stage | | | | | | | X | X | X | X |
| Acne | | | | | | | | X | X | X |
| Teach BSE | | | | | | | | X | X | X |
| Eating disorders | | | | | | | | X | X | X |
| Sports injuries | | | | | | | | X | X | X |
| Hirsutism | | | | | | | | | X | X |

*For patients at risk.
BMI: body mass index; BP: blood pressure; BSE: breast self-examination; PPD: purified protein derivative (tuberculin).

remain in the clinic for a period of 15 minutes after the injection to allow monitoring for potentially adverse effects, and particularly anaphylaxis. Should a patient develop an anaphylactic reaction, the appropriate management is an injection of epinephrine (1:1000) at a dosage is 0.1 mg/kg/dose.

After the first dose of epinephrine is administered, the patient should be monitored for 15 minutes, after which a second dose of epinephrine can be administered if needed. The patient's BP should be monitored every 5 minutes throughout the treatment period, and an oral antihistamine should be given when the patient is stable, as follows:

- **Hydroxyzine:** PO or IM at 0.5 to 1.0 mg/kg/dose

or

- **Benadryl:** PO or IM at 1 to 2 mg/kg/dose, to a maximum of 100 mg in a single dose

## Asthma, Childhood

Listed below are some recommendations from pediatric pulmonologists for the management of pediatric patients with asthma. It is essential to develop a plan of action for patients with asthma and their parents that incorporates a rescue plan and a maintenance plan for controlling asthma.

Many asthma plans are available via the Internet to help teach parents how to manage children's asthma at home. One common asthma plan uses green, yellow, and red lights to indicate different levels of urgency of asthma management, corresponding to mild intermittent, mild persistent, moderate persistent, and severe persistent asthma, with appropriate management interventions for each level.

Parents and children should be taught to use peak flow meters and nebulizers at home to help effectively manage asthma. Patient education should be provided in areas of environmental control, avoidance of allergens and infections, and control of contributing illnesses such as gastroesophageal reflux disease (GERD), sinusitis, and rhinitis. Intensive education about differences between asthma-relieving medications and asthma-controlling medications is essential to enabling parents and children to manage asthma effectively at home.

> **COACH CONSULT**
>
> The "green light approach" to an asthma management plan provides patients and parents with helpful guidance about intervention when a child's asthma state changes from one level of severity to another. The green-light component of the plan usually indicates that the child can move air on a peak flow meter at 80% to 100% of the child's own predicted best flow capacity; the yellow light component takes effect when the peak flow reading is 50% to 79% of the child's personal best peak flow capacity; and the red light component represents a peak flow of less than 50% of the child's predicted best peak flow capacity.

## Relievers

Asthma relievers, just as their name indicates, are used to relieve worsening asthma symptoms of sudden onset. When a child's asthma status changes from green to yellow or from yellow to red in the three-light intervention plan, a reliever that is a short-acting beta agonist is the first line of therapy.

Albuterol, terbutaline, sepracor, and pirbuterol are selective beta-2 agonists, and all are effective when used appropriately. The dosages are identified in the following text.

Albuterol (Proventil or Ventolin) is available as a nebulizer or a multidose inhaler (MDI). Nebulized solutions are provided as 0.5% solution, with a dosage of 0.03 cc/kg. As a MDI, albuterol is available as 90 mcg/inhalation. For children older than age 4 years, the recommended dosage is 1 or 2 puffs of the MDI every 4 to 6 hours as needed. Albuterol can also be utilized in cases of exercise induced asthma (EIA) by giving 2 inhalations of the MDI 15 minutes prior to exercise.

Terbutaline (Brethine) is available in a 2.5 mg or a 5 mg tablet, or by injectable solution of 1 mg/mL. However, the injectable is not recommended for children. For children age 12–15 years, the terbutaline dosage is 2.5 mg tablet three times a day in 6 hour intervals between doses. Children older than age 15 may be prescribed 2.5 mg or 5 mg three times a day.

Pirbuterol (Maxair) is another beta-2 agonist, available in 200 mcg/inhalation via MDI. This formulation is not recommended for children.

Sepracor (Xopenex) is available for nebulizer solutions and MDI. Nebulizer solutions vary in strength from 0.31 mg/3 mL, 0.63 mg/3 mL, and 1.25 mg/3 mL. The MDI inhaler is available as Xopenex HFA in a 45 mcg per inhalation dose. Sepracor is not recommended for children younger than 6 years of age. For children age 6 to 11 years, the recommended dose is 0.31 mg/3 mL three times a day; for children 12 years and older, the dose recommendation is 0.63 mg/3 mL given three times a day in 6 to 8 hour intervals. Older children (older than 12 years of age) may require the higher dose of sepracor (1.25 mg/3 mL) given three times a day.

Metaproterenol sulfate (Alupent) is another beta-2 agonist available in a 5% solution. For children age 6 to 12 years, the dosage is 0.1 to 0.2 mL per nebulizer three times a day. Children older than 12 years may be prescribed 0.2 mL three or four times a day.

## Controllers for Long-Term Daily Maintenance

Controllers are the second category of asthma medications and are generally used on a routine basis to maintain and control asthma. The goal in using asthma controllers is to dose them in such an effective manner that the patient will not have to use relievers for asthma exacerbations. Controllers for children include anti-inflammatory agents, long-acting beta agonists, and leukotriene modifiers.

When making decisions about which medications to select for the management of a child's asthma, the NP must consider patient symptoms, peak flow status, and pulmonary function testing. Clinical decisions are based on asthma severity, ranging from intermittent to mild persistent, moderate persistent, and severe persistent. A stepwise approach to management has been recommended by the National Asthma Education and Prevention Program. This approach includes the following treatment plans:

- **Intermittent asthma:** Use a short-acting beta agonist as needed
- **Mild persistent asthma:** Select a low-dose inhaled corticosteroid or the alternative choice of cromolyn, a leukotriene modifier, or nedocromil
- **Moderate persistent asthma:** Order a low-dose inhaled corticosteroid plus a long-acting beta agonist or a medium-dose inhaled corticosteroid. An alternative to this can be a low-dose inhaled corticosteroid plus a leukotriene modifier, theophylline, or zileuton
- **Severe persistent asthma:** Treatment involves a medium-dose inhaled corticosteroid and a long-acting beta agonist. An alternative plan would include a medium-dose inhaled corticosteroid and a leukotriene modifier, theophylline, or Zileuton. If these plans are ineffective, change to a high-dose inhaled corticosteroid and a long-acting beta agonist and consider allergy management

For any child whose asthma advances from one severity level to another, the NP may consider 5 days of treatment with an oral systemic corticosteroid, such as prednisolone (Orapred).

Examples of each of the different classes of asthma medication follow:

- Anti-inflammatory agents
  - **Inhaled corticosteroids:** Beclomethasone, budesonide, flunisolide, fluticasone, and triamcinolone
  - **Systemic corticosteroids:** For short-course use: Oral prednisone (15 mg/5 mL) at a dosage of 1 to 2 mg/kg in three divided doses per day for 5 days. Table 8–24 provides a dosing chart for oral prednisone
  - **Cromolyn sodium (Intal or Tilade):** An anti-inflammatory agent and mast cell stabilizer, available as a nasal spray solution

or as an aerosol inhalation for oral administration; may be used for children older than 5 years of age up to four times daily. The nebulizer dosage for cromolyn products is 2.0 mL per 20 mg solution three to four times a day. Dosing per MDI provides 800 mcg per actuation of the MDI and can be used two to four puffs at a time, repeated four times a day. Cromolyn sodium (Intal) is available in a MDI at 0.8 mg/actuation; nedocromil sodium (Tilade) is provided in the MDI at 1.75 mg/actuation.

- Long-acting beta-2 agonists
  - Salmeterol, fenoterol, procaterol, levalbuterol, sustained-release albuterol
- Leukotriene modifiers
  - **Zafirlukast (Accolate):** 10 mg bid for children aged 5 to 11 years; 20 mg bid for children older than 12 years.
- **Montelukast (Singulair):** Available in 4 mg and 5 mg chewable tablets, 10 mg tablets and as a 4 mg packet of oral granules; dosage for children aged 2 to 5 years is 4 mg qd; children aged 6 to 14 years should be given 5 mg qd; and those older than age 15 years should be given 10 mg qd

### *Nebulizer Treatments*

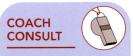

**COACH CONSULT**

Zafirlukast should be given on an empty stomach.

Nebulizer treatments can be given via face mask or mouthpiece to deliver inhaled beta-2 agonists and steroid medications effectively to children. Note that the nebulizer medications include short-acting beta agonists and corticosteroids. Use of a nebulizer is a highly effective means of delivering

## Table 8–24 Pediatric Dosing Chart for Oral Prednisone

| WEIGHT (LB) | WEIGHT (Kg) | DOSE 1 mg/kg/day | DOSE 2 mg/kg/day |
|---|---|---|---|
| 10 | 4.54 | ½ mL tid | 1 ml tid |
| 20 | 9.09 | 1 mL tid | 2 mL tid |
| 30 | 13.64 | 2 mL tid | 4 mL tid |
| 40 | 18.18 | 3 mL tid | 6 mL tid |
| 50 | 22.73 | 4 mL tid | 8 mL tid |

asthma medications to children younger than 4 years of age. If a nebulizer is unavailable, a standard metered dose inhaler with a spacer may be used. A spacer permits a child to receive the full dose of an inhaled medication more effectively than does a metered dose inhaler alone.

Clinical indications for using beta agonists and corticosteroids in nebulized form are the same as those given in the preceding section. Use a short-acting beta agonist when there is a change in the severity level of the patient's asthma on the red light, yellow light, green light scale. Two choices for short-acting beta agonists are levalbuterol (Xopenex) and albuterol sulfate (AccuNeb). Budesonide (Pulmicort), an inhaled steroid, may be ordered for a patient whose asthma reaches the mild persistent level of severity.

- Levalbuterol is a beta-2 agonist available for nebulization to treat bronchospasm in children older than 4 years of age. The solution is available in strengths of 0.31 mg/3 mL vial; 0.63 mg/3 mL vial; and 1.25 mg/3 mL vial
- Budesonide is a steroid that can be administered via nebulizer to children older than 6 months of age. It is available in strengths of 0.25 mg/2 mL vial; 0.5 mg/2 mL vial; and 1.0 mg/2 mL vial. Children 12 months to 8 years of age should be given 0.5 mg qd in two divided doses
- Albuterol, another beta-2 agonist, is available in strengths of 0.63 mg/3 mL vial or 1.25 mg/3 mL vial. Children older than 2 years of age may be given nebulizer treatments three or four times daily, with each treatment lasting 5 to 15 minutes

**COACH CONSULT**

Remind parents to clean nebulizer masks and have their child rinse his or her mouth with water after each treatment with budesonide.

## Attention Deficit-Hyperactivity Disorder

Attention deficit-hyperactivity disorder (ADHD) has become an increasingly common problem in pediatric populations. Several medications are now available for the management of ADHD. It is important to start these at a low dosage and titrate this upward as needed. After an initial treatment with an ADHD medication, the patient should be rechecked in 2 weeks to evaluate its effectiveness and make dosage adjustments if needed. Some recommendations for effective treatment of patients with ADHD include:

- Having the child's parents and teachers complete the Connors Rating Scale for ADHD

- Obtaining baseline laboratory results, including a complete blood count (CBC) and Chem-14. Sequential lab studies are to be drawn to monitor medication side effects.
- Repeating the CBC and Chem-14 every 6 months
- Obtaining a baseline electrocardiogram (ECG); this is not required if the drug of selection is atomoxetine hydrochloride (Strattera)

## Constipation

An infant with a presentation of constipation requires assessment to ensure that no physiological abnormalities are contributing to the constipation. Common physiological problems that must be considered as differential diagnoses of constipation in infants include: Hirschsprung's disease, malrotation, volvulus, intussusception, spinal cord anomalies, and inflammatory disorders of the GI tract, such as ulcerative colitis and Crohn's disease.

Infants with simple functional constipation can be treated with the addition of one tablespoon of dark Karo syrup added to each bottle of the infant's formula. If necessary, disimpaction of constipated stool can be accomplished with enemas or oral agents, such as mineral oil given twice daily for 2 or 3 days.

**ALERT**

Do not use enemas of soapsuds, tap water, or magnesium in children because of the toxicity of these solutions.

Treatments to keep children's bowels moving daily include laxatives, dietary fiber, and behavior modification. Laxative selections for children include milk of magnesia, lactulose, or mineral oil. Dietary changes include increased fluid intake and increased dietary fiber consumption as part of a healthy diet pattern, which includes fruits and vegetables as well as whole grains. Instruct the parents and child to establish regular toileting patterns, with positive reinforcements for active participation in the behavior modification plan. Once the child has an established pattern of normal bowel movements over a period of several months, begin tapering laxative use over a 1- to 2-month period.

A good history of bowel patterns will aid in proper diagnosis of the cause of constipation. Information should be assessed about stooling frequency, stool size and consistency, and unusual problems such as bleeding with defecation.

Some medications may cause constipation. Other issues to explore with the patient's parents include diet and exercise history, fluid intake, and evidence of soiling of underwear. Constipation may also be seen in children who avoid public bathrooms, experience sexual abuse, have attention deficit disorder, or have difficulties with toilet training especially if strong coercive stimulation is involved.

Along with an extensive history, a flat plate x-ray of the abdomen, as well as diagnostic laboratory tests including thyroid function tests, assays for serum electrolyte levels and lead, and testing for celiac disease antibodies, may aid in diagnosis of the cause of constipation. Children who do not respond to therapy should be referred to a pediatric gastroenterologist for further evaluation.

## Diarrhea

Young children with acute diarrhea should be evaluated for a variety of conditions that can cause this condition. Initial assessment of the child should include a detailed history of diarrhea frequency, stool color, estimated stool volume, and presence of blood or mucus in the stool. A history should include recent travel, day-care attendance, contact with pets or other animals, and recent antibiotic use. It is imperative to conduct a detailed physical examination of the child, with assessment of his or her vital signs, mental status, any evidence of malnutrition, skin color and tone, and any signs of dehydration, and a complete abdominal assessment and gentle rectal examination. Most children with acute diarrhea do not require laboratory evaluation. In cases of diarrhea of unresolved etiology, or of children with chronic diarrhea (>2 weeks duration), the following procedures should be included in the management plan:

- Collection of specimens for a CBC
- Collection of stool specimens for ova and parasites (O&P) and rotavirus cultures
- Stool culture in cases of bloody diarrhea
- Cessation of eating any dairy products
- Administration of one package of *Lactobacillus* granules (Lactinex), mixed and given twice daily until stools become firm to alter the intestinal microflora and shorten the course of diarrhea

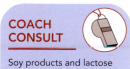

**COACH CONSULT**

Soy products and lactose free formulas may be continued.

- Administration of OTC bismuth subsalicylate, which has antimicrobial, antisecretory, and anti-inflammatory properties at doses of 100 to 150 mg/kg/dose, to decrease stool output and duration of diarrhea

- Antimicrobial therapy for acute diarrhea in children, as follows
  - *Salmonella*: Antimicrobial drugs are ineffective
  - *Shigella*: Third generation cephalosporins are highly effective
  - *Campylobacter*: Erythromycin or azithromycin are effective in some circumstances
- *Escherichia coli*: Trimethoprim-sulfamethoxazole (TMP-SMZ) is effective
- *Giardia lamblia*: Metronidazole is recommended for persistent or severe diarrhea
- Oral rehydration: Electrolyte oral solution (Pedialyte) or sports drinks to maintain hydration. The electrolyte oral solutions contain dextrose, fructose, and electrolytes to replace those lost during vomiting and diarrhea. A serving of the electrolyte solution provides 25 calories, 253 mg sodium, 6 gm carbohydrates, 2.5 mg magnesium, 152 mg potassium, 25.0 mg of calcium, and 0.1 mg of zinc.
  - A carbohydrate-to-sodium ratio of 3:1 is recommended

The most common type of chronic diarrhea in children is chronic nonspecific diarrhea. Most cases of acute diarrhea are related to infectious disease, whether viral, bacterial, or parasitic. Rotavirus causes most cases of childhood diarrhea. Other potential causes include *Salmonella, Shigella, Campylobacter jejuni, E. coli, Clostridium difficile,* and *Giardia lamblia*. Typical symptoms caused by each of these organisms are identified in Box 8–2.

## Failure to Thrive

Children younger than 2 years of age who fail to gain weight at predicted rates must be evaluated for abuse and neglect, as well as a number of physiologic problems that can interfere with metabolism and normal weight gain. A dietary history is essential in evaluating potential failure to thrive in children. Table 8–25 provides an average infant feeding schedule.

If an infant is not consuming adequate calories, it is essential to increase calorie consumption without increasing overall fluid intake. Most standard formulas provide 20 to 22 calories per fluid ounce. Infants whose growth is below the normal curve for weight gain may be given 24 or 27 calories per fluid ounce by modifying the reconstitution of their formulas. Table 8–26 provides several dilution tables for the reconstitution of infant formulas.

## Box 8–2  Common Organisms Causing Diarrhea in Children

- *Campylobacter jejuni*: Causes frequent watery stools and fever, occasionally causes bloody diarrhea. Abdominal pain is common. Transmitted by contaminated food or water
- *Clostridium difficile:* Causes antibiotic-associated diarrhea and pseudomembranous colitis; effects range from mild watery diarrhea to bloody stools to persistent diarrhea
- *Escherichia coli*: Causes traveler's diarrhea, dysentery-like illness, bloody stools, and enterohemorrhage
- *Giardia lamblia*: Most common GI parasite in the United States; transmitted by contaminated food or water or by person-to-person contact. Symptoms include loose, watery stools; abdominal cramping pains; weight loss; diarrhea for 1 to 3 weeks; fever; and in some cases grossly bloody stools
- *Rotavirus*: A common cause of diarrhea in children from 6 to 24 months of age. Causes vomiting and watery diarrhea that may lead to dehydration; fever is common
- *Salmonella*: Common in children younger than 5 years of age; transmitted by animal products; causes symptoms of gastroenteritis
- *Shigella*: Causes mild watery diarrhea with or without constitutional symptoms, and in some cases profuse watery diarrhea with fever, headache, and malaise; may cause abdominal cramping and tenderness and blood or mucus in stool. Transmitted by contaminated food or water, by contact with a contaminated object, or by flies

## Table 8–25  Average Infant Feeding Schedule

| AGE | AVERAGE NUMBER OF FEEDINGS IN 24 HOURS | AVERAGE AMOUNT PER FEEDING | AVERAGE AMOUNT PER DAY |
|---|---|---|---|
| 1–2 Weeks | 6–10 | 2–3 oz | 12–30 oz |
| 3–4 Weeks | 6–8 | 3–4 oz | 18–32 oz |
| 1–2 Months | 5–6 | 4–5 oz | 20–30 oz. |
| 2–3 Months | 5–6 | 5–6 oz | 25–36 oz |
| 3–4 Months | 4–5 | 6–7 oz | 24–35 oz |
| 4–7 Months | 4–5 | 7–8 oz | 28–40 oz |
| 7–9 months | 3–4 | 7–8 oz | 21–32 oz |
| 9–12 Months | 3 | 7–8 oz | 21–34 oz |

## Table 8–26  Dilution Tables for Calorie Increases in Infant Formula

| DILUTION | WATER (fl oz) | LEVEL UNPACKED SCOOPFUL | APPROXIMATE YIELD (fl oz) |
|---|---|---|---|
| FROM POWDER: STANDARD FORMULAS: SIMILAC ADVANCE, SIMILAC LACTOSE FREE, SIMILAC PM 60/40, ALIMENTUM POWDER, ENFAMIL, ENFAMIL LIPIL, LACTOFREE, ISOMIL, ADVANCE, PROSOBEE, NUTRAMIGEN, PROGESTIMIL | | | |
| 13 cal/fl oz | 6.3 | 2 | 7 |
| 20 cal/fl oz (standard mixture) | 2 | 1 | 2 |
| 24 cal/fl oz | 5 | 3 | 6 |
| 27 cal/fl oz | 4.25 | 3 | 5 |
| TO RECONSTITUTE SIMILAC NEOSURE, ADVANCE POWDER, AND ENFAMIL ENFACARE LIPIL | | | |
| 20 cal/fl oz | 4.5 | 2 | 5 |
| 22 cal/fl oz (standard mixture) | 2 | 1 | 2 |
| 24 cal/fl oz | 5.5 | 3 | 6.5 |
| 27 cal/fl oz | 8 | 5 | 9 |
| TO RECONSTITUTE SIMILAC, SIMILAC LACTOSE FREE, ENFAMIL, ISOMIL, ADVANCE, LACTOFREE, PROSOBEE, AND NUTRAMIGEN CONCENTRATED LIQUIDS | | | |
| 13 cal/fl oz | 2 | 1 | 3 |
| 20 cal/fl oz (standard mixture) | 1 | 1 | 2 |
| 24 cal/fl oz | 2 | 3 | 5 |
| 27 cal/fl oz | 1 | 2 | 3 |

## Gastroesophageal Reflux Disease

Many infants will experience symptoms of GERD, including frequent spitting up of formula and colicky abdominal pain with drawing up of the legs toward the abdomen. One approach to treating infant GI problems might be to change formulas, especially if there is some reason to suspect lactose intolerance. A 2-week trial of a hypoallergenic formula is the first step in treatment. If no improvement is seen, start a 2- to 3-week trial of acid suppression therapy. Another commonly used treatment approach in infants with GERD is to add rice cereal to the formula to thicken it, thus minimizing reflux activity.

If an infant is determined to have GERD, several treatment options are recommended, including:

- **Ranitidine (Zantac) syrup:** Available at 15 mg/mL; prescribe at 4 mg/kg/dose
- **Atarax syrup:** Available as preparations of 10 mg/5 mL or 25 mg/5 mL; prescribe at 2 mg/kg/day in divided doses q6-8h
- **Reglan syrup**: available at 5 mg/5 mL; prescribe at 0.1 mg/kg/dose
- **Famotidine (Pepcid)**: Prescribe 1 to 2 mg/kg/day in three divided doses
- **Axid oral solution:** Prescribe 5 mg/kg divided into two doses daily
- **Lansoprazole (Prevacid):** Prescribe 1.5 to 3.5 mg/kg/day in two divided doses

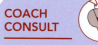

**COACH CONSULT**

Danger signs in infants with vomiting are:
- Forceful projectile vomiting
- Hematemesis
- Failure to thrive
- Onset of emesis after 6 months of age
- Diarrhea or constipation with vomiting
- Abdominal tenderness or distention
- Fever, lethargy, or both
- Hepatosplenomegaly
- Bulging fontanelles
- Seizures

**COACH CONSULT**

Be aware that in children there is an association of GERD with upper airway diseases, including apnea, asthma, laryngeal inflammation, and recurrent pneumonia. Aggressive management of GERD may prevent or alleviate such upper airway problems.

## Heart Murmurs

Four normal developmental or innocent cardiac murmurs are often encountered in children and adolescents. Innocent murmurs (systolic murmurs) include vibratory murmurs, pulmonic flow murmurs, and supraclavicular systolic murmurs, as well as the innocent venous hum. Innocent murmurs are identified in a normal clinical context, with an intensity grading of III or less, and are generally accompanied by a systolic ejection murmur. Common causes of functional murmurs include fever, anemia, and anxiety.

A 12-lead ECG may be helpful for documenting rhythm patterns. Cardiac examination should not reveal abnormalities such as a split S2, gallops, thrills, clicks, rubs, cyanosis, a hyperdynamic precordial impulse, or edema. These may be indications of pathological murmurs, which require referral to a pediatric cardiologist or further evaluation and treatment. All diastolic murmurs in children should be considered as pathological until judged otherwise by a pediatric cardiologist. A continuous murmur, beginning in systole and continuing throughout S2, may be an innocent murmur (audible with the child in a sitting position) or may be a pathological continuous murmur such as that caused by ductus arteriosus. Table 8–27 summarizes the types and features of functional heart murmurs in children.

## Hospital Admissions for Pediatric Clients
The following clinical situations necessitate hospital admission for pediatric clients:
- Age under 2 months with a fever >100.4°F
- Sickle cell anemia with fever
- Loss of consciousness after a head injury
- Vomiting after a head injury

## Jaundice
Many types of jaundice may occur in pediatric populations, and jaundice is a fairly common occurrence among breastfed newborns. To make

| Table 8–27 **Table of Functional Murmurs** | | |
|---|---|---|
| **VENOUS HUM** | **SYSTOLIC AND DIASTOLIC** | **SITTING ONLY** |
| Vibratory murmur | Midsystolic Begins directly with the first heart sound | • Musical quality<br>• Best heard over lower mid-precordium<br>• Seldom louder than grade II/VI |
| Pulmonic ejection | Ejection without a click | • Normal S2<br>• Best heard over 2nd to 3rd intercostal space just to the left of the sternal border<br>• Seldom more than grade II/VI |
| Carotid bruit | Short systolic | • Carotid area, especially on right<br>• Best heard under the right clavicle<br>• Short duration<br>• Intensity decreases significantly when child sits up with shoulders hyperextended (arms behind the patient) |
| Physiological peripheral pulmonic stenosis (seen most commonly in preterm infants) | Short systolic, bilateral | Transmitted throughout lung fields |

sure that there is no serious underlying cause for jaundice, order laboratory tests for evaluation, including measurements of direct and indirect serum bilirubin levels and a CBC with a peripheral smear, reticulocyte count, blood typing, and a direct Coombs test. Phototherapy is the first-line treatment for all cases of pathological indirect hyperbilirubinemia. The following are recommendations for the management of infants with jaundice:

- If the infant is younger than 5 days old and the bilirubin level is 13 µmol/L or less, do not change anything
- If the infant is younger than 5 days old, is breast fed, and has a serum bilirubin >13 µmol/L, supplement breast feedings with formula
- If the infant is older than 5 days and has a bilirubin >15 µmol/L, stop breastfeeding for one day and then recheck the bilirubin level after 24 hours. If the bilirubin is greater than 15 µmol/L after the 24-hour period, order a bilirubin light treatment. If the bilirubin has dropped below 15 µmol/L after the 24-hour period, no further changes are indicated
- Instruct breastfeeding mothers to feed their infants at a window with good exposure to sunlight

## Obesity, Childhood

There is a growing epidemic of obesity in adolescents, school-age children, and younger children. A combination of sedentary lifestyles and minimization of physical education in schools, coupled with high-fat fast-food choices and genetic factors, has led to this epidemic of obesity. In children, obesity can also be a result of genetic and endocrine abnormalities. All children should have regular monitoring of their height, weight, and body mass index (BMI), and these should be plotted on growth charts; children with a BMI exceeding the 85th percentile should be evaluated for obesity.

The physical examination of an obese child should focus on detecting any underlying cause as well as any complication of obesity. In addition to a complete physical examination, laboratory analyses should include a fasting lipid profile, liver function tests, a serum glucose assay, and tests of thyroid function. Family, dietary, and psychosocial factors should also be considered in seeking the source of obesity. Management of obesity requires a multidisciplinary approach, including participation by nutritionists, exercise therapists, psychologists, and medical staff members working with the child and its family to develop achievable dietary goals.

# 9 Geriatric Management Pearls

# Geriatric Management Pearls

Today there are more Americans 65 years of age and older than ever before. According to the U.S. Centers for Disease Control and Prevention (CDC), this number will double during the next 25 years because of longer lifespans and aging baby boomers. By 2030, one in five Americans will fit within the "older adult" classification. Although medical advances have extended lifespans far beyond those of past generations, there are also challenges in caring for the aging population.

Many older adults are in good health, but the proportion of those with serious medical conditions and functional problems requiring long-term care is higher than in any other age group. Long-term care entails the combination of supportive medical, personal, and social services for individuals who cannot meet their basic activities of daily living (ADL) over an extended period. These services can be provided in a variety of settings, including the home by visiting health-care agencies and within institutions. Alternative settings for long-term care, such as assisted-living facilities and elder-care communities, are growing rapidly in many states. Nursing homes are an essential component of the broad array of available long-term services and are a part of the primary care continuum.

Caring for elderly clients, especially frail, older adults, can be quite complex. Many diseases present differently in old age than they do earlier in life, and the existence of multiple chronic diseases in many older patients adds to the complexity of their management. Chronic disease states, rather than acute illnesses, are the most common reasons for medical office visits among elderly individuals, and the leading causes of death among elderly individuals are related to chronic disease states, including heart disease, cerebrovascular disease, chronic respiratory disease, and cancer.

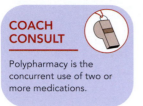

**COACH CONSULT**

Polypharmacy is the concurrent use of two or more medications.

Medications play an important role in the medical management of acute and chronic disease states in older persons. Statistics indicate that more than 30% of all prescription medications dispensed in the United States are for older persons, as are more than 40% of all over-the-counter (OTC) medications sold. A major concern for these patients is polypharmacy. Elderly patients often visit multiple care providers and specialists, and each provides new prescriptions that add to the patient's list of medications. Polypharmacy creates issues related to drug–drug interactions, increased potential for adverse drug reactions, and an increased risk for falls. Strategies for reducing polypharmacy are needed.

Many ethical issues are endemic to geriatric care. There is much that NPs can do, but in geriatric care, the key question is what should they do? As primary-care clinicians, NPs need to be skillful in discussing the patient's health care wishes with the patient. Involving patients in their own care is essential  to providing the best possible care and gives the opportunity to enhance one of the most important functions that all people desire: the right to be in command of their own destiny.

This chapter will address issues specific to the geriatric population, including issues in geriatric dermatology, depression, dementia, delirium, functional disabilities, falls, and frailty issues, and options for assisting geriatric patients with their ADL and health-care needs. Common throughout the discussion of any topic in geriatric health care should be treatment of the patient with respect and dignity. Geriatric patients need to be included in decisions about their health care and allowed to identify for themselves the quality of life they wish to have.

## Delirium

Advanced age, underlying dementia, functional impairment, and medical comorbidities are all risk factors for dementia. The hallmark of delirium is that it presents with an acute cognitive dysfunction with impaired attentiveness. This can develop suddenly or over a short time, usually hours to days. A patient with delirium experiences acute fluctuations in mental status, along with varying levels of inattention and altered levels of consciousness. Changes in memory, orientation, and abstract thinking may occur but are not diagnostic. The patient's psychomotor activity or level of arousal may also be abnormal.

Other symptoms of delirium may include hallucinations, delusions, tremor, and abnormalities in the sleep-wake cycle. In some frail elderly patients, delirium will precede the appearance of another illness and will be the only early manifestation of that illness. Delirium may persist for many weeks or months; infrequently, it never resolves completely, or it modulates into the chronic cognitive dysfunction of dementia.

Delirium can stem from a number of metabolic, infectious, and neurological disorders. Metabolic causes of delirium include:

- **Hyponatremia or hypernatremia:** Monitor the patient's serum sodium levels
- **Renal failure:** Check blood urea nitrogen (BUN) and creatinine levels
- **Hypoxia or ischemia:** Monitor oxygen saturation levels
- **Hypoglycemia or hyperglycemia:** Perform finger-stick glucose testing or a fasting glucose test
- **Hypothyroidism or hyperthyroidism:** Order thyroid function testing
- **Recreational drug use:** Order toxicology screening tests
- **Alcohol intoxication or withdrawal:** Monitor the patient's blood alcohol level and osmolarity
- **Hypercalcemia and hypermagnesemia:** Monitor laboratory values for calcium and magnesium
- **Hypophosphatemia:** Check the patient's serum phosphate levels

Infectious causes of delirium include:

- **Sepsis:** Perform cultures, check the patient's complete blood count (CBC), and obtain a urinalysis report
- **Meningitis:** Order a lumbar puncture, cerebrospinal fluid (CSF) and blood cultures, and a CBC

Neurological causes of delirium include:

- **Subarachnoid hemorrhage:** Order a computed tomographic (CT) scan of the patient's brain and a lumbar puncture
- **Cerebral infarction:** Order a CT scan or magnetic resonance imaging (MRI) of the patient's brain
- **Seizures, postictal state:** Order a brain CT scan or MRI and an electroencephalogram (EEG)

The diagnosis of delirium consists of two elements: (1) establishing the presence of delirium and (2) if possible, establishing its underlying cause. In as many as 80% of cases, delirium is undiagnosed or misdiagnosed, but this is much less likely with an interdisciplinary approach and input from physicians, nurses, and significant others who know the patient well, such as family members.

The diagnostic criteria for delirium include:

- Disturbance of consciousness, including a reduced ability to focus or maintain attention
- Cognitive changes, including disorientation, language disturbances, and perceptual disturbances
- Acute onset and with an identifiably precise time of onset; onset over a period of hours to days; and an onset that fluctuates during the course of the day

A thorough history is required to determine both the frequency and duration of changes in mental status as well as other clinical features of delirium. The history recorded by the NP should include a complete medication review that focuses on changes in the patient's drug regimen, such as additions, deletions, and dosage changes that may have precipitated the delirium. Medications that may precipitate changes in mental status include:

- Psychoactive drugs, especially sedative-hypnotics, and including lithium, barbiturates, antiparkinsonian drugs, benzodiazepines, antipsychotics, and tricyclic antidepressants
- Antidepressants
- Anticholinergics
- Opioids
- Cimetidine, ranitidine
- Digitalis
- Clonidine
- Alcohol use
- OTC medications

The physical examination of the patient with delirium can be challenging. Important etiological clues can be provided by vital signs and oxygen saturation levels. Thorough cardiac, respiratory, abdominal, neurological, and mental status examinations should be performed.

**COACH CONSULT**

Delirium may result from medical conditions, substance overuse or abuse, and substance withdrawal. Symptoms of delirium are generally worse at night (sundowning) than during the day.

**ALERT**

Remember to ask about OTC medications and herbal medications, because these are frequently used by elderly patients before seeking medical care.

**COACH CONSULT**

Differential diagnosis should include depression and dementia because both may coexist with delirium.

Patients with delirium are especially vulnerable to iatrogenic problems, predominantly those caused by physical or chemical restraints. Bowel and bladder retention or incontinence are common and can contribute directly to delirium. Patients with delirium who are bedridden are prone to atelectasis, pressure sores, and deconditioning. These conditions can be reduced by mobilization, such as by having the patient sit up in a chair. Acute malnutrition may result from the inability to attend to eating. To prevent this, close attention must be given to the patient's nutritional intake, and manualassistance with eating should be provided when necessary.

**ALERT**

Delirium is a medical emergency. Identify its underlying cause and treat it if this is within your scope of practice. Remember that the most common causes of delirium in the elderly are related to fluid and electrolyte imbalances, infections, and medications. If the cause is not readily identifiable, refer the patient for further evaluation.

## Dementia

The prevalence of dementia is a growing public health problem. Dementia is an acquired syndrome marked by a decline in memory and at least one other cognitive dysfunction. In primary care settings, 6% of patients 65 years of age and older have dementia. Among primary care patients diagnosed as having dementia, 70% suffer from Alzheimer's disease, 5% have vascular dementia (VaD), and 22% have mixed disease with both Alzheimer's disease and VaD. Various types of dementia are described in the following:

- **Alzheimer's disease:** Patients with Alzheimer's disease present with a progressive decline in intellectual or cognitive function caused by damage to the hippocampus, amygdala, and other areas of the brain. Typical symptoms include:
  - Recent memory loss, disorientation
  - Impaired judgment and reasoning
  - Poor attention span
  - Communication and speech difficulties
  - Insomnia and daytime sleepiness
  - Hyperactivity, wandering, and restlessness
  - Mood disturbances and emotional outbursts
  - Urinary and fecal incontinence
  - Paranoia, hallucinations, and delusions

- **VaD:** Patients with VaD generally have better verbal memory and poorer performance in executive function than patients with Alzheimer's disease. There are four subtypes of VaD:
  - Cortical or multi-infarct VaD, which presents with stepwise deterioration
  - Subcortical VaD, which presents with progressive cognitive decline and executive dysfunction
  - VaD from single strategic vascular insults, which has a sudden onset followed by a plateau of stability
  - VaD from generalized severe cerebral hypoperfusion
- **Dementia of the Lewy body type:** Characterized by fluctuating cognitive defects, Parkinsonian symptoms, delirium-like attention deficits, and visual hallucinations
- **Dementia of Parkinson's disease:** Dementia of Parkinson's disease generally occurs in the later phases of the disease, usually at least 12 months after original diagnosis of the disease

More rare types of dementia include:

- **Frontotemporal dementia:** A very rare dementia, with symptoms of personality changes, apathy, and executive dysfunction
- **Primary progressive aphasia:** Characterized by progressive expressive aphasia and abnormalities of hand/motor function
- **Normal pressure hydrocephalus:** The typical presentation of dementia resulting from normal pressure hydrocephalus includes the triad of progressive dementia, urinary incontinence, and apraxic gait
- **Huntington's disease:** Characteristics of this disease include jerking, uncontrollable movements of the limbs, trunk, and head; progressive cognitive decline; and behavioral symptoms
- **Creutzfeldt-Jakob disease:** This is a rapidly progressive and fatal dementia disorder related to an infectious disease and is more typically seen in younger patients
- **Dementia related to AIDS:** This disorder is fairly common in patients with established HIV

Early signs of dementia may be subtle and difficult to identify. Often the patient denies symptoms. Family members or caregivers may be needed to provide a more objective history. The NP should realize that even family members may overlook or compensate for symptoms of dementia. The ability of the NP to obtain a comprehensive history of the patient is paramount to making an accurate diagnosis of dementia. When recording the history of a patient suspected of having dementia, look for the following:

- A history of previous medical and psychiatric illnesses
- Chronic diseases such as diabetes mellitus, hypertension, heart disease, chronic obstructive pulmonary disease (COPD), liver or renal diseases, previous strokes, Parkinson's disease, and cancer
- Recent acute illness, infection, hospitalization, or surgery
- Previous experiences of anxiety, depression, or other psychiatric illnesses
- Alcohol use
- A history of head trauma
- A history of the onset, duration, and course of the patient's current symptoms of dementia

Symptoms present in dementia include:

- Difficulty in learning or retaining new information
- Repetitive conversation or behaviors
- Difficulty with short-term memory
- Difficulty with complex tasks
- Disorientation to person, time, place, or events
- Difficulty in finding words
- Personality changes including increased irritability, increased suspiciousness, and decreased self-directedness
- Changes in personal presentation, including changes in dress and hygiene

**COACH CONSULT**

A history of previous medical and psychiatric illness is essential for the diagnosis of dementia.

## Assessment of Dementia

Assessment of the patient with dementia requires a complete physical examination to rule out metabolic or physiological events as its possible cause. Note that most patients with dementia will have normal findings in a neurological examination. The patient may show some disturbances in gait that are commonly attributed to extrapyramidal disorders or VaD. Once the physical findings have been assessed, the patient should be screened for symptoms of depression, using either the Beck Depression Inventory, the Hamilton Depression Rating Scale, or Geriatric Depression Scale.

Diagnostic evaluation of the patient with dementia is important for ruling out metabolic or physiological causes of cognitive impairment. The focus of the diagnostic work-up is to identify any treatable etiologies of dementia. A good diagnostic work-up for patients with dementia should include:

- Laboratory studies
  - CBC, erythrocyte sedimentation rate (ESR), antinuclear antibody (ANA) assay, complete metabolic panel, liver function tests, thyroid panel, anemia panel including folate levels, vitamin B12 levels, syphilis serology, and urinalysis
  - Assays for drug levels if appropriate
  - Testing for the gene that encodes apolipoprotein E4, a gene on chromosome 19 that correlates with and increases the risk of developing Alzheimer's disease
- Oxygen saturation level and arterial blood gas analysis to rule out metabolic causes of dementia
- Electrocardiogram (ECG) to rule out cardiac causes of dementia, such as silent myocardial infarction (MI)
- Imaging studies to rule out other causes of dementia
  - CT scan of the head
  - MRI if VaD is suspected
  - EEG if the patient has a history of seizure disorder or if it is suspected, or for patients with rapidly progressing dementia
  - Lumbar puncture for suspected central nervous system (CNS) infection, systemic lupus erythematosus (SLE), multiple sclerosis (MS), or hydrocephalus

### *Cognitive Assessment of Dementia*

One of the most commonly utilized cognitive assessment tools is the Mini-Mental State Examination. This evaluation assesses language, word-finding skills, judgment, and short-term memory. Remember that the MMSE is a screening tool and not a diagnostic tool and may yield false-positive results, depending on the patient's level of education. As a screening tool, the MMSE may be utilized in sequential visits to periodically monitor changes in a patient's cognitive status.

The MMSE can be useful in the staging of dementia. The three stages of progression in dementia are early, middle, and late, each marked by a greater level of cognitive decline than the preceding stage. Symptoms of early-stage dementia are often subtle, and may go undetected. They may include some forgetfulness, difficulty in learning new material, slowed reaction times, and indecisiveness. As the patient progresses to the middle stage, symptoms are more pronounced with confusion, fearfulness, easy frustration, inability to follow simple directions, difficulty with word finding, difficulty with calculations, and changes in physical activity such as pacing, wandering, and sleep disturbances. In the late stages of dementia, patients exhibit total dependence for ADL, including inability to feed themselves, incontinence, and inability to communicate. They are often bedbound and do not recognize family or friends. Patients with early-stage dementia have an MMSE score >17 points. An MMSE score ranging from 11 to 17 points indicates middle-stage dementia. Patients with severe or late-stage dementia score 10 or lower on the MMSE.

**COACH CONSULT**

Functional assessment is critical in patients with dementia. Observe the patient's ability to transfer from a chair to the examination table. Assess the patient's ability to undress and dress. Consider safety issues relevant to independent living status.

### Differentiating Delirium from Dementia

Differentiating between delirium and dementia is not always easy because features of the two syndromes sometimes overlap. The onset of delirium is rapid, whereas dementia usually develops slowly. In delirium the ability to focus attention is primarily affected. In early-stage dementia, memory rather than attention is affected. In late-stage dementia attention may be severely impaired. Delirium is often caused by toxic or metabolic factors that impair brain-cell function and is often regarded as potentially reversible; conversely, because dementia is usually caused by damage to or loss of brain cells, it is permanent. The duration of cognitive decline is therefore probably the clearest way to differentiate these disorders. Although most individuals with delirium recover fully, some do not. In addition, some persons have dementia of a reversible cause and may recover. The diagnosis of dementia should not be made until all appropriate treatments have been tried and several months have passed to allow for recovery. Table 9–1 compares features of dementia, delirium, and depression in elderly persons.

## Treatment of Dementia

When treating a patient with dementia, follow these guidelines:

- Identify triggers of demented behavior and eliminate them if possible
- Provide caregiver support
- Simplify tasks related to personal hygiene, dressing, toileting, and feeding.
- Monitor the patient for wandering and safety issues
- Monitor the patient for signs of fluid and electrolyte disturbances, including dehydration, constipation, hunger, and thirst

## Table 9–1 Comparison of Dementia, Delirium, and Depression

| CLINICAL FEATURE | DELIRIUM | DEMENTIA | DEPRESSION |
|---|---|---|---|
| Onset | Acute, sudden | Gradual | Sudden or brief |
| Course | Short; diurnal fluctuations; symptoms worse at night and on awakening | Lifelong; symptoms progressive and irreversible | Diurnal effects, typically worse in morning; situational fluctuations, but less pronounced than with acute confusion |
| Progression | Abrupt | Slow but uneven | Variable, rapid, or slow, but steady |
| Duration | Hours to less than 1 month, seldom longer | Months to years | At least 2 weeks, can last from several months to years |
| Alertness | Fluctuates, lethargy or hypervigilance | Generally normal | Normal |
| Attention | Decreased | Generally normal | Normal |
| Orientation | Generally impaired but reversible | May be impaired as disease progresses | Possible disorientation |
| Memory | Recent and immediate memory impaired | Recent and remote memory impaired | Selective or patchy impairment |
| Thinking | Disorganized, distorted, and fragmented | Difficulty with abstraction; impoverished thoughts, impaired judgment, difficulty in finding words | Intact, with themes of hopelessness, helplessness, or self-deprecation |
| Perception | Distorted, with illusions, delusions, and hallucinations; difficulty in distinguishing reality from misperceptions | Misperceptions usually absent | Intact, without delusions or hallucinations except in severe cases |
| Speech | Incoherent, either slow or accentuated | Dysphasia as disease progresses, aphasia | Normal, slow, or rapid |

| Table 9–1 Comparison of Dementia, Delirium, and Depression—cont'd | | | |
|---|---|---|---|
| CLINICAL FEATURE | DELIRIUM | DEMENTIA | DEPRESSION |
| Psychomotor behavior | Variable: hypokinetic, hyperkinetic, and mixed | Possible apraxia | Variable, with psychomotor agitation or retardation |
| Sleep and wake cycles | Altered | Fragmented | Insomnia or somnolence |
| Affect | Variable affect; anxiety, restlessness, and irritability; reversible | Superficial, inappropriate, and labile; attempts made to conceal deficits in intellect; possible personality changes, aphasia, and agnosia; lack of insight | Depression, dysphoric mood with exaggerated and detailed symptoms; preoccupation with personal thoughts; insight present; verbal elaboration |

Adapted from McCann, J. (ed.). *Portable Signs and Symptoms.* Philadelphia: Lippincott Williams & Wilkins, 2008.

- Observe the patient for skin-care needs issues related to episodes of incontinence
- Suggest community resources including home health care, adult day care centers, palliative care, and nursing home placement

Medications used to treat dementia include:

- Cholinesterase inhibitors: Have positive effects on cognitive ability, and possible effects on declines in ADL and on aggression and agitation, depression, and apathy
- Memantines: Have very positive effects on cognitive ability and on declines in ADL, aggression and agitation, and symptoms of depression
- Neuroleptics: May be helpful with aggression and agitation of dementia, as well as with some features of psychosis
- Antidepressants: Helpful for patients exhibiting depression and apathy
- Anticonvulsants: May provide assistance in the management of aggressive and agitated states related to dementia

# Depression

Age- and life-related changes that many elderly individuals face can lead to depression, especially in those who are without a strong support system. The death of a spouse and medical problems are changes that have been identified as causes of depression. According to the National Institutes of Health, approximately 2 million Americans 65 years of age or older suffer from severe depression and another 5 million suffer from less severe forms of psychiatric illness. Although depression is not a necessary or normal part of the aging process, it is a common problem in the elderly population. Major depression in older adults may involve little overt dysphoria; more often, apparent mental confusion dominates, demonstrating the vulnerability of the brain to an illness that is increasingly viewed as physical.

Depression in older adults is often difficult to diagnose. It may even be overlooked. Persons in this age group are often isolated, with few people around them to notice that they may be in distress. On the other hand, some individuals assume that elderly persons have legitimate reasons to be downcast or sad. Some health care providers ignore depression in older patients and concentrate on physical complaints, and many seniors are reluctant to discuss their feelings or ask for help.

Depression that persists without recognition carries the risk of serious consequences, including abuse of alcohol and prescription drugs, increased mortality, and suicide. Causes and risk factors that contribute to depression in the elderly include:

- **Loneliness and isolation:** Living alone; a dwindling social circle from deaths or relocations; decreased mobility from illness or loss of driving privileges
- **Reduced sense of purpose:** Feelings of purposelessness or loss of identity from retirement or physical limitations on activities
- **Health problems:** Illness and disability; chronic or severe pain; cognitive decline; damage to body image from surgery or disease
- **Medications:** Many prescription medications can trigger or exacerbate depression. Table 9–2 presents a list of medications that can cause symptoms of depression
- **Fears:** Fear of death or dying; anxiety about financial problems or health issues

## Table 9–2 Medications That May Cause Depressive Symptoms

| DRUG CLASS | SPECIFIC MEDICATIONS |
|---|---|
| Antihypertensives | Clonidine, hydralazine, guanethidine, methyldopa propranolol, reserpine |
| Analgesics | Narcotic: Morphine, codeine, meperidine, pentazocine, propoxyphene<br>Non-narcotic: Indomethacin |
| Antiparkinsonism drugs | Levodopa |
| Antimicrobials | Sulfonamides, isoniazid |
| Cardiovascular drugs | Digitalis, diuretics, lidocaine |
| Hypoglycemic agents | Psychotropic drugs,<br>Sedatives: Barbiturates, benzodiazepines, meprobamate<br>Antipsychotics: Chlorpromazine, haloperidol, thiothixene<br>Hypnotics: Chloral hydrate, flurazepam |
| Steroids | Corticosteroids, estrogens |
| Others | Cimetidine, chemotherapy agents, alcohol |

Adapted from Ham, R., Sloane, P., and Warshaw, G. *Primary Care Geriatrics,* ed. 5. St. Louis: Mosby, 2007.

- **Recent bereavement:** The death of friends, family members, and pets; the loss of a spouse or partner

## Assessment of Depression in the Elderly

Many reliable tools are available for identifying and assessing depression, including the Hamilton Depression Rating Scale, Beck Depression Inventory, Center for Epidemiologic Studies Depression Scale (CES-D), and Geriatric Depression Scale. Many of these are available from local pharmaceutical representatives in pad form. Patients or their family members can fill out the form while waiting for the NP in the latter's office. Scores on these tools are easily tabulated, allowing the NP to readily assess the answers and review the tool with the patient.

**COACH CONSULT**

When assessing an elderly patient for depression, look for these symptoms:
- **Sadness:** Usually present but may be masked by other symptoms
- **Fatigue:** A common depressive symptom among the elderly
- **Cognitive impairment:** May be marked and may even mimic dementia
- **Aches and pains:** May include other physical, somatic symptoms

The Geriatric Depression Scale has 15 questions with yes or no answers. Scores between five and nine suggest depression; scores above nine indicate depression. Table 9–3 presents questions and scoring for the Geriatric Depression Scale Short Form.

### Assessment of Suicide Potential

Data suggest that 80% of patients who commit suicide had visited their primary care provider within the month before suicide. Twenty percent of suicide victims had been to their provider within 24 hours before committing suicide. Practitioners must be vigilant in monitoring elderly persons for potential suicidal ideation and tendencies. When assessing for suicide potential, follow these tips:

- Always ask the patient direct questions about suicidal ideation and plans
- Inquire about the patient's access to means for committing suicide
- Identify the availability of family, friends, or social support systems for the patient

| Table 9–3  **Geriatric Depression Scale** | | |
|---|---|---|
| Are you basically satisfied with your life? | Yes | No* |
| Have you dropped many of your activities and interests? | Yes* | No |
| Do you feel that your life is empty? | Yes* | No |
| Do you often get bored? | Yes* | No |
| Are you in good spirits most of the time? | Yes | No* |
| Are you afraid that something is going to happen to you? | Yes* | No |
| Do you feel happy most of the time? | Yes | No* |
| Do you often feel helpless? | Yes* | No |

Table 9–3 **Geriatric Depression Scale—cont'd**

| | | |
|---|---|---|
| Do you prefer to stay at home rather than going out and doing new things? | Yes* | No |
| Do you feel you have more problems with memory than most? | Yes* | No |
| Do you think it is wonderful to be alive now? | Yes | No* |
| Do you feel pretty worthless the way you are now? | Yes* | No |
| Do you feel full of energy? | Yes | No* |
| Do you feel that your situation is hopeless? | Yes* | No |
| Do you think that most people are better off than you are? | Yes* | No |

Each answer indicated by an asterisk counts as one point. Add the points together.

Scoring:

      12–15 Severe depression

      8–11 Moderate depression

      5–8 Mild depression

      0–4 Normal

Source: Yesavage, J.A., Brink, T.L., Rose, T.L., et al. Development and validation of a geriatric depression screening scale: A preliminary report. *J Psychiatr Res* 17:37–49, 1983.

## Dermatological Issues

Cumulative exposure to ultraviolet (UV) sunlight, particularly in Caucasian persons, will lead to a typical pattern of photoaging that presents as deep wrinkling; irregular pigmentation; telangiectasias; yellowing; and a dry, leathery appearance of sun-exposed areas of the skin. Over time, exposure to sunlight increases the risk of actinic keratoses, basal cell cancer, squamous cell cancer, and malignant melanoma. Geriatric patients may also present with a number of nonmalignant skin lesions. Table 9–4 provides an overview of typical skin lesions seen in geriatric practices.

Xerosis is a very common skin condition in elderly patients. Xerotic skin looks dry, rough, and scaly. This appearance is pronounced on the anterior surfaces of the legs and extensor aspects of the arms and forearms.

## Table 9–4 Skin Lesions in Geriatric Patients

| COLOR OF LESISON | NAME OF LESION | LESION DESCRIPTION | MALIGNANCY STATUS |
|---|---|---|---|
| Skin-colored | Actinic keratosis | Multiple, flat, or slightly elevated rough, scaly macule, on hyperemic base; 0.2–1.5 cm diameter; on sun-exposed areas of skin | Premalignant |
| | Basal cell carcinoma | Nodular or ulcerative; begins as small papule, enlarges with central depression and pearly border; overlying telangiectatic vessels on sun-exposed areas of skin | Malignant |
| | Dermal nevi | Fleshy, elevated , slightly pigmented papules, may have extending terminal hairs<br>Shape may change over time as lesion progresses; pigmentation may vary | Nonmalignant |
| | Epidermoid | Cysts containing blood or pus, usually in a non-hairy part of body; may occur in pierced areas of skin | Nonmalignant |
| | Lipoma | Soft, moveable, fatty-tissue tumor | Nonmalignant |
| | Keratoacanthoma | Slightly reddish; bud-shaped; grows rapidly from hair follicle | Nonmalignant |
| | Molluscum contagiosum | Umbilicated pearly papule; single or multiple lesions | Nonmalignant |
| | Seborrheic keratoses | Brown/black; "stuck on" appearance; not related to sun exposure;" postage stamp lesions | Nonmalignant |

Table 9–4 **Skin Lesions in Geriatric Patients—cont'd**

| COLOR OF LESSION | NAME OF LESSION | LESSION DESCRIPTION | MALIGNANCY STATUS |
|---|---|---|---|
| | Squamous cell carcinoma | Variable presentation; commonly single, keratotic nodule on erythematous base; often arises from actinic keratosis | Malignant |
| | Warts | Verrucous, small rough lesion, often on hands or wrists | Nonmalignant |
| Brown | Dermatofibroma | Pink or brown firm lesion, often on legs; associated with immunological diseases | Nonmalignant |
| | Nevus: Compound, dysplastic, junctional | Brown lesions derived from either vascular or connective tissue, melanocytes, or epidermal tissues | Nonmalignant Premalignant: Dysplastic nevus |
| | Freckles | Flat macules | Nonmalignant |
| | Lentigines | Brown spots; pigmented circumscribed macules; may develop into lentigo-maligna melanoma over many years | Nonmalignant |
| Blue | Blue nevus | Blue tinted papular lesion, usually nonprogressive | Nonmalignant |
| | Nodular malignant melanoma | Dark brown to black papule or nodule; may break down to ulcer; common on legs, trunk, earlobes | Malignant |
| | Kaposi's sarcoma (can be red or brown) | Red, brown, or black papular lesions on skin, but may also appear in mouth, GI tract; associated with HIV infection | Malignant |

*Continued*

## Table 9–4 Skin Lesions in Geriatric Patients—cont'd

| COLOR OF LESSION | NAME OF LESSION | LESSION DESCRIPTION | MALIGNANCY STATUS |
|---|---|---|---|
| | Venous lakes | On lower lips and ears; soft, compressible, flat, bluish red lesions of 4–6-mm diameter | Nonmalignant |
| Red | Cysts (inflamed) | Fluid-filled, raised lesions; may be on erythematous base | Nonmalignant |
| | Cherry hemangiomas | Bright red papules of 1–5 mm diameter | Nonmalignant |
| | Erythema nodosum | Tender erythematous nodules of sudden bilateral eruption; occur in patches on knees, shins, ankles, as well as trunk. Associated with IBD, sarcoidosis, TB, and streptococcal or fungal infections | Nonmalignant |
| | Erythema ab igne | "Redness from the fire"; due to prolonged exposure to heat; hyperpigmented hypopigmentated; telangiectasis and atrophy of skin may be seen | Nonmalignant |
| | Urticaria | Wheals, raised irregular-shaped eruptions | Nonmalignant |
| | Erythema multiforme | Urticarial, red-pink, iris-shaped lesion; localized. May occur as drug reaction | Nonmalignant |
| | Herpes zoster | Vesicular rash preceded by erythema; occurs along a dermatome in a linear pattern; painful | Nonmalignant |

Table 9–4 **Skin Lesions in Geriatric Patients—cont'd**

| COLOR OF LESSION | NAME OF LESSION | LESSION DESCRIPTION | MALIGNANCY STATUS |
|---|---|---|---|
| | Seborrheic dermatitis | Redness and scaling on scalp, around ears, nose, and eyebrows | Nonmalignant |
| White | Milia | White epidermal cysts of 1 mm diameter; common on face and periorbital skin. Advise patients to use soap-free cleansers (Cetaphil) | Nonmalignant |
| | Tinea versicolor | Superficial, scaling plaques on trunk; may look tan on light skin and light on dark skin | Nonmalignant |
| | Vitiligo | Chronic skin condition with irregularly shaped areas of hypopigmentation | Nonmalignant |
| Yellow | Sebaceous hyperplasia | Single or multiple soft, yellowish papules on face or chest, from sebaceous glands | Nonmalignant |
| | Xanthomas | Fat buildup under the skin, commonly on joint areas, feet, ankles | Nonmalignant |

GI: gastrointestinal; HIV: human immunodeficiency virus; IBD: inflammatory bowel disease; TB: tuberculosis.

Adapted from Ham, R., Sloane, P., and Warshaw, G. *Primary Care Geriatrics*, ed. 5. St. Louis: Mosby, 2007.

It is more commonly seen in the winter months and in climates with low humidity, dry heat, and windy weather. Excessive bathing contributes to the condition.

Xerosis is compounded by intense pruritus, which leads to chronic rubbing and scratching, both of which cause lichenification of the skin. In severe cases this may result in superinfection or cellulitis.

Xerosis may be attributed to a number of causes, including contact dermatitis, medication or food allergies, scabies, diseases of the liver or biliary

**COACH CONSULT**

Some common products that are helpful as moisturizers include Aveeno, hydrophilic ointment, Vaseline, Eucerin, or Moisturel.

ducts, metabolic diseases, and drug reactions, as well as psychogenic causes. These situations must be ruled out before treating for xerosis.

Treatment of xerosis includes humidification; limited soaking of affected areas of skin in hot water; use of mild moisturing soaps; and consistent use of skin moisturizers. If the skin is cracking or inflamed, a short course of a moderate- or high-potency topical corticosteroid may be helpful.

## Functional Assessment of Elderly Patients

The functional assessment of elderly patients should be done regularly at least every 6 months, but more often if indicated by changes in cognitive and physical health. Basic ADLs essential to independent living include the ability to provide food for oneself, to bathe, and to meet one's toileting needs. Decline in the ability to maintain independent activities of daily living (IADL) is often subtle and difficult to identify. It may be necessary to include children or other family members in identifying an elderly persons problems with shopping, paying bills, cleaning, doing the laundry, keeping medical appointments, maintaining a home or apartment, and keeping a safe living environment.

### Falls and Frailty Issues

Falls are the leading cause of accidental death in older adults. Falls in the elderly may produce a range of injuries, from minor soft-tissue injuries to lacerations, bruises, fractures, and head trauma. Every fall should be evaluated for the history of events that preceded it, as well as for any circumstances that contributed to it. Risk factors for falls include medications, chronic illness, acute medical illness, and changes in cognitive or functional status. Extrinsic risk factors for falls include effects of polypharmacy; environmental issues such as lighting, loose rugs, slippery floors, and poor-fitting shoes; and situational factors, such as stairs, tripping over clutter, rapid movements, reaching overhead, and climbing ladders.

The physical examination of an elderly person who has experienced a fall should include a complete cardiovascular evaluation, a thorough neurological examination, and an assessment of gait and balance. Assess the patient's muscle strength in the upper and lower extremities and the patient's deep-tendon reflexes, and measure the patient's vital signs in the orthostatic position.

Potential risk factors for falls in elderly individuals include:

- Anemia
- Arrhythmias
- Arthritis
- Carotid sinus hypersensitivity
- Cataracts
- Cervical myelopathy
- Dementia
- Depression
- Foot problems such as bunions, calluses, and nail abnormalities
- Hypoglycemia
- Hyponatremia
- Hypothyroidism
- Impaired cognition
- Macular degeneration
- Parkinson's disease
- Postprandial hypotension
- Postural hypotension
- Previous cerebrovascular accident (CVA)
- Weakness
- Vertebrobasilar insufficiency
- Visual disturbances, including spatial and dark/light perception

## Assessing the Risk for Falls

To assess an elderly patient's potential for falls, the NP could utilize the "Get Up and Go Test" as a part of a routine evaluation. Observations of gait and balance are critical to identifying frailty and disturbances in gait. The NP should observe any patient who reports having fallen while the patient performs the tasks in the "Get Up and Go" test.

Patients who present with a history of multiple falls require more intensive assessment and evaluation to identify any underlying medical disorders. A work-up for elderly patients who have had multiple falls should include a:

- Detailed history and physical examination
- CBC, blood chemistry tests, and thyroid function tests
- Serum drug assays

**COACH CONSULT**

For the "Get Up and Go Test," instruct the patient to:
- Stand from a sitting position without use of the arms of the chair for support
- Walk several paces, turn, and return to a sitting position
- Sit back without using the arms for support

Inability to perform any of these tasks without faltering indicates that the patient may be at risk for falling.

- Urinalysis
- An ECG, echocardiography, and Holter monitoring if cardiovascular problems are suspected
- A CT scan or MRI of the brain or cervical spine if neurological problems or gait disturbances are noted
- Referral to an ophthalmologist for visual disturbances

## Preventing Falls

Any elderly or frail patient should consider the use of a home medical alert system. Some examples of such systems for senior citizens include the Life Guardian, Lifeline, Life Link, and Medic Alert System. These systems utilize a necklace, watch, or bracelet that the wearer can activate with the push of a button in case of a fall or medical emergency. Medical alert bracelets that include vital information about the patient's health and medications should be recommended for any elderly, frail patient.

# Mistreatment and Neglect of Elderly Persons

Abuse and neglect of an elderly person may be difficult to identify. Victims are often embarrassed to admit that their family members have taken advantage of them. Often, fear of being moved from their homes to a long-term care facility keeps a victim of abuse from confronting the perpetrator or reporting the abuse. Patients with dementia and depressive disorders are common targets of abuse. The perpetrators are often close family members, are depressed or have other mental illness, exhibit dependence on alcohol or substances, and are financially connected to the victim in some way.

Nurse practitioners who suspect elder abuse should contact the nearest office of the Adult Protective Services Association and the police. It is not a violation of the Health Insurance Portability and Accountability Act (HIPPA) to share medical information with the police or with an Adult Protective Services representative when abuse is suspected. Documentation of office visits should include reports of findings such as bruises and abrasions. Photographs or diagrams are helpful to support documentation of abuse. The record should also include any statements made by the victim. Indicators of possible abuse include:

- Unexplained weight loss
- Dehydration
- Poor hygiene
- Elongated toenails

- Inappropriate attire for current weather
- Lacerations or abrasions
- Hematomas
- Traumatic alopecia
- Bruises in unusual locations
- Welts
- Burns
- Pressure ulcers
- Rectal or vaginal bleeding
- Signs of sexually transmitted diseases

## Disorders Related to Alcohol Use by Elderly Persons

Older adults who drink have higher blood alcohol levels for the amount of alcohol they consume than do their younger counterparts. Sensitivity of the CNS to alcohol increases with age. The concomitant consumption of alcohol may also adversely influence the effects of many medications, including the following instances:

- Histamine H2 blockers and aspirin may raise blood alcohol levels
- Alcohol may increase the sedative effects of benzodiazepines, tricyclic antidepressants, narcotics, barbiturates, and antihistamines and impair psychomotor functioning
- Alcohol with aspirin or other nonsteroidal anti-inflammatory drugs (NSAIDs) may increase bleeding times or induce gastric inflammation
- Combined use of alcohol and metronidazole, sulfonamides, or long-acting oral hypoglycemic agents may cause severe nausea and vomiting
- Concurrent use of alcohol with reserpine, Aldomet, nitroglycerine, or hydralazine may cause hypotension
- Hepatotoxicity may result from combining alcohol with acetaminophen, isoniazid, or phenylbutazone
- The use of alcohol with antihypertensive, antidiabetic, or antiulcer drugs; gout medicines; or heart medicines may exacerbate the underlying disease state
- Consumption of alcohol may alter the metabolism of benzodiazepines, narcotics, barbiturates, warfarin, propranolol, isoniazid, and tolbutamide

**COACH CONSULT**

Consumption of alcohol in the elderly may trigger or worsen the following conditions:
- Liver problems, cirrhosis, gastrointestinal bleeding, and GERD
- Gout, hypertension, or diabetes
- Insomnia and gait disorders
- Depression, anxiety, or other mental disorders

**COACH CONSULT**

When assessing a patient for a disorder related to use of alcohol, remember that all of the following are equivalent to one another:
- 12 ounces of beer
- 4 to 6 oz of wine
- 1.5 oz of liquor/spirits
- 4 oz of sherry, liqueur, or aperitif

**COACH CONSULT**

A blood alcohol level >100 mg/dL without intoxication suggests tolerance.

## Risk Factors Related to Use of Alcohol by the Elderly

Elderly patients at risk for disorders related to use of alcohol may present with symptoms including memory loss; cognitive impairment; depression; anxiety; changes in appetite; nutritional deficits; sleep disturbances; poor control of hypertension, diabetes or seizure disorders; impaired gait and balance; recurrent gastritis; poor control of warfarin dosing; and neglect of personal hygiene and appearance.

## Assessment of Disorders of Alcohol Use

Initial questions for elderly patients are aimed at quantifying alcohol use. Ask the patient how often he or she has a drink containing alcohol. This can be followed with a more specific inquiry, such as "On a typical day when you drink, how many drinks do you have?" If these questions raise concerns about possible alcohol abuse, use the CAGE questions to further assess the situation:

- Have you ever felt that you should CUT down on your drinking?
- Have people ever ANNOYED you by criticizing your drinking?
- Have your ever felt GUILTY about your drinking?
- Have you even had a drink (EYE OPENER) as you first act upon awakening in the morning, to steady your nerves or get rid of a hangover?

The NP should explore positive responses on any of the CAGE questions with the patient, to determine potential problems with the use of alcohol.

The following laboratory studies may help in assessing disorders related to the use of alcohol:

- Elevated gamma-glutamyl transpeptidase
- Mean corpuscular volume (MCV) to aid in identification of microcytic, normocytic, or macrocytic anemias commonly seen in chronic alcohol abuse

- Carbohydrate-deficient transferring (CDT), which is a serum protein marker for liver disease associated with alcohol abuse

**ALERT**

The use of Disulfram in the treatment of elderly patients with alcohol use disorder must be done with caution because of possible cardiac effects.

## Treatment of Alcohol Abuse

When treating a patient for a disorder in the use of alcohol, follow these guidelines:

- Provide personalized feedback
- Establish sensible drinking limits
- Make a drinking agreement in the form of a prescription
- Instruct the patient about self-help groups, motivational counseling, and family therapy
- Provide treatment for concurrent depression or anxiety states

# Options for Alternative Care

Most elderly patients are cognitively and physically able to remain independently in their homes throughout their lifetimes, enjoying a high quality of life. For those who have physical or cognitive problems, alternative care options are available, including palliative care, home health services, hospices, and nursing homes. The role of the NP is explored in the following sections for each of these alternative health care options.

## Palliative Care

Palliative care is an interdisciplinary approach to care focused on the relief of suffering and attainment of the best possible quality of life for patients and their families during an illness. Palliative care can be provided concomitantly with life-prolonging therapies to identify and ameliorate functional and cognitive impairment, reduce caregiver exhaustion, and reduce the burden of symptoms. This approach to care goes with the patient as the patient moves from one level of care to another.

## Home Health Services

Home health services often utilize NPs in the role of home health administrators who direct and organize the daily operations of these services. This can involve marketing, budgeting, new product analysis, quality assurance programs, addressing issues of regulatory compliance, and staff evaluation. The NP engaged in home health care can evaluate the independent living needs of patients and plan for their general welfare.

The federal statutes governing reimbursement for home health services require that a physician certify the need for the services. The physician must also review the plan of care within the time guidelines designated by the U.S. Centers for Medicare and Medicaid Services (CMS). Nurse practitioners and physician assistants (PAs) can bill Medicare for oversight of a care plan. Included in this oversight are such activities such as discussing management of the patient with the home care nurse or physical therapist, reviewing consultant reports, and medical decision making. CMS will reimburse for these services if they require more than 30 minutes per patient in a calendar month.

## Hospice Care

The purpose of hospice care is to provide high quality compassionate care and support for patients with life-limiting illnesses. Hospice care is covered by Medicare, Medicaid, and most private insurance companies. Life-limiting illnesses included in hospice guidelines include cancer, congestive heart failure (CHF), COPD, dementia, end-stage renal disease, and other diseases in which there is a prognosis of 6 months of survival or less. The attending physician must certify a terminal diagnosis or a prognosis of 6 months of survival or less. The attending physician may also recertify any diagnosis or prognosis of terminal illness.

Nursing home residents who are not in a skilled nursing facility are eligible for hospice services while in the nursing home. Medicare provides hospice benefits for two 90-day periods and for an unlimited number of 60-day periods for the remainder of a patient's life.

Nurse practitioners may be designated as attending physicians for hospice patients, but their Medicare reimbursement for this is 85% of the usual and customary fee. Nurse practitioners cannot certify a diagnosis or prognosis of 6 months of survival or less or recertify a diagnosis or prognosis of terminal illness. However, NPs may see, treat, and write orders for hospice patients if their state nursing practice act permits this. Nurse practitioners may be employed by a hospice agency.

## Nursing Home Care

Geriatric nurse practitioners (GNPs) have been employed in nursing homes since 1970. In some situations, the GNP also serves as the director of nursing for a nursing home. Specific advantages to patients cited for advanced practice nurses in the nursing home include:

- Increased accessibility and efficiency of health care provider to the patient

- Availability of the NP to handle minor medical problems as they arise in the nursing home setting
- Cost containment
- Increased health education and counseling provided to the patient by more availability of the NP health provider on site in the nursing home
- Better quality of care
- Greater resident and family satisfaction

Among federal guidelines for nursing home management of patients by NPs are that:

- An initial visit after admission is not required, because admission to a nursing home implies physician contact in the period before admission
- Routine visits must be made every 30 days for the first 90 days after admission, and every 60 days thereafter. A visit must be made within 10 days after the date by which the visit was required
- Visits for acute care may be made whenever medically necessary

Nurse practitioners may be employed by a nursing home, work for an affiliated physician or physician group, or be contracted to work by a managed care organization. They provide sick/urgent, preventive, end-of-life, and wound care services in nursing home settings. The CMS has established regulations for mid-level NPs in both skilled nursing facilities and nursing homes:

- NPs and PAs may provide medically necessary services to residents within the scope of practice defined by the state
- In skilled nursing facilities, the initial full comprehensive visit to a patient must be completed by a physician
- PAs may not sign initial certification or recertification documents in skilled nursing facilities, but an NP who is not an employee of a skilled nursing facility may sign a certification or recertification document if permitted by state requirements
- A physician may delegate alternate follow up visits (30- or 60-day evaluations) to a collaborating NP or PA in a skilled nursing facility

In nonskilled nursing facilities, wide latitude is generally given to NPs and PAs to substitute for the physician and make an initial comprehensive visit, make subsequent required visits, and provide certification and recertification, as long as the NP or PA is not an employee of the facility, is working in collaboration with a physician, and is subject to the individual state regulations governing the NP or PA.

# 10 Tools

# CHAPTER 10

# Tools

## Abbreviations

| | |
|---|---|
| AAA: | Abdominal aortic aneurysm |
| ACE: | Angiotensin-converting enzyme |
| ACTH: | Adrenocorticotropic hormone |
| ADHD: | Attention deficit-hyperactivity disorder |
| ADLs: | Activities of daily living |
| ADR: | Adverse drug reaction |
| AF: | Atrial fibrillation |
| AIDS: | Acquired immunodeficiency syndrome |
| ALL: | Acute lymphoblastic leukemia |
| ALT: | Alanine aminotransferase |
| AML: | Acute myeloid leukemia |
| ANA: | Antinuclear antibody |
| AP: | Anteroposterior |
| ASA: | Acetylsalicylic acid (aspirin) |
| ASD: | Atrial septal defect |
| AST: | Aspartate aminotransferase |
| AUC: | Area under the curve |
| AV: | Atrioventricular |
| BBB: | Bundle branch block |
| BMI: | Body mass index |
| BMP: | Basic metabolic panel |
| BP: | Blood pressure |
| BPH: | Benign |
| BUN: | Blood urea nitrogen |
| CAD: | Coronary artery disease |

| | |
|---|---|
| CBC: | Complete blood count |
| CDC: | Centers for Disease Control and Prevention |
| CES-D: | Center for Epidemiologic Studies-Depression Scale |
| CFS: | Chronic fatigue syndrome |
| CH: | Cluster headache |
| CHF: | Congestive heart failure |
| CMS: | Centers for Medicare and Medicaid Services |
| CNS: | Central nervous system |
| COPD: | Chronic obstructive pulmonary disease |
| CPAP: | Continuous positive airway pressure |
| CPK: | Creatine phosphokinase |
| CPT: | Current Procedural Terminology |
| CR: | Controlled-release |
| CSF: | Cerebrospinal fluid |
| CT: | Computed tomography |
| CVA: | Cerebrovascular accident |
| CVAT: | Costovertebral angle tenderness |
| CYP450: | Cytochrome P450 |
| DEA: | Drug Enforcement Administration |
| DIC: | Disseminated intravascular coagulation |
| DTR: | Deep tendon reflex |
| ECG: | Electrocardiogram |
| EEG: | Electroencephalogram |
| E/M: | Evaluation and management |
| ENT: | Ear, nose, throat |
| EOS: | Eosinophil |
| ER: | Extended-release |
| ESR: | Erythrocyte sedimentation rate |
| FAP: | Functional abdominal pain |
| FDA: | U.S. Food and Drug Administration |
| $FEV_1$: | Forced expiratory volume in one second |
| FT4: | Free thyroxine |
| FVC: | Forced expiratory vital capacity |
| GAD: | Generalized anxiety disorder |
| GCS: | Glasgow Coma Scale |
| G6PD: | Glucose-6-phosphate dehydrogenase |
| GERD: | Gastroesophageal reflux disease |
| GI: | Gastrointestinal |
| GNP: | Geriatric nurse practitioner |
| GnRH: | Gonadotropin releasing hormone |

| | |
|---|---|
| GU: | Genitourinary |
| HAV: | Hepatitis A virus |
| HBcAg: | Hepatitis B core antigen |
| HBe: | Hepatitis B e-antigen |
| $Hb_{1Ac}$: | Hemoglobin $1_{AC}$ (glycosylated hemoglobin) |
| HBsAg: | Hepatitis B surface antigen |
| HBV: | Hepatitis B virus |
| hCG: | Human chorionic gonadotropin |
| Hct: | Hematocrit |
| HDL: | High-density lipoprotein |
| Hgb: | Hemoglobin |
| HIPAA: | Health Insurance Portability and Accountability Act of 1996 |
| HIV: | Human immunodeficiency virus |
| HLA-B27: | Human leukocyte antigen-B27 |
| HMG-CoA: | Hydroxymethylglutaryl-coenzyme A |
| HPI: | History of the present illness |
| HTN: | Hypertension |
| IADL: | Independent activities of daily living |
| IBD: | Inflammatory bowel disease |
| IBS: | Irritable bowel syndrome |
| ICD: | International Classification of Diseases |
| IDA: | Iron deficiency anemia |
| IgA: | Immunoglobulin A |
| IGF-1: | Insulin-like growth factor-1 |
| INR: | International Normalized Ratio |
| IPSS: | International Prostate Symptom Score |
| IUD: | Intrauterine device |
| JVP: | Jugular venous pressure |
| LA: | Long-acting |
| LAHB: | Left anterior hemiblock |
| LDH: | Lactate dehydrogenase |
| LDL: | Low-density lipoprotein |
| LES: | Lower esophageal sphincter |
| LGL: | Lown–Ganong–Levine syndrome |
| LLQ: | Left lower quadrant |
| LPHB: | Left posterior hemiblock |
| LSD: | Lysergic acid diethylamide |
| LUQ: | Left upper quadrant |
| LVH: | Left ventricular hypertrophy |

| | |
|---|---|
| MAO: | Monoamine oxidase |
| MAOI: | Monoamine oxidase inhibitor |
| MB: | Myoglobin |
| MCH: | Mean corpuscular hemoglobin |
| MCV: | Mean corpuscular volume |
| MI: | Myocardial infarction |
| MMSE: | Mini-Mental Status Examination |
| MRCP: | Magnetic resonance cholangiopancreatography |
| MRI: | Magnetic resonance imaging |
| MRSA: | Methicillin-resistant *Staphylococcus aureus* |
| MSSA: | Methicillin-sensitive *Staphylococcus aureus* |
| NIH: | National Institutes of Health |
| NP: | Nurse Practitioner |
| NPI: | National Provider Identifier |
| NSAID: | Nonsteroidal anti-inflammatory drug |
| O&P: | Ova and parasites |
| OM: | Otitis media |
| OTC: | Over the counter |
| PA: | Physician assistant |
| PCP: | Phencyclidine |
| PFSH: | Past family and social history |
| PID: | Pelvic inflammatory disease |
| PS: | Pulmonary stenosis |
| PSA: | Prostate-specific antigen |
| PT: | Prothrombin time |
| PTT: | Partial thromboplastin time |
| RA: | Rheumatoid arthritis |
| RAD: | Right axis deviation |
| RBC: | Red blood cell |
| RDA: | Recommended Daily Allowance |
| RDW: | Red cell distribution width |
| RLQ: | Right lower quadrant |
| ROS: | Review of body systems |
| RUQ: | Right upper quadrant |
| RVH: | Right ventricular hypertrophy |
| SGOT: | Serum glutamic oxaloacetic transaminase |
| SGPT: | Serum glutamic pyruvic transaminase |
| SLE: | Systemic lupus erythematosus |
| SNRI: | Serotonin–norepinephrine reuptake inhibitor |
| SR: | Sustained-release |

| SSRI: | Selective serotonin reuptake inhibitor |
| STD: | Sexually transmitted disease |
| TB: | Tuberculosis |
| TCA: | Tricyclic antidepressant |
| Td: | Tetanus and diphtheria vaccine |
| TF: | Tetralogy of Fallot |
| TIBC: | Total iron binding capacity |
| TM: | Tympanic membrane |
| TMP–SMX: | Trimethoprim–sulfamethoxazole |
| TSH: | Thyroid stimulating hormone |
| T3: | Triiodothyronine |
| URI: | Upper respiratory infection |
| UTI: | Urinary tract infection |
| UV: | Ultraviolet |
| VaD: | Vascular dementia |
| VREF: | Vancomycin-resistant *Enterococcus faecalis* |
| WBC: | White blood cell |
| WPW: | Wolff–Parkinson–White syndrome |

## Anatomical Landmarks

### Anterior View with Landmarks

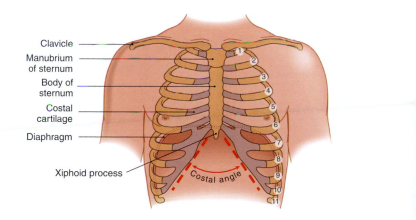

## Left Lateral View with Landmarks

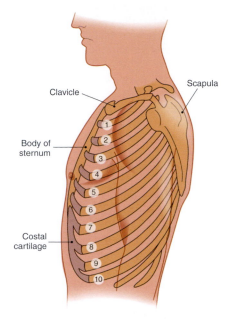

Clavicle

Scapula

Body of
sternum

1
2
3
4
5
6
7
8
9
10

Costal
cartilage

## Structure of the Heart

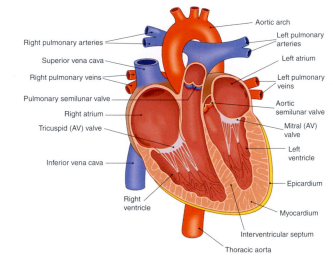

Aortic arch

Right pulmonary arteries

Left pulmonary
arteries

Superior vena cava

Left atrium

Right pulmonary veins

Left pulmonary
veins

Pulmonary semilunar valve

Aortic
semilunar valve

Right atrium

Mitral (AV)
valve

Tricuspid (AV) valve

Left
ventricle

Inferior vena cava

Epicardium

Right
ventricle

Myocardium

Interventricular septum

Thoracic aorta

# Abdominal Organs and Structures

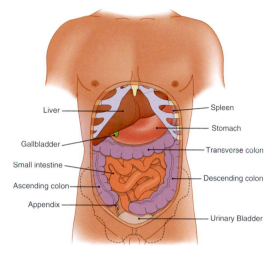

Liver

Gallbladder

Small intestine

Ascending colon

Appendix

Spleen

Stomach

Transverse colon

Descending colon

Urinary Bladder

# Internal Female Genitalia

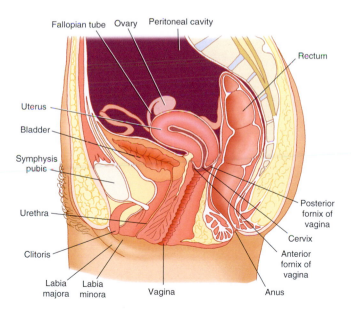

Fallopian tube   Ovary   Peritoneal cavity

Rectum

Uterus

Bladder

Symphysis pubis

Urethra

Clitoris

Labia majora   Labia minora   Vagina

Posterior fornix of vagina

Cervix

Anterior fornix of vagina

Anus

## Internal Male Genitalia

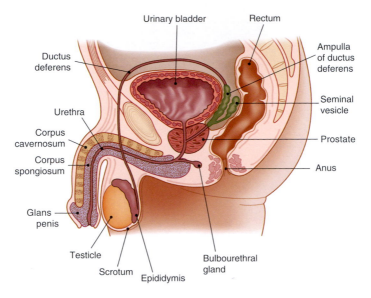

Urinary bladder

Rectum

Ductus
deferens

Ampulla
of ductus
deferens

Seminal
vesicle

Urethra

Corpus
cavernosum

Prostate

Corpus
spongiosum

Anus

Glans
penis

Testicle

Scrotum    Epididymis

Bulbourethral
gland

# Cross-Section of Musculoskeletal System

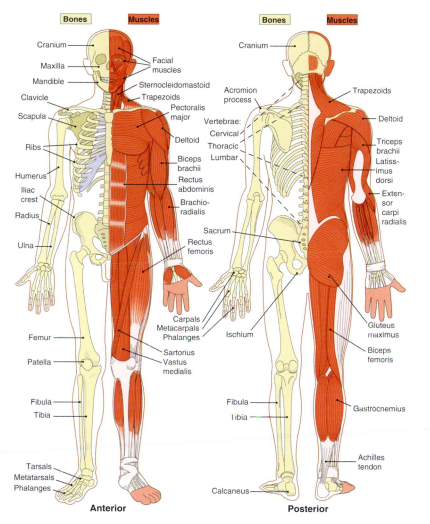

**Anterior**

Bones | Muscles

- Cranium
- Maxilla
- Mandible
- Clavicle
- Scapula
- Ribs
- Humerus
- Iliac crest
- Radius
- Ulna
- Femur
- Patella
- Fibula
- Tibia
- Tarsals
- Metatarsals
- Phalanges

- Facial muscles
- Sternocleidomastoid
- Trapezoids
- Pectoralis major
- Deltoid
- Biceps brachii
- Rectus abdominis
- Brachioradialis
- Rectus femoris
- Carpals
- Metacarpals
- Phalanges
- Sartorius
- Vastus medialis

**Posterior**

Bones | Muscles

- Cranium
- Acromion process
- Vertebrae:
- Cervical
- Thoracic
- Lumbar
- Sacrum
- Ischium
- Fibula
- Tibia
- Calcaneus

- Trapezoids
- Deltoid
- Triceps brachii
- Latissimus dorsi
- Extensor carpi radialis
- Gluteus maximus
- Biceps femoris
- Gastrocnemius
- Achilles tendon

## Lobes of the Brain

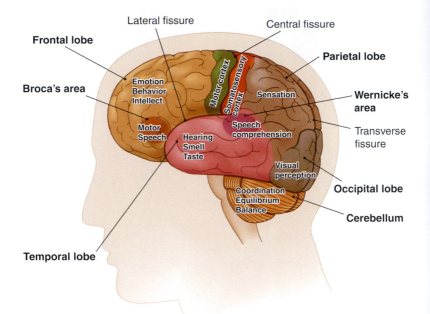

Lateral fissure

Central fissure

**Frontal lobe**

**Parietal lobe**

**Broca's area**

Emotion
Behavior
Intellect

Motor cortex

Somatosensory cortex

Sensation

**Wernicke's area**

Transverse fissure

Motor
Speech

Hearing
Smell
Taste

Speech comprehension

Visual perception

**Occipital lobe**

Coordination
Equilibrium
Balance

**Cerebellum**

**Temporal lobe**

# Origin of Cranial Nerves

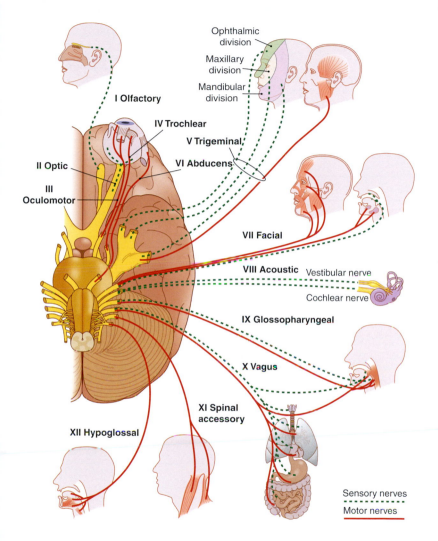

Ophthalmic division
Maxillary division
Mandibular division

**I Olfactory**

**IV Trochlear**

**II Optic**

**III Oculomotor**

**V Trigeminal**

**VI Abducens**

**VII Facial**

**VIII Acoustic**  Vestibular nerve

Cochlear nerve

**IX Glossopharyngeal**

**X Vagus**

**XI Spinal accessory**

**XII Hypoglossal**

- - - - Sensory nerves
———— Motor nerves

## General Chemistry

<u>Note:</u> Reference ranges vary according to brand of laboratory assay materials used. Check normal reference ranges from your facility's laboratory when evaluating results.

| LABORATORY ASSAY | CONVENTIONAL UNITS OF MEASUREMENT | STANDARD INTERNATIONAL UNITS |
|---|---|---|
| Albumin | 3.5–5.0 g/100 mL | 35–50 g/L |
| Aldolase | 1.3–8.2 U/L | 22–137 nmol sec$^{-1}$/L |
| Alkaline phosphatase | 13–39 U/L, infants and adolescents up to 104 U/L | 217–650 nmol sec$^{-1}$/L, up to 1.26 µmol/L |
| Ammonia | 12–55 µmol/L | 12–55 µmol/L |
| Amylase | 4–25 U/mL | 4–25 arbitrary units |
| Anion gap | 8–16 mEq/L | 8–16 mmol/L |
| AST (SGOT) | Male: 8–46 U/L | 0.14–0.78 µkat/L |
| | Female: 7–34 U/L | 0.12–0.58 µkat/L |
| Bilirubin, direct | Up to 0.4 mg/100 mL | Up to 7 µmol/L |
| Bilirubin, total | Up to 1.0 mg/100 mL | Up to 17 µmol/L |
| BUN | 8–25 mg/100 mL | 2.9–8.9 mmol/L |
| Ca$^+$ (calcium) | 8.5–10.5 mg/100 mL | 2.1–2.6 mmol/L |
| Calcitonin | Male: 0–14 pg/mL | 0–4.1 pmol/L |
| | Female: 0–28 pg/mL | 0–8.2 pmol/L |
| Carbon dioxide ($CO_2$) | 24–30 mEq/L | 24–30 mmol/L |
| Chloride ($Cl^-$) | 100–106 mEq/L | 100–106 mmol/L |
| Cholesterol | <200 mg/dL | <5.18 mmol/L |
| Cortisol | (AM) 5–25 mcg/100 mL | 0.14–0.69 µmol/L |
| | (PM) <10 mcg/100 mL | 0–0.28 µmol/L |

# General Chemistry—cont'd

| LABORATORY ASSAY | CONVENTIONAL UNITS OF MEASUREMENT | STANDARD INTERNATIONAL UNITS |
|---|---|---|
| Creatine | Male: 0.2–0.5 mg/dL | 15–40 µmol/L |
| | Female: 0.3–0.9 mg/dL | 25–70 µmol/L |
| Creatine kinase (CK) | Male: 17–148 U/L | 283–2467 nmol · sec$^{-1}$/L |
| | Female: 10–79 U/L | 167–1317 nmol · sec$^{-1}$/L |
| Creatinine | 0.6–1.5 mg/100 mL | 53–133 µmol/L |
| Ferritin | 10–410 ng/dL | 10–410 µg/dL |
| Folate | 2.0–9.0 ng/mL | 4.5–20.4 nmol/L |
| Glucose | 70–110 mg/100 mL | 3.9–5.6 mmol/L |
| Ionized calcium | 4.25–5.25 mg/dL | 1.1–1.3 mmol/L |
| Iron (Fe) | 50–150 mcg/100 mL | 9.0–26.9 µmol/L |
| Iron binding capacity | 250–410 mcg/100 mL | 44.8–73.4 µmol/L |
| K$^+$ (potassium) | 3.5–5.0 mEq/L | 3.5–5.0 mmol/L |
| Lactic acid | 0.6–1.8 mEq/L | 0.6–1.8 mmol/L |
| LDH | 45–90 U/L | 750–1500 nmol · sec$^{-1}$/L |
| Lipase | 2 U/mL or less | Up to 2 arbitrary units |
| Magnesium | 1.5–2.0 mEq/L | 0.8–1.3 mmol/L |
| Mg$^{++}$ (magnesium) | 1.5–2.0 mEq/L | 0.8–1.3 mmol/L |
| Na$^+$ (sodium) | 135–145 mEq/L | 135–145 mmol/L |
| Osmolality | 280–296 mOsm/kg water | 280–296 mmol/kg |
| Phosphorus | 3.0–4.5 mg/100 mL | 1.0–1.5 mmol/L |
| Potassium (K$^+$) | 3.5–5.0 mEq/L | 3.5–5.0 mmol/L |

*Continued*

## General Chemistry—cont'd

| LABORATORY ASSAY | CONVENTIONAL UNITS OF MEASUREMENT | STANDARD INTERNATIONAL UNITS |
|---|---|---|
| Prealbumin | 18–32 mg/dL | 180—320 mg/L |
| Protein, total | 6.0–8.4 g/100 mL | 60–84 g/L |
| PSA | <4.0 ng/mL | <4 mcg/L |
| Pyruvate | 0–0.11 mEq/L | 0–0.11 mmol/L |
| Sodium (Na$^+$) | 135–145 mEq/L | 135–145 mmol/L |
| T3 | 75–195 ng/100 mL | 1.16–3.00 nmol/L |
| T4, free | Male: 0.8—1.8 ng/dL | 10–23 pmol/L |
| | Female: 0.8—1.8 ng/dL | 10–23 pmol/L |
| T4, total | 4–12 mcg/100 mL | 52–154 nmol/L |
| Thyroglobulin | 3–42 ng/mL | 3–42 μg/L |
| Triglycerides | 40–150 mg/100 mL | 0.4–1.5 g/L |
| TSH | 0.5–5.0 μU/mL | 0.5–5.0 arbitrary units |
| Urea nitrogen | 8–25 mg/100 mL | 2.9–8.9 mmol/L |
| Uric acid | 3.0–7.0 mg/100 mL | 0.18–0.42 |

AST: aspartate aminotransferase; BUN: blood urea nitrogen; CK: creatine kinase; LDH: lactate dehydrogenase; PSA: prostate specific antigen; SGOT: serum glutamic oxaloacetic transaminase; T3: triiodothyronine; T4: thyroxine; TSH: thyroid stimulating hormone.

## Metric Conversions

| WEIGHT | | TEMPERATURE | | HEIGHT | | |
|---|---|---|---|---|---|---|
| lbs | kg | °F | °C | cm | inches | ft/in |
| 300 | 136.4 | **212*** | **100*** | 142 | 56 | 4′ 8″ |
| 275 | 125.0 | 107 | 42.2 | 145 | 57 | 4′ 9″ |
| 250 | 113.6 | 106 | 41.6 | 147 | 58 | 4′ 10″ |
| **225** | **102.3** | 105 | 40.6 | 150 | 59 | 4′11″ |
| **210** | **95.5** | 104 | 40.0 | 152 | 60 | 5′ 0″ |
| **200** | **90.9** | 103 | 39.4 | 155 | 61 | 5′ 1″ |
| **190** | **86.4** | 102 | 38.9 | 157 | 62 | 5′ 2″ |
| **180** | **81.8** | 101 | 38.3 | 160 | 63 | 5′ 3″ |
| **170** | **77.3** | 100 | 37.8 | 163 | **64** | 5′ 4″ |
| **160** | **72.7** | 99 | 37.2 | 165 | **65** | 5′ 5″ |
| **150** | **68.2** | **98.6** | **37.0** | 168 | **66** | 5′ 6″ |
| **140** | **63.6** | 98 | 36.7 | 170 | **67** | 5′ 7″ |
| **130** | **59.1** | 97 | 36.1 | 173 | **68** | 5′ 8″ |
| **120** | **54.5** | 96 | 35.6 | 175 | **69** | 5′ 9″ |
| **110** | **50.0** | 95 | 35.0 | 178 | **70** | 5′ 10″ |
| **100** | **45.5** | 94 | 34.4 | 180 | **71** | 5′ 11″ |
| 90 | 40.9 | 93 | 34.0 | 183 | **72** | 6′ 0″ |
| 80 | 36.4 | 92 | 33.3 | 185 | 73 | 6′ 1″ |
| 70 | 31.8 | 91 | 32.8 | 188 | 74 | 6′ 2″ |
| 60 | 27.3 | 90 | 32.1 | 191 | 75 | 6′ 3″ |
| 50 | 22.7 | **32†** | **0†** | 193 | 76 | 6′ 4″ |

*Continued*

## Metric Conversions—cont'd

| WEIGHT | | TEMPERATURE | | HEIGHT | | |
|---|---|---|---|---|---|---|
| *lbs* | *kg* | *°F* | *°C* | *cm* | *inches* | *ft/in* |
| 40 | 18.2 | | | 196 | 77 | 6' 5" |
| 30 | 13.6 | | | | | |
| 20 | 9.1 | | | | | |
| 10 | 4.5 | | | | | |
| 5 | 2.3 | | | | | |
| **2.2** | **1** | | | | | |
| 2 | 0.9 | | | | | |
| **1** | **0.45** | | | | | |
| lb = kg x 2.2     or     kg = lb x 0.45 | | | | | | |
| °F = (°C x 1.8) + 32   or     °C = (°F − 32) x 0.556 | | | | | | |
| Inches = cm x 0.394   or     cm = inches x 2.54 | | | | | | |

*Boiling point.
†Freezing point.

## FIGURE CREDITS

Figure 3-2 is from Jones, S. A. (2006). *ECG notes*. Philadelphia: F.A. Davis Company.

Figures 4-1 and 4-2 are © Dr. Benjamin Branklin, 2007, all rights reserved.

Figure 4-3 is from Wilkinson, J. M., & Van Leuven, K. (2008). *Fundamentals of nursing.* Philadelphia: F.A. Davis Company.

The figures in Chapter 10 are from Dillon, P. M. (2007). *Nursing health assessment: A critical thinking, case studies approach* (2nd ed.). Philadelphia: F.A. Davis Company.

### References
Centers for Disease Control and Prevention. www.cdc.gov

Desai, S. (2001). *Clinician's guide to diagnosis.* Cleveland, OH: Lexi-Comp Inc.

Dillon, P. M. (2007). *Nursing health assessment: A critical thinking, case studies approach* (2nd ed.). Philadelphia: F.A. Davis, p. 410.

Fauci, A. S., et al. (2009). *Harrison's principles of internal medicine* (17th ed.). New York: McGraw-Hill.

Ferri F. F. (2009). *Ferri's clinical advisor 2009.* St. Louis: Mosby.

Ham, R., Sloane, P., Warshaw, G. (2007). *Primary care geriatrics* (5th ed.). St. Louis: Mosby.

Hancock, J. (2001). *The practitioner's pocket pal ultra rapid medical reference.* Miami, FL: Medmaster.

Hollier, A. (2006). *Adult and family NP certification review book.* Lafayette, LA: APEA Publishers.

Jones, S. A. (2006). *ECG notes.* Philadelphia: F.A. Davis, p. 78.

Kernick, I. (2007) *How to read that 12 lead EKG: A primer for electrocardiographic interpretation using the 12 lead EKG.* Shreveport, LA: Schumpert Hospital.

Lee, B. (2009). *Medical notes.* Philadelphia: F.A. Davis.

McCann, J. (ed). *Portable signs and symptoms.* (2008). Philadelphia: Lippincott Williams & Wilkins.

Monthly Prescribing Reference. New York: Haymarket Media: http://www.empr.com

National Data Bank for Rheumatic Diseases. www.arthritis-research.org

Nemeroff, C., Schatzberg, A. (1999). *Recognition and treatment of psychiatric disorders.* Washington DC: American Psychiatric Press, Inc.

Nurse Practitioners' Prescribing Reference Winter 2008–2009. New York: Haymarket Media Publications.

Olson, L., DeWitt, T., First, L., Zenel, J. (2008) *Pediatrics.* St. Louis: Elsevier Mosby.

U.S. Food and Drug Administration. www.fda.gov

Wasson, J. (2001). *The common symptom guide* (5th ed.). New York: McGraw Hill.

Wilkinson, J. M., Van Leuven, K. (2008). *Fundamentals of nursing,* vol. 1. Philadelphia: F.A. Davis, p. 817.

World Health Organization. www.who.int

Yesavage, J. A., Brink, T. L., Rose, T. L., et al. (1983). Development and validation of a geriatric depression screening scale: A preliminary report. *Journal of Psychiatric Research,* 17:37–49.

# Index

Note: Page numbers followed by "t" and "b" indicate tables and boxes, respectively.